THE
MEDICAL
DICTIONARY
OF CONDITIONS AND DISEASES

Dr Judith O'Malley-Ford

Foreword by Professor Major General John Pearn

GW00685840

First published in 2012 by New Holland Publishers
London • Sydney • Cape Town • Auckland

86 Edgware Road London W2 2EA United Kingdom
1/66 Gibbes Street Chatswood NSW 2067 Australia
Wembly Square First Floor Solan Street Gardens Cape Town 8000 South Africa
218 Lake Road Northcote Auckland New Zealand

www.newhollandpublishers.com
www.newholland.com.au

A record of this book is held at the National Library of Australia

ISBN 978178009 2256

Publisher: Fiona Schultz and Patsy Rowe
Publishing Manager: Lliane Clarke
Medical Reviewers: Dr Richard Bailey and Dr John Hollingsworth
Designer: Barbara Cowen
Production Manager: Olga Dementiev

Printer: Toppan Leefung Printing Limited

10 9 8 7 6 5 4 3 2 1

Keep up with New Holland Publishers on Facebook and Twitter http://www.
facebook.com/NewHollandPublishers

Twitter: @NewHollandpub
and::   @NewHollandAU

DEDICATION

I wandered lonely as a cloud

That floats on high o'er vales and hills,

When all at once I saw a crowd,

A host, of golden daffodils;

Beside the lake, beneath the trees,

Fluttering and dancing in the breeze.

For oft, when on my couch I lie

In vacant or in pensive mood,

They flash upon that inward eye

Which is the bliss of solitude;

And then my heart with pleasure fills,

And dances with the daffodils.

William Wordsworth

1770-1850

CONTENTS

Foreword   6

Introduction—How to use this book   7

Summary of conditions by system   8

A–Z of conditions and diseases   **14**

Quick reference list of conditions   345

FOREWORD

Our health is our most precious possession. As individuals, as parents and partners, and as friends and neighbours; in our relationships with all these, issues of health are so important.

Everyone needs a convenient reference text, authoritative and concise, to answer the frequent questions which arise about disease and injury. This reference medical dictionary, written for all irrespective of one's calling, trade or profession, admirably satisfies this need. Parents will find it invaluable because an inescapable role of parenthood is the regular management of illness and injury in our children. Partners will find it invaluable, as one so often has to make decisions about whether symptoms should lead one to seek medical advice. Colleagues at work will find it helpful, as sick leave in a team member necessarily involves others.

A strength of *The Medical Dictionary of Conditions and Diseases* is the clear discussion of common symptoms, in addition to the descriptions of important diseases. Another strength is the explanation of Doctors' jargon. So often, after a medical or health-clinic visit, one needs to return home to look up the meaning of a technical term. The meaning of such medical terms is often taken for granted by others. The topics covered herein range from lice to lung cancer, from prostate cancer to the problems of puberty. I commend this book and will keep a copy of it on my own shelves.

Emeritus Professor Major General John Hemsley Pearn

MD, PhD (*London*), DSc, FRCP, FRACP, DCH, AM, AO.

INTRODUCTION: HOW TO USE THIS BOOK

The Medical Dictionary of Conditions and Diseases is intended as a quick and handy reference guide for the causes, symptoms, diagnostic tests and treatments for the most commonly occurring medical conditions.

The book is written from my own professional point of view—that of a general practitioner who works with patients every day. I have outlined the conditions I most commonly encounter and present them to the reader as a snapshot of causes, symptoms, diagnoses and possible treatment regimes. This will help both health professionals and the general reader whose first point of contact is their GP.

I've included a Summary of System Symptoms to help the reader locate medical disease and illness.

At the back of the book I have included a Quick Reference List of Conditions to help the reader navigate this dictionary.

Dr Judith O'Malley-Ford

MBBS, JP, MPH, FRACGP.

SUMMARY OF CONDITIONS BY SYSTEM

In medicine, the body is divided into systems with specific symptoms which relate to each of the systems and act as hallmarks for disease and illness. When doctors question patients about their symptoms, a positive response may indicate a potential medical problem is present. All the conditions that appear in the book are listed below under the area of the body where symptoms will be felt.

Cardiovascular

Abdominal aortic aneurysm • Abdominal lumps • Abdominal pain • Aneurysm • Angina • Arm and hand pain • Arrhythmia • Atherosclerosis • Back pain • Bleeding • Blindness or loss of vision • Blood pressure • Cardiomyopathies • Cardiopulmonary resuscitation • Cardiovascular system problems • Chest pains • Cholesterol • Confusion • Coordination • Coronary artery disease and atherosclerosis • Coronary syndrome • Cough • Coughing blood (haemoptysis) • Dizziness • Endocarditis • Foot pain • Heart attack • Heart failure • Hypertension • Hypotension • Leg pains • Mesenteric artery occlusion • Myocardial infarction • Neck pain • Obesity • Pain • Palpitations and arrhythmias • Platelet dysfunction abnormalities • Renal vascular disorders • Smoking • Thrombophlebitis • Tiredness • Travel medicine problems • Travel sickness • Valvular disorders of the heart • Vision, sudden loss of • Weight management problems • X-rays • Xanthelasma

Respiratory

Asthma • Back pain • Bad breath (halitosis) • Bleeding • Bronchiectasis • Bronchiolitis • Bronchitis • Brucellosis • Chest pains • Children, common problems • Chlamydia • Chronic obstructive airway disease • Colds and flu or viral upper respiratory infection • Cough • Coughing blood (haemoptysis) • Croup • Crying baby • Cystic fibrosis • Emphysema (chronic obstructive airway disease) • Erectile dysfunction or impotence • Fever • Flu • Haemophylus influenza B • Infections • Influenza (flu) • Lung abscess • Lung cancer • Lung function tests, abnormalities • Occupational lung diseases • Pain • Pleurisy • Pneumococcus • Pneumonia • Pneumothorax • Respiratory system • Respiratory system cancer (cancer of the nasopharynx, larynx, tonsil and tongue) • Smoking • Tiredness • Travel medicine problems • Travel sickness • Tuberculosis • X linked conditions • X-rays

Central nervous system

Aneurysm • Arm and hand pain • Bells' Palsy or facial weakness • Blindness or loss of vision • Brain tumours • Coma • Confusion • Convulsions • Coordination • Disturbed patients • Insomnia • Pain • Smoking • Stroke • Transient ischaemic attack (TIA) • Tremor • X-rays

Infectious diseases

Abscess • Adenitis, mesenteric • Anal pain • Anorexia • Bacterial infections • Bed wetting (enuresis) • Belching, bloating • Bladder problems • Blisters • Blood disorders • Blood in the urine • Boils • Breastfeeding • Cervical cancer • Chest pains • Chickenpox • Childhood infectious diseases • Chlamydia • Cholera • Cold sores • Colds and flu or viral upper respiratory infection • Coma • Confusion • Convulsions • Corneal ulcer • Cough • Coughing blood (haemoptysis) • Crying baby • Cryptosporidium • Cytomegalovirus • Dengue fever • Dermatitis, eczema • Diarrhoea • Diphtheria • Dysuria (pain on passing urine) • Fever • Fevers in children • Flu • Foot odour • Genital herpes, herpes simplex infection • Glandular fever • Gonorrhoea • Haemophylus influenza B • Hand, foot and mouth disease • Hepatitis • Herpes simplex virus (lips or genital area) • Herpes zoster (shingles) • HPV • Human immunodeficiency virus • Human papillomavirus (HPV) • Immunisation for childhood infectious diseases • Infections • Infectious diseases of adults • Influenza (flu) • Ingrown toenails • Leptospirosis • Malaria • Measles • Meningococcal disease • Mumps • Mycoplasma pneumoniae infection • Needle stick injury • Osteomyelitis • Pain • Papillomavirus • Pneumococcus • Polio • Q fever • Rabies • Ross River virus • Rubella • Scabies • Scarlet fever • Septic arthritis • Septic shock • Sexually transmitted disease • Shingles (herpes zoster) • Staphylococcus aureus • Syphilis • Tetanus • Thrombophlebitis • Thrush • Tiredness • Toxic shock • Travel medicine • Travel medicine problems • Travel illness • Tuberculosis • Typhoid • Urinary tract infections • Vaginal discharge • Viral infections • Warts or human papilloma virus (HPV) • Whooping cough • Yellow fever

Immunology and allergic disorders

Allergic reactions and hypersensitivity disorders • Anaphylaxis, allergic reactions • Blindness or loss of vision • Blood disorders • Crohn's disease • Fever • Headache • Immune response • Immunisation • Pain • Polymyalgia rheumatica • Rheumatoid arthritis • Systemic lupus erythematosus • Temporal arteritis • Temporomandibular joint • Tension headache • Transplantation • Vision, sudden loss of

Gastroenterology

Abdominal lumps • Abdominal pain • Alcohol abuse • Anaemia • Anal itch • Anal pain • Anorexia • Appendicitis • Back pain • Bad breath (halitosis) • Belching, bloating • Bleeding • Bowel motions, black • Bowel obstruction, large • Bowel obstruction, small • Chest pains • Children, common problems • Cholera • Cirrhosis of the liver • Coeliac disease • Colic, baby • Colon cancer • Colon cancer, colonic polyps • Colon problems • Constipation • Cough • Coughing blood (haemoptysis) • Crohn's disease • Crying baby • Cystic fibrosis • Diarrhoea • Diverticular disease • Fever • Flatulence • Gastro-oesophageal reflux • Gastroenteritis • Gastroenteritis, viral • Giardia • Haematemesis • Haematemesis and Melena • Haemorrhoids • Haemochromatosis • Hangover • Heartburn • Helicobacter pylori infection • Hernia • Infections • Inflammatory bowel disease • Irritable colon/bowel • Ischaemic colitis • Melaena (black bowel motions) •

Oesophagitis, gastro oesophageal reflux • Oesophagus, problems • Pain • Peptic, perforated or gastric ulcer • Piles • Pseudomembranous colitis • Rectal bleeding • Stomach • Stomach cancer • Tiredness • Travel medicine problems • Travel sickness • Vomiting blood (haematemesis)• Weight management problems • X-rays

Liver and biliary

Abdominal lumps • Abdominal pain • Anorexia • Back pain • Belching, bloating • Biliary colic • Bleeding • Bruising • Cholesterol • Cirrhosis of the liver • Coma • Depression • Gallbladder problems • Hepatitis • Jaundice • Liver problems • Pain • Pancreatic cancer • Pancreatitis • Spleen disorders • Weight management problems • X-rays

Nutrition

Alcohol abuse • Amenorrhoea (no period) • Anaemia • Angina • Anorexia • Atherosclerosis • Bad breath (halitosis) • Belching, bloating • Bleeding • Body odour • Breastfeeding • Cholesterol • Cirrhosis of the liver • Constipation • Coordination • Coronary artery disease and atherosclerosis • Coronary syndrome • Cramps • Hangover • Heart attack • Iron deficiency • Myocardial infarction • Obesity • Osteoporosis • Tiredness • Weight management problems • Xanthelasma

Endocrine

Addison's disease • Adrenal crisis • Adrenal gland, problems • Adrenal virilism (adrenogenital syndrome) • Aldosteronism (Conn's syndrome) • Amenorrhoea (no period) • Arrhythmia • Bladder problems • Carpal tunnel syndrome • Confusion • Coordination • Cushing syndrome • Depression • Diabetes • Erectile dysfunction or impotence • Foot pain • Goitre • Grave's disease • Hyperpituitarism • Hyperthyroidism • Hypopituitarism • Hypothyroidism • Paget's disease • Phaeochromocytoma • Pituitary gland abnormalities • Platelet dysfunction abnormalities • Testosterone, low (hypogonadism) • Thyroid cancer • Thyroid problems • Thyrotoxicosis • Tiredness • Toxic diffuse goitre • Toxic nodular goitre • Weight management problems • X-rays

Haematology and oncology

Abdominal lumps • Alcohol abuse • Anaemia • Angina • Arrhythmia • Blood disorders • Bruising • Cancer • Factor V Leiden • Headache • Hodgkin's disease • Iron deficiency • Leukaemia • Nose bleed • Pain • Smoking • Thalassaemia • Tiredness • X linked conditions

Musculoskeletal and connective tissue diseases

Abdominal pain • Ankylosing spondylitis • Arm and hand pain • Arthritus • Back pain • Bruising • Calluses, corns • Carpal tunnel syndrome • Chest pains • Congenital dislocation of the hip • Cramps • Ewing's tumour • Foot odour • Foot pain • Foot strain • Fractures and dislocations • Ganglion, wrist, forearm • Gout • Groin pain • Heel pain • Hernia • Hip pain • Ingrown toenails • Injuries to the ligaments • Knee pain • Leg pains • Lymphoma • Neck pain • Osgood Schlatter disease • Osteoarthritis • Osteomyelitis • Osteoporosis • Pain • Perthe's disease • Septic arthritis

• Slipped femoral epiphysis • Sprains • Tarsal tunnel syndrome • Tension headache • Thoracic outlet syndrome • Weight management problems • X-rays

Neurological

Arm and hand pain • Blindness or loss of vision • Coma • Convulsions • Coordination • Cramps • Deafness and hearing loss • Dizziness • Epilepsy • Hangover • Impotence • Jetlag • Meningitis • Migraine headache • Multiple sclerosis • Pain • Parkinson's disease • Smoking • Tremor

Psychiatric

Amenorrhoea (no period) • Anorexia nervosa • Anxiety • Belching, bloating • Confusion • Depression • Disturbed patients • Domestic violence • Eating disorders • Insomnia • Obsessive compulsive disorder • Panic disorder • Psychiatric conditions • Schizophrenia • Travel medicine problems • Tiredness • Weight management problems

Genito–urinary

Abdominal pain • Atrophic vaginitis • Back pain • Balanitis • Bed wetting (enuresis) • Bladder cancer • Bladder problems • Bleeding • Blood in the urine • Children, common problems • Chlamydia • Dialysis • Dysuria (pain on passing urine) • Erectile dysfunction or impotence • Fever • Genital herpes, herpes simplex infection • Genital warts • Glomerulonephritis • Gonorrhoea • Groin pain • Haematospermia • Haematuria (blood in the urine) • Herpes simplex virus (lips or genital area) • Impotence • Incontinence • Infections • Infertility, male • Intercourse, problems • Kidney cancer • Kidney disorders • Kidney/renal failure • kidney stones • Libido • Male reproductive system • Pain • Penile disorders • Peyronie's disease • Phimosis paraphimosis • Premature ejaculation • Priapism • Prostate cancer • Prostate infection or prostatitis and prostate abscess • Prostatic hyperplasia/benign • Renal stones • Renal colic • Renal dialysis • Renal failure, chronic • Renal vascular disorders • Retention of urine, acute • Scrotal mass • Scrotal pain • Sexually transmitted disease • Testicular and epididymis infections • Testicular cancer and tumours • Testis torsion • Testosterone, low (hypogonadism) • Undescended testes • Urinary incontinence • Urinary tract infections • X-rays

Gynaecological

Abdominal lumps • Abdominal pain • Amenorrhoea (no period) • Atrophic vaginitis • Bladder problems • Bleeding • Breast cancer • Breast cysts and lumps • Breast discharge • Breastfeeding • Breast infection and abscess (mastitis) • Breast pain and tenderness • Cervical cancer • Contraception • Contraception, emergency—morning after pill • Dysmenorrhoea (painful periods) • Ectopic pregnancy • Endometriosis • Enuresis • Female reproductive system • Fever • Genital herpes, herpes simplex infection • Gonorrhoea • Groin pain • Herpes simplex virus (lips or genital area) • Human papillomavirus (HPV) • Incontinence • Infertility, female • Intercourse, problems • In vitro fertilisation • Iron deficiency • Libido • Mastitis • Menopause problems • Menorrhagia (heavy periods) • Morning after pill • Morning sickness • Neck pain

• Oral contraceptives • Osteoporosis • Ovarian cancer • Ovarian cyst, acute torsion • Ovarian cyst, ruptured • Ovarian follicles • Pain • Papillomavirus • Pelvic adhesions • Pelvic inflammatory disease • Period problems • Periods, painful • Pill, the • Polycystic ovary syndrome • Pregnancy, associated problems • Retracted nipples • Rheumatic fever • Sexually transmitted disease • Thrush • Tiredness • Urinary incontinence • Urinary tract infections • Vaginal bleeding • Vaginal discharge • Vaginitis atrophic • X-rays

Paediatric

Adolescent health, problems • Asperger's syndrome • Asthma • Autism • Baby, problems • Balanitis • Bed wetting (enuresis) • Breastfeeding • Breath holding • Cerebral palsy • Chickenpox • Child abuse • Childhood infectious diseases • Children, common problems • Colic, baby • Congenital dislocation of the hip • Constipation • Convulsions • Cough • Crying baby • Dermatitis, eczema • Diarrhoea • Diphtheria • Eating disorders • Enuresis • Fever • Fevers in children • Floppy baby • Hand, foot and mouth disease • Immunisation • Intussusceptions • Knock knees • Mumps • Nappy rash • Pain • Pigeon toes • Puberty problems • Pyloric stenosis • Smoking • Sudden infant death syndrome • Tantrums • Teething • Undescended testes • Urinary incontinence • Urinary tract infections • X-rays

Ear, nose and throat

Bad breath (halitosis) • Bleeding • Children, common problems • Cough • Coughing blood (haemoptysis) • Deafness and hearing loss • Ear infections • Ear lobes, infected (perichrondritis) • Ear pain • Ear wax • Ears, pressures problems • Epistaxis (bleeding nose) • Eyes, red, unilateral (one eye) • Fever • Hay fever (rhinitis) • Hearing • Infections • Influenza (flu) • Laryngitis • Mastoiditis • Meibomian cyst • Meniere's disease • Meningitis • Nose bleed • Otitis externa • Otitis media • Pain • Perichrondritis • Respiratory system cancer (cancer of the nasopharynx, larynx, tonsil and tongue) • Sinusitis • Smoking • Snoring and sleep apnoea • Thrush • Tonsillitis • Tropical ear • X-rays

Eye

Bed sores • Bells' Palsy or facial weakness • Blepharitis • Blindness or loss of vision • Cataract • Children, common problems • Conjunctivitis • Corneal ulcer • Dermatitis, eczema • Ectropion • Entropion • Eye inflammation • Eye or eyelid infection • Eye trauma • Eyes • Eyes, pressure in • Eyes, red, bilateral (two eyes) • Fever • Flashes and floaters (in the eyes) • Genital herpes, herpes simplex infection • Glaucoma • Herpes zoster (shingles) • Infections • Meibomian Cyst • Pain • Pressure in the eye • Red eyes • Refractive error • Stye • Tearduct blockage • Vision, sudden loss of • Visual acuity, problems • X-rays

Skin and hair

Abscess • Acne • Alopecia (hair loss) • Anal itch • Bites and stings • Bleeding • Blisters • Body odour • Boils • Bruising • Burns • Calluses, corns • Cellulite • Children, common problems • Dandruff • Dry hair • Dry skin • Eczema • Fever • Folliculitis • Head lice • Impetigo • Infections • Insect bites • Jock itch/rash • Keloid scar • Keratoacanthoma • Keratoses (skin conditions) • Lice • Melanoma • Molluscum contagiosum • Pain • Paronychia • Psoriasis • Seborrhoeic keratoses • Skin problems • Smoking • Solar keratoses • Sunburn • Sweating • Tinea •

Dental

Bad breath (halitosis) • Dental problem • Gingivitis • Headache • Mouth ulcers • Pain • Salivary gland, stone • X-rays

abdominal aortic aneurysm *(AAA)*

See *aneurysm*

Cause

An abdominal aortic aneurysm (AAA) occurs when a weakness in the blood vessel wall allows it to balloon out, producing a lump in the abdomen. As an abdominal aortic aneurysm increases in size, the risk of rupture is related to the rate of increase in the diameter of the vessel.

Symptoms

Pain is a common presenting symptom of an AAA. Sometimes an abdominal aortic aneurysm may be found incidentally when investigating other complaints or during an abdominal ultrasound, CT or MRI scan. These investigation techniques may also be used for monitoring the size and progress of the AAA. If a patient with a known abdominal aortic aneurysm suddenly collapses, this may indicate that the aneurysm has ruptured. This requires urgent medical attention and an ambulance for immediate transportation to hospital.

Treatment

Treatment for abdominal aortic aneurysm requires surgical intervention. Before surgery occurs, monitoring of the size of the aneurysm may occur. Early treatment of an AAA reduces the likelihood of acute rupture, a medical emergency with a high mortality rate.

abdominal lumps

See *abscess*
See *aneurysm*
See *bladder problems*
See *cancer*
See *Crohn's disease*
See *hernia*
See *Hodgkin's disease*
See *liver problems*
See *lymphoma*
See *pregnancy*
See *spleen disorders*

Abnormal abdominal lumps are commonly found by patients and doctors and are always a cause for concern until a serious cause is excluded.

abdominal pain

See *pain*

In children and infants

See *adenitis, mesenteric*
See *colic, baby*
See *immunisation for childhood infectious diseases*
See *intussusception*
See *pyloric stenosis*

In adults

See *abdominal aortic aneurysm*
See *appendicitis*
See *biliary colic*
See bowel obstruction, large
See *bowel obstruction, small*
See *diverticulitis*
See *gall bladder problems*
See *infectious diseases of adults*
See *pancreatitis*
See *pancreatic cancer*
See *renal colic*

Lower abdominal pain in adults

See *ectopic pregnancy*
See *endometriosis*
See *ovarian cyst*
See *ovarian follicles*
See *pelvic adhesions*
See *testis, torsion*

Cause

Abdominal pain is one of the most common presentations, particularly in general practice and may indicate a problem with any of the abdominal organs, vessels or nerves. These organs may include the liver, spleen, bladder, gut, uterus, ovaries and pancreas. Abdominal pain may also be due to inflammation of lymph nodes in the abdomen, as well as problems with arteries, veins, muscles, ligaments and bony structures.

The nature of the pain is important in determining the cause of the pain. Pain may be described as being sharp or dull, colicky or constant. The location of the pain is also important in determining the cause such as whether it occurs in the upper abdomen, around the umbilicus (navel), in the groin area or on the left or right sides of the body.

Symptoms

Pain may be accompanied by nausea and vomiting, constipation or menstrual periods; or may be increased by eating, passing urine or passing faeces.

Investigations

Determining the cause of abdominal pain may require further investigations, including tests on the blood, urine or faeces, as well as X-rays, CT, MRI and ultrasound scans, endoscopy, colonoscopy and cystoscopy. The last three of these investigations involves placing a camera on the end of a fibre-optic lens into the upper gut or lower gut or bladder. An endoscopic retrograde cysto-pancreatogram (ERCP) may be necessary to investigate problems involving the pancreas. Sometimes investigation of abdominal pain may require surgical intervention.

abscess

Cause

An abscess is a collection of pus that can occur anywhere, including in the abdominal cavity, as a result of infection. The most common sites of infection in the abdominal cavity are in the appendix, fallopian tubes and gall bladder, or as a result of a penetrating wound or following an operation.

Symptoms

The symptoms of an abscess in the abdominal cavity will result in pain in the abdomen. Sometimes it may be difficult to localise the abscess. The patient may feel unwell, complain of nausea and vomiting and have an elevated temperature. Often the patient is significantly unwell and requires immediate admission to hospital.

Treatment

Treatment for an abscess in the abdominal cavity involves locating the abscess, draining the pus and then surgically washing out the area containing the pus. This may involve inserting a draining mechanism from the wound to the exterior to allow ongoing drainage. The patient may then require oral or intravenous antibiotics for a period of time. Treatment for appendicitis invariably requires removal of the appendix. Similarly, for infection in the gall bladder, removal of the gall bladder is the treatment of choice. Following an infection in the fallopian tubes, the fallopian tubes may become blocked and the patient may become infertile. The assistance of a fertility specialist may be required in order to achieve pregnancy.

acne

Cause

Acne, also called pimples, is the result of blockage of tiny glands in the skin which are commonly found on the face, but may also occur on the neck and on the back. Once the pores of the glands are blocked, the glands become filled with thick, oily material followed by surrounding inflammation of the skin. This results in a localised infection which will eventually burst. The oily substance in the glands is called sebum and is often accentuated by the hormonal changes of puberty. The severity of acne in an individual, more commonly in teenagers, often depends on the severity of acne in their parents. Acne is often a strongly inherited condition and usually subsides after the teenage years.

Other causes of acne include hormonal changes before a menstrual period, menopause and stress. Restrictive clothing around the neck may also aggravate the problem.

Treatment

There are many and varied treatments for acne. Some of them may be obtained over the counter at a chemist and some as prescription items from your local doctor. In women, some oral contraceptive preparations will improve acne symptoms.

Topical treatments are also useful, e.g. benzoyl peroxide gel, topical Clindamycin, Cetaphil wash and topical antibiotic gels. Once treatment has begun, it should be reviewed after three months to assess progress. Often recurrences will occur and treatment needs to be reviewed. Oral antibiotics are also useful at times for severe outbreaks, e.g. tetracycline, doxycycline or minocycline. The medications should be used for four weeks (or a maximum of 10 weeks) if responses slow. Severe cystic acne may require referral to a dermatologist who may prescribe Roaccutane. Treatment of facial scars following severe cystic acne may require collagen injections in the sunken scar. This may be carried out by some dermatologists or, alternatively, by medical practitioners in cosmetic surgery clinics.

Addison's disease

See *adrenal gland, problems*
See *adrenal crisis*

Cause

Addison's disease, named after the London physician Thomas Addison, is caused by underactivity of the adrenal cortex. It produces a deficiency of the hormones cortisol and aldosterone. In most instances the cause of Addison's disease is unknown, but it is thought to be due to a autoimmune self-destructive process. Other possible causes include the effects of tuberculosis, adrenal tumour, amyloidosis, haemorrhage or an inflammatory process in the gland.

Symptoms

Symptoms of Addison's disease include a feeling of weakness and fatigue, hypotension (low blood pressure), postural hypotension (low blood pressure upon standing) and low blood sodium. Increased pigmentation (tanning) of skin exposed to sunlight may occur, especially on scars and the palmar creases and, to a lesser extent, tanning may also occur in parts of the body not exposed to sunlight. Other symptoms include loss of appetite, nausea, vomiting, diarrhoea, weight loss, dehydration and dizziness. On occasions, fainting episodes may also occur along with cold intolerance, slowing of the metabolic rate and hypoglycaemia (low blood sugar) after episodes of fasting or reduced food intake. This is because of the body's inability to generate glucose due to the hormonal deficiency. If not given additional amounts of hormones, such as cortisol, to help them cope, people with Addison's disease are in danger of collapse and even death when faced with stressful physiological situations such as infection, operations and trauma.

Treatment

Treatment of Addison's disease consists of replacement of the hormones which are lacking. The body normally produces cortisol hormones with a diurnal (daily) variation, with the maximal production in the morning and becoming less as the day wears on. Hydrocortisone is administered in the morning and fludrocortisone in the afternoon or evening to replace aldosterone. During times of illness, particularly infections, patients with Addison's disease require greater amounts of these hormones. If the patient is unable to take these preparations orally, then administration by injection is mandatory.

With Addison's disease, a condition called adrenal crisis may occur under conditions of physiological stress, e.g. following surgery, during infection or other illness or injury. Failure to recognise or treat an adrenal crisis could prove fatal. Symptoms of adrenal crisis include abdominal pain, low back pain and/or leg pain, hypotension (low blood pressure) and either lowering or elevation (fever) of body temperature. Administration of intravenous hydrocortisone and fluid replacement as well as correction of electrolyte balance, is mandatory for these patients.

adenitis, mesenteric

Cause

Mesenteric adenitis is an inflammation of the lymph nodes of the lining of the abdominal wall. It is sometimes a difficult problem to diagnose as it may be confused with acute appendicitis because the history of the two conditions is very similar.

Symptoms

The localisation of the pain in mesenteric adenitis is not as definite as in appendicitis and high temperatures may be present. A child may have little appetite and may also present with nausea and vomiting. The illness may last for about five days, after which recovery is rapid.

Treatment

Treatment for the condition is mainly symptomatic, with pain relief, adequate fluid intake and rest.

adolescent health, problems

See *acne*
See *anorexia nervosa*
See *depression*

During adolescence, some people are prone to adjustment disorders. Symptoms such as increased self-consciousness, self-awareness, self-centredness and lack of self-confidence are typical hallmarks. Both male and female adolescents need time and space to adjust during this developmental phase. During this time of adolescence, each individual is in the process of establishing their own identity, self-image, independence from family, as well as increasing self-reliance. They will need privacy, confidentiality, security in a stable and loving home, acceptance by their peers, and the ability to form special relationships with trusted adults.

Adolescence is a time for developing appropriate adult sexual roles and personal moral codes, decision-making regarding future career paths and vocational choices.

Emotional problems during adolescence are common and must be handled sensitively and sympathetically. Anxiety and depression, sex, stress, self-esteem, eating disorders such as anorexia and bulimia, drug-taking for recreational purposes, and anxieties regarding their future life are all important issues for adolescents.

Depression is common during the adolescent years and suicide must always be considered as a risk when a young person presents with depressive symptoms such as increasing isolation at home or deterioration in their school performance. Male adolescents are four times more likely to commit suicide than female adolescents; however females are more likely to attempt suicide unsuccessfully.

adrenal crisis

See *Addison's disease*
See *adrenal gland, problems*

Cause

Adrenal crisis may occur during times of physiological stress. Failure to recognise or treat an adrenal crisis may prove fatal.

Symptoms

Symptoms of adrenal crisis include abdominal pain, low back pain and/or leg pain, hypotension (low blood pressure) and either lowering or elevation (fever) of body temperature.

Treatment

Administration of intravenous hydrocortisone and fluid replacement as well as correction of electrolyte imbalance is mandatory.

adrenal gland, problems

See *Addison's disease*
See *adrenal virilism*
See *aldosteronism*
See *Cushing's syndrome*

The adrenal glands are a pair of glands situated on the upper pole of each kidney and form part of the endocrine system. The adrenal glands consist of two portions called the cortex and medulla. The adrenal cortex is responsible for producing glucocorticoids or cortisol, mineralocorticoids or aldosterone (which regulates electrolyte control, particularly that of sodium and potassium in the kidney) and androgens (primarily dehydroepiandrosterone or DHEA).

The adrenal medulla is composed of cells that produce and secrete adrenaline substances, including histamine, serotonin and neuropeptide hormones. The adrenaline substances are those responsible for arming the body with the ability to respond to the classic flight, fright or fight response.

Hyperactivity (overactivity) of the gland results in a medical problem called Cushing's syndrome. Hypoactivity (underactivity) of the gland results in a medical problem called Addison's disease. Both of these conditions are directly related to the amount of corticosteroid produced by the glands.

adrenal virilism *(adrenogenital syndrome)*

See *adrenal gland, problems*

Cause

This condition results from exposure of the patient to excessive amounts of adrenal androgens (male sex hormones) resulting from a tumour of the adrenal glands.

Symptoms

The extent to which patients will develop symptoms depends on the early diagnosis of the condition, as well as the age and sex of the patient. Symptoms include hirsutism (or increased facial hair), baldness, acne, deepening of the voice and increased libido (sexual drive).

Treatment

Treatment for adrenal virilism is the administration of dexamethasone. However, monitoring of the dosage of dexamethasone is important in order to prevent a secondary effect causing Cushing's syndrome. For those patients where a tumour of the adrenal gland results in Cushing's syndrome, removal of the tumour is also recommended.

If the condition remains untreated or unrecognised in young people, premature or sexual maturation may occur. In female infants the condition may be suspected in the presence of ambiguous genitalia and, in particular, enlargement of the clitoris. Older females may experience cessation of periods, as well as a decrease in the size of the uterus, breasts and skeletal muscles. In adult men, the increased amounts of adrenal androgens may suppress testicular function, thus causing infertility.

alcohol abuse

See *anxiety*
See *cirrhosis of the liver*
See *depression*

Cause

Alcohol abuse may present as frequent or infrequent bouts of excessive alcohol consumption. This may be in response to situations of stress or anxiety or may be due to the influences of peer pressure resulting in episodes of binge drinking. When the consumption of alcohol starts to interfere with a person's daily life, this may be regarded as problem drinking or alcoholism.

Excessive alcohol intake over a prolonged period of time can lead to significant health problems. In order to reduce alcohol intake, people often require professional counselling and treatment.

Symptoms

The symptoms of alcoholism include drinking alone, hiding one's drinking habits from others, alcohol consumption which interferes with work and social commitments, craving alcohol at any time of the day or night and episodes of bingeing on alcohol. The symptoms of alcohol excess are increased by the fact that alcoholics often fail to eat proper food and drink alcohol in preference to food which becomes a source of 'empty' kilojoules. The long-term effects of alcohol abuse include cirrhosis of the liver, brain damage with symptoms of depression, irrational behaviour and mental deterioration (Wernicke-Korsakoff syndrome or psychosis). This is related to vitamin B deficiency, particularly vitamin B1 or thiamine. Degeneration of parts of the brain may also occur, resulting in coordination difficulties with the hands and walking. Damage to the nerves supplying the legs might also occur, causing muscle cramps, the sensation of pins and needles and muscle aches and pains. If alcohol is suddenly withdrawn from someone who is chronically addicted to large amounts of alcohol, these people may experience acute withdrawal effects known as the DTs or delirium tremens. During this time, people may experience hallucinations and epileptic fits, and may even die.

Treatment

Treatment is available for helping an addict withdraw from excessive alcohol intake. Patients will require additional vitamin B1 supplements, regular meals, social support and medications in order to prevent the DTs and overcome the craving for alcohol intake. Detoxification (detox) centres are available for managing treatment programs for alcoholics who are significantly addicted to alcohol. Detox centres are also available for people addicted to various forms of over-the-counter, prescription and illegal medications. Patients may require sedation, e.g. diazepam, in order to prevent the DTs. Medication called acamprosale calcium is also available to reduce the craving effect of excessive alcohol and may be obtained on authority prescription from a local doctor or from medical staff in detox centres.

aldosteronism *(Conn's syndrome)*

See *adrenal gland, problems*

Cause

This condition is caused by the production of increased amounts of aldosterone from the adrenal cortex due to the presence of either hypoplasia of the cortex, tumour formation or carcinoma of the gland. Secondary hypo-aldosteronism may occur in the presence of renal artery stenosis or blockage of the artery supplying the kidney.

Symptoms

Symptoms of this condition include weakness, elevation in blood pressure and electrolyte imbalance involving low potassium levels.

Treatment

Removal of the tumour is recommended. If hypoplasia of the gland is detected, treatment consists of administration of spironolactone.

allergic reactions and hypersensitivity disorders

See *asthma*
See *conjunctivitis*
See *glomerulonephritis*
See *immune response*
See *hay fever (rhinitis)*
See *systemic lupus erythematosus*

Allergic reactions and hypersensitivity disorders are caused by an exaggerated form of activation of the immune response which is unrelated to infection or injury.

Hypersensitivity reactions may be classified as Type 1 to 4:

Type 1 hypersensitivity results when immunoglobulin called IgE binds to an antigen (an allergic substance such as peanuts or pollen) and triggers the release of substances which include histamine, proteases, prostaglandins, leucotrines and also platelet activating factor

(PAF). These substances produce dilatation of the vessels, increase the permeability of the capillaries, increase mucus production, produce smooth muscle spasm and result in infiltration of the area with eosinophils (white cells specifically associated with allergic reactions), helper 2 T cells and other inflammatory cells. This process is basic to conditions such as asthma, hay fever (rhinitis), conjunctivitis and food allergies.

Type 2 hypersensitivity reactions present when an antibody binds to cell or tissue antigens. The antigen–antibody complex activates killer T cells or macrophages and complement (an enzymatic protein found in the blood), leading to cell and tissue damage. This reaction is termed cell-mediated cytotoxicity. Type 2 hypersensitivity reactions are found in rejection of transplanted organs, haemolytic anaemias, Hashimoto's thyroiditis and Goodpasture's syndrome.

Type 3 hypersensitivity reactions are caused by an acute inflammatory response to circulating antigen–antibody complexes in blood vessels or tissues. Type 3 hypersensitivity reactions include serum sickness, SLE (or systemic lupus erythematosus), rheumatoid arthritis, certain forms of vasculitis and certain types of glomerulonephritis.

Type 4 hypersensitivity reaction is a delayed hypersensitivity reaction involving T cells that have become sensitised to an antigen by prior exposure. These T cells activate when re-exposed to the same antigen and an inflammatory reaction occurs designed to oppose the antigen—like an army fighting the enemy. Like in war, there are innocent casualties and the attempt of the body to deal with the offending allergen results in body tissue damage. Hypersensitivity reactions are thought to play a role in the following conditions: autoimmune haemolytic anaemia, autoimmune thrombocytopenia purpura, Goodpasture's syndrome, Graves' disease, Hashimoto's thyroiditis, insulin resistance, myasthenia gravis, pemphigus, systemic lupus erythematosus (SLE), some cases of diabetes mellitus, glomerulonephritis, Addison's disease, some cases of infertility, connective tissue disease, pernicious anaemia, polymyositis, rheumatoid arthritis, Sjögren's syndrome, chronic active hepatitis, endocrine gland failure, primary biliary cirrhosis, atopic dermatitis, urticaria, asthma, vasculitis, vitiligo. Type 4 hypersensitivity reactions include drug hypersensitivity and contact dermatitis.

Drug hypersensitivity is an immune-mediated reaction to a drug. Some drugs are able to stimulate antibody production directly; however most drugs bind to cellular proteins and this drug–protein complex stimulates anti-drug antibody production via T cells.

The way that primary sensitisation occurs and how the innate immune system is initially involved is unclear. However, once a drug stimulates an immune response, cross reactions between drug classes may then occur. Symptoms of drug hypersensitivity may vary from mild to severe skin rashes. The most severe of drug hypersensitivity reactions are called anaphylactic reactions and serum sickness.

Treatment

Treatment for drug hypersensitivity reactions includes withdrawing of the drug causing the reaction, desensitisation, as well as antihistamine medications and corticosteroids. Sometimes, for severe life-threatening reactions, drug hypersensitivity reactions may require the administration of subcutaneous adrenaline. Skin testing for drug hypersensitivity may be undertaken, in particular, skin testing for penicillin allergy. However it has been reported that only 10 to 20 per cent of patients who report penicillin allergy have positive skin-testing reactions. Skin testing in this way is unreliable because it detects only the presence of IgE-mediated reactions and therefore is of no value in investigating other types of hypersensitivity reactions such as those occurring in haemolytic anaemias and kidney damage. For patients who require a definite diagnosis of penicillin allergy, the skin prick test is used as the first test of choice. If the prick test is negative, intradermal testing is the next option. If the skin test is positive, treating the patient with penicillin would produce an anaphylactic reaction and endanger the person's life.

alopecia *(hair loss)*

See *hypothyroidism*

Cause

Hair growth has a cyclical pattern of growing and falling out and a normal healthy adult may lose up to a hundred hairs per day from the head. If excessive amounts of hair loss continue over a period of time, this may be regarded as abnormal and becomes a concern for males and females alike. Hair may be lost in patches (alopecia areata) or in large amounts (alopecia totalis or baldness) or there may be loss of hair from all over the head. The most common type of hair loss is male pattern baldness, which is often an inherited trait and may commence as early as the late teens. Since it is inherited, male pattern baldness responds poorly to treatment in the long term. This form of baldness is, as the name suggests, much more common in males but can also occur in females and in these cases, a cause should be sought. Diffuse hair loss in women may be related to the menstrual cycle, with hair loss occurring at certain times of the month. Other causes for hair loss include stress and anxiety, menopause and myxoedema, the sudden loss of weight either as a result of diet or exercise and/or after pregnancy. Hair loss after pregnancy is often related to changes in hormonal levels after delivery, breast development related to milk production and the stress of having a newborn in the household.

Symptoms

The density of hair tends to decrease with age and older people—both men and women—will often have fewer hair follicles in the growing phase compared to younger people.

Sometimes total body hair loss may occur. This may be related to extreme stress, psychiatric disturbance or as the result of administration of some drugs. Total hair loss is common during chemotherapy (a treatment for cancer). Patients on anticoagulants such as warfarin may also experience hair loss. Some diseases may contribute to increased hair loss, e.g. diabetes, thyroid abnormalities, pituitary gland abnormalities and abnormalities of the sex hormones. A group of diseases called autoimmune conditions may also contribute to hair loss, e.g. systemic lupus erythematosus (SLE). Rare causes of hair loss include liver and kidney failure, cancer, syphilis and hair pulling (trichotillomania).

Treatment

There are some treatments available which may reduce the rate of hair loss, e.g. in male pattern baldness Regain is a topical preparation used. Its effects continue only for the duration of application. It may take up to six months to see any improvement in the rate of hair loss and even longer periods of time in which to see some new hair growth. For men, finasteride may be administered in tablet form. Hair transplantation may be considered; however this treatment is often costly and the quality of service depends on the experience of the operator.

amenorrhoea *(no period)*

See *pregnancy*

Cause

Amenorrhoea or the absence of periods in women, may occur as a result of delayed puberty or a chromosomal abnormality. It may be primary, i.e. not commence at all. In the case of chromosomal abnormalities and congenital adrenal hyperplasia, the periods have never started. More common is secondary amenorrhoea, when periods start but cease due to excessive dieting and weight loss, excessive exercise, stress factors in a person's lifestyle, the presence of a polycystic ovary (which may be accompanied by increased facial hair and being overweight), pituitary dysfunction, thyroid problems, chronic liver disorder or obesity.

Investigations

Menstrual periods normally start between 12 and 15 years of age. If periods have not commenced by the age of 16, investigation to determine the cause should be undertaken. Usually in the cases of chromosomal abnormalities and congenital adrenal hyperplasia, these diagnoses will have been made long before the age of 12 years. Investigations of secondary amenorrhoea (periods have started and then stopped) include testing for pregnancy as the first-line measure. A pelvic ultrasound in combination with hormone testing may be required to determine the presence of a polycystic ovary.

Treatment

Treatment for amenorrhoea is directed at the cause of the problem.

anaemia

Cause

Anaemia is a decrease in the number of red cells and, therefore, haemoglobin (protein that carries oxygen) in the blood. Anaemia is a description, not a diagnosis and means having a low haemoglobin level and/or red cell count. The red cell mass is a balance between production and destruction of the red cells, which circulate in the blood and have a limited lifespan. Anaemia may be caused by blood loss, excessive destruction of red cells, or inadequate replacement of red cells during new red cell production in the bone marrow. Iron deficiency is the most common form of anaemia resulting from blood loss. Blood loss may be acute or chronic.

There are various types of anaemia which are classified according to the size of the red blood cell. The red blood cell may be either too small (microcytic anaemia) or too large (macrocytic anaemia). The causes of microcytic anaemia include iron deficiency, inherited conditions, e.g. thalassaemia, which is more prevalent in some races than others (such as people from Mediterranean backgrounds). Chronic disease states may also cause microcytic anaemia. Macrocytic anaemia may be caused by vitamin deficiencies, in particular vitamin B12, folate deficiency or cytotoxic drugs used during treatment for cancer. People may also become acutely anaemic due to sudden or chronic blood loss and chronic renal disease.

Symptoms

Anaemia develops in stages. Initially, the body's iron requirements exceed the dietary intake, which then causes a reduction in iron stores. As the iron stores are depleted, a compensatory absorption of dietary iron occurs from the diet, assuming an adequate dietary intake. As the deficiency in iron becomes more pronounced, red blood cell production becomes impaired. This may contribute to feelings of fatigue (tiredness) and poor endurance (sporting or other performance), inflammation of the tongue, concave fingernails and sometimes pain on swallowing. People who are anaemic may often feel tired, lethargic, run down and have no energy. People who experience sudden blood loss may feel faint or light-headed and may even collapse. These patients will require urgent medical treatment and investigations to determine the cause of their anaemia and blood loss.

Treatment

The treatment for anaemia is first to diagnose and then treat the specific cause. In the case of iron deficiency, iron replacement is the best treatment option. Replacement of blood volume will also correct anaemia due to blood loss. This is the most common treatment in situations where inadequate replacement of red cells is the cause of the anaemia, e.g. with varying forms of leukaemia or anaemia due to chronic disease.

anal itch

See *gonorrhoea*
See *haemorrhoids*
See *molluscum contagiosum*
See *syphilis*
See *vaginal discharge*

Cause

Anal itch, also known as pruritus ani, is associated with irritation around the anal sphincter. This may be associated with using harsh toilet papers, excessive sweating or localised inflammation. The itch may also be the result of haemorrhoids around the anal area; small cracks in the anal area; skin diseases such as dermatitis, eczema, psoriasis, skin tags; vaginal discharges; and poor hygiene.

Itching of the anal area might also be produced by some infections, e.g. fungal infections, intestinal worms, molluscum contagiosum, gonorrhoea and syphilis.

Treatment

The treatment for anal itch involves using soft toilet tissues, soothing creams and sometimes may require mild steroid creams in order to relieve the itch. Treatment of the haemorrhoids will also improve anal itching.

anal pain

See *haemorrhoids*

Cause

Anal pain may be due to anal fissures (cracks or small tears in the anal area), peri-anal haematomas or haemorrhoids, strangulated haemorrhoids, or because of an abscess around the anus or pelvic floor.

Treatment

Anal fissures or superficial cracks may become acute or chronic. The treatment involves prevention of constipation and healing the fissure aggravated by the passing of bowel motions. Local analgesia or pain relief will relieve the symptoms and also help heal the fissure. Creams and suppositories are available as treatment for haemorrhoids; however, often more immediate relief is gained by incision of the peri-anal haematoma and draining clotted blood from inside the vessels. In order to do this, the area is injected with local anaesthetic then an incision is made and the blood clot is removed.

An abscess around the anal canal, referred to as a peri-anal abscess, is extremely painful and requires careful assessment. Sometimes this may require treatment by a specialist surgeon under anaesthetic in hospital, and post-operative antibiotics.

anaphylaxis *(acute allergic reaction)*

See *allergic reactions and hypersensitivity disorders*

Cause
Anaphylaxis is a severe form of acute allergic reaction and may be life-threatening in some individuals, e.g. peanut allergy in some children, as well as allergies to strawberries, shellfish and iodine.

Acute allergic reactions may be localised or generalised. Localised reactions may appear as hives or a reddening of the skin. Local allergic reactions may be caused by an insect bite or, alternatively, by ingesting, inhaling or contact on the skin with the substance that has caused the allergy.

Symptoms
Acute allergic reactions are often intensely itchy, causing the skin to become red and inflamed looking and often raised from the surrounding skin. Some people with more severe reactions may experience difficulty breathing and swelling in or around the mouth. This becomes a medical emergency. Some patients may experience problems with breathing, called bronchospasm or wheezing.

Treatment
Treatment of an acute allergic reaction depends on the severity of the reaction. For minor skin reactions, simple antihistamine medications may be sufficient, e.g. for bites and stings. For more severe allergic reactions, the administration of subcutaneous adrenaline may be required. In some instances, administration of oral or injected hydrocortisone (steroid) may be required. For patients with documented acute allergic reactions, the local doctor may recommend providing an Epipen, which will be dispensed by the chemist. A special authority prescription is required when prescribing an Epipen for acute allergic reactions. Provision of an Epipen is recommended for children who are allergic to peanuts or who have other life-

threatening allergies. If bronchospasm occurs during an acute allergic reaction, administration of salbutamol and/or subcutaneous hydrocortisone may be recommended in hospital.

aneurysm

See *abdominal aortic aneurysm*
See *heart attack*
See *stroke*

Cause

An aneurysm may form in an artery when the wall of the artery balloons out to a point where it may rupture. An aneurysm may occur in any artery of the body. Where an aneurysm forms in the aorta—a major vessel leading out of the heart and distributing blood to the rest of the body—a mass may occur. This can be felt by examining the abdomen. If the mass is large enough to be felt, it will pulsate in synchrony with the heartbeat. If an aneurysm forms in the vessels of the brain or in the vessels leading away from the heart, the person may be in imminent danger of heart attack, stroke or even sudden death.

Symptoms

Symptoms of an aneurysm may include pain, abdominal discomfort, headache or sudden collapse.

Treatment

The best mode of treatment for an aneurysm is surgical repair before major symptoms occur. This applies not only to abdominal aneurysms but also to aneurysms which occur in the vessels supplying the brain.

angina

See *heart attack*

Cause

Angina is caused by lack of oxygen being delivered to the tissues of the heart. This may occur during exercise or at rest.

Symptoms

Symptoms of an angina attack include chest pain which may radiate to the arm, more commonly the left and may also involve the jaw.

Investigations

Investigations of angina pain may involve an electrocardiogram (ECG) or cardiac catheterisation to assess the level of blockage in one or more of the coronary vessels. Clinical examination may indicate the possibility of musculoskeletal chest wall pain, the possibility of gallstones or even gastro-oesophagial problems, including reflux. Chest X-ray may reveal a fracture or an injury or a chest infection causing pain.

Treatment

Symptoms of angina may be relieved by the administration of some medications, including glyceryl trinitrate and short- and long-acting versions of beta-blocker medications. Angina may be described as stable or unstable, where the above medications may be prescribed. Angina may also be described as refractory, where imminent risk of coronary artery occlusion (heart attack) may occur. The administration of soluble aspirin may help to relieve the pain and blockage of the coronary vessel and is standard procedure in acute onset of chest pain where it is thought the pain is related to blockage of the coronary artery or arteries. The presence of ongoing pain may require admission to hospital with further stabilisation. If it is determined that one or more of the coronary arteries are blocked then stenting (a procedure where a mesh cylinder is placed in the artery and dilated with a balloon) or, alternatively, coronary artery bypass graft surgery (often referred to as bypass surgery) may be indicated to relieve symptoms.

ankylosing spondylitis

See *arthritis*

Cause

The cause of ankylosing spondylitis is unknown, but it is an uncommon cause of arthritis which selectively affects the joints in the vertebra in the spine.

Symptoms

Whatever the cause of the arthritis, the symptoms are the same, namely pain, swelling of the involved joints, tenderness, stiffness and the joints feeling hot to the touch.

Treatment

The principles of treatment for arthritis are the same irrespective of the cause. These include a balance between rest and exercise; heat packs to painful joints; reduction of weight if overweight; gentle exercise; physiotherapy; simple analgesics e.g. paracetamol; and non-steroidal anti-inflammatory medications (NSAIDs), e.g. ibuprofen. At times referral to a rheumatologist or specialist orthopaedic surgeon will be necessary.

anorexia

See *adolescent health problems*
See *anorexia nervosa*

Cause

Anorexia describes the state where a person does not experience a normal hunger drive from the eating centre in the hypothalamus situated in the brain. It very commonly occurs in those in states of worry and mental depression, but also in other forms of illness. It can also occur as part of a normal response, e.g. not feeling hungry or in emergency situations, such as having to flee for one's life. Anorexia is a symptom which may be associated with any acute illness or may present as a chronic medical problem with other medical co-morbidities. Acute illness (either viral or bacterial) may accompany anorexia, e.g. acute respiratory infections, gastroenteritis, urinary tract infections, malignancy and terminal disease. Anorexia is common in elderly patients and sometimes in children in the 'terrible twos' phase.

Treatment

Treatment for the condition is symptomatic and supportive management is indicated depending on the cause.

anorexia nervosa

See *amenorrhoea*
See *anorexia*
See *anxiety*
See *depression*

Cause

Anorexia nervosa is a condition which is characterised by patients being significantly underweight and who have a fear of gaining excess weight. These patients are usually female, with the condition commonly commencing in their teens or sometimes even earlier. Less commonly it occurs in males. The cause of this disorder is not really known.

Symptoms

The condition is characterised by a pathological fear of being fat and attempts are made by the patient to maintain a low food intake at all costs. This includes employing secretive methods of concealing their food intake. Women may experience coexistent depression, anxiety and amenorrhoea. Denial that there is a problem is a common feature of this disorder. Some of these patients even refuse to be weighed for fear that they might learn that they have gained a kilo or two. A body mass index (weight in kilograms divided by height in metres squared) of 18 or less is considered to be significantly underweight.

Treatment

Treatment for the condition has mixed long-term results and is achieved with cognitive behaviour therapy, general support and with anti-depressant medication. Ongoing management with the assistance of the general practitioner, a psychiatrist, a psychologist, a counsellor and a dietitian is commonly required. Sometimes nasogastric feeding in hospital is required to maintain weight.

anxiety

See *adolescent health problems*
See *depression*
See *menopause*

Cause

Anxiety, by definition, is an uncomfortable feeling of fear of an imminent disaster. Anxiety and depression often go hand in hand. Anxiety may be classified as general anxiety disorder, panic disorder, phobias, obsessive-compulsive disorder and post-traumatic stress disorder. Some anxiety may be regarded as a normal reaction to the situation, e.g. nervousness prior to examinations.

Symptoms

The symptoms may be related to a specific problem in the person's daily life, e.g. financial difficulty, marital or work disharmony, worry about children, an overactive thyroid or a phobia (a situation or something which causes disproportionate fear in a person, e.g. fear of heights, spiders or aeroplanes).

Treatment

Patients suffering from anxiety and/or depression require reassurance and explanation. Treatment of general anxiety disorders may require specific psychotherapy; however, much of this treatment may be able to be provided by the local doctor and/or counselling services. Discussing stress management techniques may improve coping abilities. For acute anxiety, small amounts of intermittent benzodiazepines may be helpful and may improve the symptoms. As benzodiazepines are drugs of dependence, their unsupervised use is to be discouraged.

Sometimes people may experience acute anxiety when having to make a presentation to a gathering of people. If making such presentations is part of a person's occupation, the symptoms of anxiety may be improved by intermittent administration of a medication called a beta blocker, which is designed to overcome feelings of a racing heart and hence improve a feeling of anxiety. Drugs such as beta blockers are often used and antidepressants alone or in combination may be used for this purpose. Treatment of panic disorders may be improved by cognitive behaviour therapy, where the aim is to teach patients how to identify, evaluate, control and modify their negative and fearful thoughts and behaviour. This may require referral to a psychologist or psychiatrist. Treatment of phobic states involves psychotherapy and behaviour modification. Obsessive-compulsive disorders are best managed by a combination of psychotherapy, various forms of relaxation techniques including the use of hypnotherapy and meditation and medication. Post-traumatic stress disorder is a difficult condition to treat and symptoms may appear long after the traumatic event has passed. The aim of treatment is to desensitise the patient to the events which caused the trauma.

appendicitis

See *abscess*

Cause

Appendicitis is the most common surgical emergency. Acute appendicitis is mainly a condition of young adults, especially those 20 to 30 years of age, but it may affect all ages. It is uncommon under the age of three years and should be regarded with suspicion in anyone over the age of 50 years. For a patient over the age of 50 years presenting with abdominal pain in this area, the most likely diagnosis will be one of malignancy, which must be excluded by clinical examination and investigations and not necessarily acute appendicitis.

Symptoms

Initially, the symptoms of acute appendicitis start with pain around the umbilicus (navel). The person may also experience nausea and vomiting and later this tenderness will become more localised on the lower right side of the abdomen. The patient may present with fever. Sometimes the appendix may burst before the diagnosis is made and the person will become very sick and develop peritonitis—a severe infection of the membrane called the peritoneum, inside the abdominal cavity.

Treatment

Treatment of acute appendicitis is an appendicectomy (surgical removal of appendix). If the patient develops peritonitis (inflammation of the membrane lining the abdominal cavity), they will require treatment with additional antibiotics and also may require a drain to be inserted in the abdominal wall to allow the escape of any accumulating pus.

arm and hand pain

See *heart attack*
See *osteoarthritis*

There are many causes of arm and hand pain, including problems with the cervical spine, shoulder, elbow, wrist (including carpal tunnel syndrome), tennis elbow, osteoarthritis, heart problems (including acute heart attack), lung cancer, some infections and tendonitis of the hand. Uncommon causes include dislocated elbow in children, foreign bodies in the arm, polymyalgia rheumatica and thoracic outlet syndrome (compression of the nerves in the neck).

arrhythmia

See *heart attack*
See *palpitations and arrhythmias*

Cause

The heartbeat originates in the specialised group of cells in the right atrium (one of the top chambers of the heart). The wave of electrical activity passes along a specialised system, called the conducting system, to all areas of the heart simultaneously. This results in a coordinated contraction of all the muscle fibres and blood being pumped out into the main arteries and being distributed to all parts of the body. Arrhythmias are conditions where this process does not occur normally, resulting in the heart beating either faster than normal, slower than normal or irregularly. These disorders, which include tachycardias, bradycardias and heart block, may be congenital (present from birth) and relate to the presence of heart disease. They may also result from electrolyte abnormalities (e.g. low potassium and magnesium), lack of oxygen to the heart, hormonal imbalances (i.e. thyroid disease) and/or drugs (i.e. alcohol and caffeine).

Symptoms

Major cardiac symptoms include chest pain or discomfort, shortness of breath, weakness and fatigue, palpitations (awareness of the heart beating; regular or irregular), discernible irregularities of the heart, a feeling of light-headedness or a feeling of being about to faint. These symptoms may occur in cardiovascular as well as other non-cardiac disorders.

Investigations

Heart rate and rhythm may be examined by performing an ECG or electrocardiograph, (a device used to record the transmission of the cardiac impulse through the heart muscle), a Holter monitor or cardiac stress testing. A Holter monitor is a device which the patient wears in order to record in a minicomputer every heartbeat for a 24-hour period. The patient has a diary in which he or she records any significant event or cardiac symptoms during this period of time. In a stress test, the patient walks or runs at increasing speeds as well as increasing levels of difficulty and gradient on a treadmill, while the heart rate, blood pressure and ECG are carefully monitored.

Treatment

The exact nature of a cardiac arrhythmia needs to be identified before a treatment plan is put into place. Once a cardiac arrhythmia is diagnosed and treatment deemed necessary, stabilisation of an arrhythmia may occur using medication, surgical ablation (i.e. burning or freezing) of abnormal electrical conduction pathways in the heart or cessation of the causative or aggravating agents, e.g. smoking and caffeine. ECG tracing, exercise stress testing, stress echocardiogram or cardiac catheritisation may be required under the management of a cardiologist.

arthritis

See *ankylosing spondylitis*
See *gout*
See *Osgood-Schlatter disease*
See *osteoarthritis*
See *osteomyelitis*
See *psoriasis*
See *rheumatoid arthritis*
See *systemic lupus erythematosus*

Cause

Arthritis is an inflammatory process that can affect any joint in the body. Every joint is surrounded and supported by ligaments, tendons and muscles. The ends of the bones are covered by cartilage, which helps the joints move smoothly. There are many causes for painful joints, and some diseases which affect the body in other ways may also produce sore joints.

Symptoms

Whatever the cause of the arthritis, the symptoms are mainly pain, swelling of the involved joints, tenderness, stiffness and/or the joints feeling hot to the touch.

Treatment

The principles of treatment are the same irrespective of the cause and include a balance between rest and exercise, heat packs for painful joints, reduction in weight if overweight, gentle exercise, physiotherapy, simple analgesics (e.g. paracetamol), non-steroidal anti-inflammatory medications (NSAIDS) such as ibuprofen. Splinting of joints may be required in some cases of rheumatoid arthritis and at times referral will be necessary to a specialist orthopaedic surgeon or rheumatologist. Septic arthritis, either blood-borne or post-operative, may need aspiration or drainage.

Asperger's syndrome

See *autism*

asthma

See *hay fever*
See *respiratory system*

Cause

Asthma is a lung condition characterised by hyper-reactivity of the airways and narrowing of the small airways in the lung (called bronchoconstriction), causing entrapment of air in the lung. Asthma is an inflammatory disease of the respiratory tract. It is often associated with a positive family history, allergy, hay fever and eczema. In young children under the age of two years, asthma-like symptoms are referred to as bronchiolitis.

Symptoms

The symptoms of asthma include cough, shortness of breath (both resting and after exercise), wheezing, waking in the night short of breath (commonly around 2 am) and production of bronchial secretions, which are clear or white. Because of the entrapment of air, the patient finds it difficult to fully expel all the air out of the lung with normal respiration. Expiration is accompanied by the sound of wheezing. If the asthma is severe and the patient is complaining of severe breathlessness or can only speak in monosyllables and the wheezing disappears, this indicates that the patient needs to be referred to an emergency department straightaway. Asthma may be associated with exercise (exercise-induced asthma), cigarette smoking (either by the asthmatic or another member of the household or office), change in climatic conditions (commonly asthma will increase with the sudden change in temperature in autumn or spring with warm days and cold nights or very cold conditions), windy weather, alcohol consumption, laughing or allergens, e.g. pollens, foods, perfumes. Not uncommonly, asthma is accompanied by other atopic conditions such as eczema, dermatitis or hay fever. In fact hay fever may be considered to produce the same reaction in the upper airways that asthma produces in the lower airways.

Investigations

Investigations for asthma include spirometry (breathing test) and peak flow estimations, as well as allergy skin testing to determine allergic trigger reactions. Desensitisation for allergic reactions may be considered, where a weekly or fortnightly subcutaneous injection of small amounts of modified allergens of varying strengths are injected over a period of time, usually monthly or even fortnightly. The aim of this is to acclimatise the body to the allergens, thus reducing the body's reactions to these substances. Desensitisation for allergic reactions may also be considered for problematic hay fever. A chest X-ray or sometimes a bronchoscopy may be needed where it is suspected that a child may have inhaled a foreign body into the windpipe or trachea.

Occupational asthma also occurs i.e. when a patient is exposed to allergens as part of their work, with the result being asthma. Patients with asthma are more prone to bronchitis, pneumonia and sinusitis.

Treatment

There are two main groups of medications used in the treatment of asthma: relievers and preventers. Relievers are administered by inhalation either as a puffer or as a nebuliser.

Preventer medications may be administered alone or in the form of combination therapy, i.e. relievers and preventers in the same device. Treatment of an acute asthma attack involves administration of salbutamol either in a spacer or by nebuliser with oxygen at a rate of 8L per minute, along with hydrocortisone given by inhalation, intramuscularly (by injection into muscles) or intravenously (by injection into the blood veins). Respiratory function may be estimated using a spirometer or a peak flow meter or by estimating oxygen concentration in the blood by using a pulse oximeter. In severe cases of asthma, adrenaline may be administered and referral to a hospital is mandatory.

atherosclerosis

See *heart attack*
See *stroke*

atrophic vaginitis

See *menopause, problems*
See *vaginitis, atrophic*

autism

Cause

Autism is a neurodevelopmental disorder, the cause of which is unknown. The disorder sometimes runs in families. For example, Rhett's syndrome, a subtype of autism, is thought to be caused by a mutation on one of the X chromosomes.

Symptoms

Autism is characterised by impaired social interaction and communication. It is associated with repetitive types of behaviour and is often accompanied by intellectual disability. A number of other types of autism may occur, including Asperger's syndrome, which is characterised by social isolation, clumsiness, repetitive movements or behaviour, increased sensitivity to sensory stimuli, and difficulty recognising humour and jokes. Children with Asperger's syndrome may have less disability than children with other subtypes of autism and even display normal or above average intelligence. Another subtype of autism is Rhett's syndrome, which will usually start to appear after the age of six months of normal development and is associated with impaired growth and social interactions, mental retardation, loss of speech, purposeful hand movements, epilepsy, autistic features, ataxia (failure or irregularity of muscle coordination) and is found exclusively in females. While Rhett's syndrome is found in girls, another inherited disorder Fragile X syndrome is found mainly in boys and also causes learning difficulties. It is thought that 1 in 10 autistic children have a genetic (i.e. inherited) abnormality such as Rhett's syndrome or Fragile X syndrome.

Treatment

Treatment for the spectrum of autism disorders is based on behavioural management and support of therapy for additional medical problems, e.g. epilepsy.

baby, problems

See *breastfeeding*
See *colic, baby*
See *crying baby*
See *floppy baby*
See *immunisation for childhood infectious diseases*
See *intussusception*
See *pyloric stenosis*

back pain

See *osteoarthritis*

Cause

Back pain is a common presentation in medical practice. The most common reasons for back pain include back strain, prolapsed vertebral disc, ligament and muscle strain due to injury, arthritis, sciatica, osteoporosis, urinary tract infections and stones, period pain, secondary deposits from cancer, cancer of the bones of the vertebra, an aortic aneurysm which is increasing in size and scoliosis.

Symptoms

The site of the pain, the age of the patient or a history of trauma—including participation in sporting activities—gives a clue to the problem causing back pain. A detailed history from the patient is important when looking for a cause for back pain. Pain may be worse when sitting, standing or walking, and may be accompanied by stiffness. A history of fever or strong-smelling urine may indicate the presence of a kidney infection or the presence of a kidney stone. Recurrent symptoms for urinary infections originating in the kidney are investigated with ultrasound or an intravenous pyelogram or even a CT (computerised tomography) scan.

Treatment

Treatment of back pain is first to establish a cause. The basic approach to treating back pain caused by injury or trauma includes rest (less than two days), pain relief, hot or cold compression packs, mobilisation exercises, physiotherapy or referral to a back specialist. Surgical intervention for treating prolapsed discs is uncommon. In cases where fractures are evident and need to be stabilised, surgery is indicated; or in cases where an acute fracture has occurred in the presence of osteoporosis, stabilisation of the vertebral fracture may be achieved by the use of injectable material into the substance of the vertebrae. Most people with back pain will also require education to learn how to manage the problem and minimise their symptoms. Pilates and yoga are also useful tools for chronic back pain management.

bacterial infections

See *infections*

Cause

Bacteria are micro-organisms consisting of double stranded deoxyribonucleic acid or DNA with cell walls. Some bacteria may have additional protection with the addition of an enclosed capsule which protects them from being destroyed by the body's defence mechanisms. Some bacteria require the presence of air (termed aerobic) whereas other bacteria do not (termed anaerobic). Still others may grow and flourish with or without the presence of air and are termed facultative bacteria. Bacteria may live and replicate intracellularly (inside cells) or extracellularly (outside cells).

Symptoms

Symptoms of bacterial infection include fever, malaise, discharge (including sputum production and pus), inflammation of the area concerned, redness, pain and discomfort.

Treatment

Drugs which are used to combat bacterial infections are derived from either the bacteria itself or moulds, or are generated in a laboratory. The term antibiotic originally referred to bacteria-fighting agents that were derived from either bacteria or moulds.

Antibacterial agents or antibiotics have a number of action mechanisms to fight infection. These mechanisms include inhibiting cell wall synthesis of the organism, increasing cell wall permeability of the organism and interfering with protein synthesis and nucleic acid metabolism of the organism.

Antibiotics are often similar to one another and may be classified into certain classes or groups of drugs; however small changes in their biochemical structure may confer on them different properties for fighting bacterial infections. The use of antibiotics for viral illnesses is felt to be inappropriate. The reason for this is that it subjects the patient to the possibility of drug complications without any specific benefit and also enables bacteria to gain resistance to the antibacterial agents.

Resistance to antibiotics may be achieved by mutations of specific organisms through acquisition of those organisms of genes from another organism that encode the antibiotic resistance. The mechanisms for achieving bacterial resistance are related to the properties of the organism themselves and the enzyme reactions which they are able to produce or induce.

Antibiotics may sometimes interact with other drugs, either raising or lowering their degree of efficiency, e.g. the oral contraceptive pill is metabolised more quickly in the presence of antibiotic administration. The effects of Warfarin, digoxin and phenytoin are enhanced by many medications, most commonly those of antibiotics.

bad breath *(halitosis)*

See *dental problems*
See *gastro-oesophageal reflux*
See *tonsillitis*

Cause

Causes of bad breath include smoking; poor dental hygiene; throat infections and sinus infections; poor diet; medical conditions such as kidney failure, liver failure, diabetes; and some drugs.

Bad breath is caused by the residue left behind from cigarettes, which are left behind not only in the mouth but also in the tissues of the lungs. The particles which are left behind from cigarettes are then exhaled as the person breathes out and can be detected by other people in close contact. Poor dental hygiene is a result of accumulation of bacteria around the teeth and gums, dental caries and abscesses. These bacteria may cause infection of the gums, called gingivitis, retraction of the gums from around teeth, loss of bony material in the jaw (called osteoporosis of the jaw) and toothache. There is even an increased association between poor dental hygiene and an increase in heart attacks.

The presence of bacteria in the throat and sinusitis also give off odours which may be detected by the patient and by the examining practitioner. Some dietary intakes also give off volatile gases which may be detected. A common example of this is excess garlic which is evident on the breath and may also be excreted in perspiration.

Patients with end-stage kidney failure also give off a characteristic odour which may be detected by an observant experienced medical practitioner. The breath of some diabetics may smell sweet and fruity and is characteristic of this disease. Some medications, e.g. those used for treating angina, depression, fungal infections and some antibiotics may be detected on the breath.

Symptoms

Bad breath is a symptom in itself and may accompany symptoms of other diseases listed, depending on the cause.

Treatment

Treatment for some of these conditions is obvious, i.e. treat the cause. Bad breath and smoking may be cured by stopping smoking. Good dental hygiene is the aim for everyone. Not only is regular brushing and regular flossing of the teeth important, but a yearly visit to the dentist is important for thorough cleaning and the scaling of teeth. This is particularly important for older people and those on medication which increases the scaly deposits on the teeth around the gum line and leads to gum disease.

balanitis

Cause

Balanitis is an inflammation of the foreskin and glans penis. This may be caused by poor hygiene or fungal infection (candida) or it may be caused by diabetes.

Symptoms

The symptoms of balanitis include pain and tenderness, irritation on urinating and pain on retraction of foreskin.

Treatment

Treatment of balanitis includes washing of the area and taking a swab to check for bacterial infection. Prescribing an antibiotic medication for balanitis will depend on which organisms are identified. Treatment may include clotrimazole cream and antibiotics such as Chloromycetin. If the condition continues, circumcision may be indicated.

bed sores

Cause

Bed sores are a problem for people who spend long amounts of time in bed, either at home or in a nursing home or those with poor mobility who are confined to wheelchairs or recliner chairs. The key to prevention of bed sores is good nursing care, frequent turning or moving of the patient, adequate attention to urine and faecal incontinence, good nutrition and nutritional supplementation if necessary.

Symptoms

Inflammation, redness and ulceration and infection of the skin on pressure areas of the body, most commonly the lower back and pressure points on the bony prominences of the lower limbs.

Treatment

Bed sores will require intensive nursing and medical attention to help minimise the effects of broken skin and associated infection. Regular dressing of wounds is essential and general hygiene important. For elderly, infirm or disabled patients who are confined to home, assistance may be sought from domiciliary nursing services. On occasions, patients with difficult-to-heal or extensive bed sores may require antibiotics, a period of hospitalisation and surgical intervention.

bed-wetting (enuresis)

See *urinary incontinence*

Cause

Bed-wetting is often due to a maturational problem between bladder and nerve control and is a common occurrence in children up to the age of five years of age. Bed-wetting is often a source of stress in the family, with disturbed sleep at night and constant washing of bed linen. Often it takes longer for boys to become dry at night than it does for girls. Enuresis or bed-wetting involves a complex series of reflexes between the bladder, the brain and back to the bladder, instructing the bladder whether to empty or not. A urinary tract infection may also increase episodes of bed-wetting.

Other causes for bed-wetting include urinary tract infections, abnormalities of the bladder, irritable bladder syndrome, stressful situations at home or at school in children, developmental delay in children, diabetes, epilepsy.

Bed-wetting may sometimes be a problem in adult women and men. Stress incontinence may be a cause of bed-wetting, paticularly in women who have had children, pregnant women and post-menopausal women.

Investigations

It is important to exclude a urinary tract infection as the cause for enuresis. Micro-urine, a full blood count, blood sugar levels and an ultrasound of the urinary tract are important investigations to perform.

Treatment

Treatment of any underlying cause may improve the bed-wetting. If no specific cause can be found, parents may choose to try a liquid-sensitive pad and buzzer mechanism. Medication is available to help control bed-wetting, e.g. desmopressin, available either in spray or tablet form and may be titrated to a dose which suits the individual. Other forms of medication include a low dose of imipramide. This medication may be used at times for the treatment of depression and its side effects are the retention of urine; however in the treatment of bed-wetting much lower doses are used.

Women with incontinence should be instructed in ways to improve the tone of their pelvic floor muscles. This may be done by tightening the pelvic floor muscles as if to stop the flow of urine from the bladder in normal urination. This process is repeated in cycles of five to 10 exercises every day. These exercises may be performed throughout the normal course of the day and will improve the muscle tone of the pelvic floor. They can be performed while doing other activities either at work or at home or even while travelling in a car or bus to or from work. Solifenacin and Oxybutynin medication may also improve these symptoms for women and stabilise bladder tone.

For men, investigations regarding prostate problems would be undertaken and treated accordingly.

belching, bloating

See *anxiety*
See *gastroesophageal reflux*
See *helicobacter pylori infection*

Cause

Belching is the name given to forced expulsion of air from the stomach. It often entails extensive swallowing of air either as a result of ingesting fizzy drinks, eating too quickly and swallowing air with meals or excessive use of chewing gum. Bloating may also be a symptom associated with belching and may be due to excessively large meals, the regular intake of high-fibre food, gassy drinks or an infection called helicobacter pylori.

Symptoms

Other symptoms may accompany belching and bloating and include indigestion, nausea and abdominal discomfort. Belching and bloating symptoms may be accompanied by symptoms of gall bladder problems.

Treatment

Often the patient needs to be made aware of the cause of belching. If a patient complains of excess of belching and bloating, they should be screened for the presence of helicobacter pylorus.

Bell's palsy or facial weakness

See *stroke*
See *transient ischaemic attack*

Cause

Bell's palsy is caused by inflammation of or damage to the facial nerves.

Symptoms

Most commonly it occurs spontaneously on either the right or left side of the face, with weakness of the facial muscles and drooping of the eyelid.

Treatment

Treatment for Bell's palsy includes administration of oral steroids commencing with a high dose reducing over the following seven days. Attention should be paid to protect the cornea (the clear covering over the coloured part of the eye) from drying out, which may be done by taping the eyelids shut at night or the frequent administration of artificial tears. In most cases Bell's palsy patients will recover fully; however, in some cases, drooping of the eyelids and weakness of the facial muscles may persist. This can be improved by exercises to the facial muscles. The assistance of a speech therapist may be required for this.

In some cases where full recovery of the facial weakness does not occur, plastic surgery may be needed to improve the appearance of the facial muscles.

benign prostatic hyperplasia *(BHP)*

See *prostatic hyperplasia, benign*

biliary colic

See *abdominal pain*

Cause

Biliary colic is severe upper-abdominal right-sided pain caused by the passage of gallstones as they move from the liver and gall bladder down the ducts to the intestines.

Symptoms

The symptoms of biliary colic are severe pain which may radiate through to the back, associated with nausea and sometimes vomiting. Inflammation or infection of the gall bladder, called cholecystitis, is made worse by eating fatty foods.

Treatment

The treatment of biliary colic is to relieve the pain. If biliary colic recurs, cholecystectomy will usually be recommended. These days cholecystectomy can be done by keyhole surgery, usually with an overnight stay in hospital and minimal inconvenience to the patient and a much shorter convalescence compared to the past. There are still occasions when an open procedure is required due to difficulties in accessing the gall bladder by keyhole surgery.

bipolar disorder

See *anxiety*
See *depression*

Bipolar disorder is often considered in the differential diagnosis of depression. Not all patients with depression will exhibit bipolar symptoms, but patients with bipolar disorder will often describe phases of depression with or without manic episodes. The depressive phase of the biploar disorder may not be distinguishable from depression. The presence of both depressive and manic components makes the diagnosis of biploar disorder more likely.

Symptoms

Symptoms of depression with hypersomnia and overeating occur in bipolar disorder. This may be combined in a cyclical fashion with symptoms of increased levels of social functioning where the person with bipolar disorder is described as the 'life of the party'; reduced amounts of sleep; episodes of reckless; and overspending in the absence of need.

Treatment

Patients with bipolar disorder may require more than one form of medication to stabilise their mood and reduce problematic symptoms. A mood stabiliser such as lithium carbonate may be required in conjunction with an antipsychotic medication such as risperadone.

bites and stings

Cause

Bites and stings may be the result of a minor incident, such as stings from mosquitoes or bites from midges, or may be more serious such as stings or bites from bees, wasps, spiders, domestic or marine animals, or snakes.

Symptoms

The symptoms resulting from bites and stings may include localised reddening in the area, with or without the presence of a puncture wound or wounds. If no puncture wounds can be found, it is more than likely that the bite or sting has resulted from a less dangerous cause. Some people however and in particular young children, are very sensitive even to minor bites and stings from insects. The red marks which result from bites and stings may last for some days and may become infected due to constant scratching by the child due to irritation of the area.

Treatment

Treatment of minor bites and stings may require minor first aid in the form of washing the area and applying simple topical treatments. Some people are particularly sensitive to bee stings and may even require the provision of emergency adrenaline using an Epipen. Adequate instruction should be given to anyone who carries an Epipen or caregivers of young children responsible for administering the device. It is not difficult to learn the technique and even children may be trained in the use thereof.

Bites from domestic animals are best treated by washing the affected area, ensuring that the person's immunisation to tetanus is current, applying a sterile dressing to the wound. Seek medical attention if at all concerned. Often bites from domestic animals do not need suturing.

Marine bites and stings are potentially serious. Of most concern is the sea box jellyfish. First aid measures include removing the person from any further danger, checking for respiration and heartbeat, commencing cardiac pulmonary resuscitation if necessary, applying copious amounts of vinegar to the tentacles and seeking urgent transportation to a hospital. Pain relief will be necessary either in the form of oral or injectable analgesics, with or without the application of ice. Holidaymakers should enquire about the possibilities of the presence of marine stingers and should always seek to bathe between the yellow and orange flags and follow the directions of the lifesavers.

bladder cancer

Cause

Bladder cancer is associated with smoking, chronic irritation of the bladder and with people involved in the processing of rubber products.

Symptoms

Symptoms of bladder cancer include blood in the urine, pain on passing urine, frequency of passing urine and chronic infection of the bladder. A palpable bladder mass may be detected.

Treatment

If detected early treatment of bladder cancer is possible with trans-urethral resection of the bladder lesion, but for lesions that are well advanced total removal of the bladder may be necessary, with radiation and urinary diversion.

bladder problems

See *enuresis*
See *incontinence*
See *menopause*
See *pregnancy problems*
See *prostate infection or prostatis and prostate abscess*
See *urinary incontinence*

Cause

Some women may experience bladder problems particularly at night. This may be due to an irritable bladder, urinary infection, pressure on the bladder from fibroids of the uterus, increasing size of the uterus due to pregnancy or the onset of menopause. Men may experience bladder problems at night due to pressure from an increase in size of the prostate gland.

Symptoms

Women may find that this is a problem particularly at night and may need to empty the bladder frequently, thus disturbing their sleep. This is more common for women who have given birth vaginally, and around the time of the menopause.

Treatment

Frequent pelvic floor exercises—squeezing the pelvic floor as if holding a flow of urine and faeces and releasing—repeated numerous times throughout the day helps. Some physiotherapists are trained to provide help for women to retrain their pelvic floor muscles. Medication is also available to help prevent symptoms from this problem, e.g. Solifenacin and Oxybutynin. Tamsulosin hydrochloride may improve symptoms for men, but inevitably assessment of the prostate by a urologist will be necessary

bleeding

See *aortic aneurysm*
See *bladder cancer*
See *bronchitis*
See *colon cancer, colonic polyps*
See *haemorrhoids*
See *lung cancer*
See *menopause problems*
See *period problems*
See *pneumonia*
See *pregnancy*
See *stomach cancer*
See *tuberculosis*
See *urinary tract infection*

Cause

Bleeding may be described as normal, as in the case of the menstrual cycle or abnormal. Causes of abnormal bleeding include clotting disorders, e.g. haemophilia (factor VIII deficiency), Christmas disease (factor IX deficiency), platelet deficiency, vitamin K deficiency and medication used to thin the blood, e.g. anticoagulants.

Abnormal bleeding may occur in the form of bleeding from the bowel, nose or gums. Excessive blood loss may occur through the bowel in cases of colonic polyps and cancer of the bowel. Blood loss may also occur from ulcers in the stomach and oesophagus, and vomiting of blood may occur. The term applied to this condition is called haematemesis. Haematemesis may also occur as a result of bleeding oesophageal varicose veins. Bleeding may occur from the bladder, even in simple cases of urinary tract infections, but may also present in cases of tumours of the bladder. Bleeding may also occur as a result of serious injury and excessive loss of blood can be a result of an autoimmune disease.

In women, bleeding between periods is considered abnormal and requires medical investigation. Menstrual blood loss may increase during menopause. If this occurs, this may be regarded as abnormal and require medical intervention, e.g. curette, an endometrial ablation or hysterectomy. Post-menopausal bleeding should always be regarded as abnormal until otherwise proven.

Excessive bleeding may occur at the time of giving birth which is often a very dramatic presentation and requires immediate emergency medical intervention, sometimes a blood transfusion or, at the very least, postnatal administration of iron supplementation.

Bleeding may occur during severe respiratory infections (called haemoptysis), where the patient will cough up varying amounts of bright red blood. Sometimes bleeding from the lungs may be excessive, as in the case of patients with tuberculosis where tuberculosis lesions erode into a major vessel, resulting in massive amounts of bleeding from a lung. This could result in sudden death. Sometimes severe bronchitis or pneumonia may result in coughing up blood. Lung cancer should be excluded.

Symptoms

The symptoms associated with abnormal bleeding include anaemia, tiredness, fatigue and easy bruising. In haemophilia, symptoms may include bleeding into joints and soft tissues of the body. Excessive amounts of blood loss during the menstrual cycle may produce symptoms of tiredness, fatigue, no energy and even result in symptoms of reduced exercise tolerance, weakness and fainting. In cases of excessive bleeding from the bowel, patients may complain of black bowel motions (malena) or bright red blood appearing at the time of passing bowel motion. In cases of urinary tract infections, patients might observe blood in the urine. Loss of blood from the lungs may be accompanied by coughing and pain on respiration.

Investigations

If a patient presents with signs and symptoms as above, investigations which may determine a cause for bleeding should be undertaken by the general practitioner. A full blood count including haemoglobin level, red cell count, platelet numbers, urine testing and genetic screening for diseases such as haemophilia should be undertaken. Investigations by a haematologist may include a bone marrow biopsy.

In most instances a family history of such inherited conditions will be forthcoming and assist in making a diagnosis of a bleeding disorder. In cases where bleeding from the bowel is suspected, endoscopy and colonoscopy should be undertaken. Other investigations may include chest X-ray, bronchoscopy (looking into the lung with a fibre-optic camera, in much the same way as doing an endoscopy or colonoscopy) or even lung biopsy and sputum cultures.

Treatment

Treatment begins with establishing a diagnosis for the blood loss. Once a diagnosis has been made, steps may be undertaken to rectify further blood loss. In cases of trauma, compression to the bleeding area should be undertaken as a first aid treatment in order to prevent further bleeding.

blepharitis

See *eye or eyelid infection*

Cause

By definition, blepharitis is an inflammation or infection of the outer eyelids, which may be caused by a bacterial infection or an eczema-type condition called seborrhoea.

Symptoms

The symptoms of blepharitis include a sore, itchy and red eyelid margin.

Treatment

The treatment of blepharitis includes adequate attention to eyelid hygiene, the provision of artificial tears and sometimes antibiotic treatment or treatment using mild shampoo on an application stick.

blindness or loss of vision

See *migraine*
See *transient ischemic attack*

Cause

Blindness is defined as loss of vision. Technically speaking, a person may be defined as being legally blind if they are unable to read the largest letter on the eye chart at the top of the page, when the vision is tested by a general practitioner or eye specialist. This degree of loss of vision is called 6/60 vision, meaning the person is only able to read at 6 metres what a person with normal vision can read at 60 metres.

Loss of vision may be temporary or permanent.

Temporary loss of vision may be due to the effects of migraine or may be a warning that a migraine is about to occur. In this case, the loss of vision may not be total and may come and go gradually during an episode of migraine. Temporary loss of vision could be due to small pieces of material, either cholesterol deposits or portions of blood clots, coming from one of the main arteries in the neck called the carotid artery. This requires investigation either from the local doctor or by the eye specialist and is called amaurosis fugax.

When sudden total loss of vision occurs this represents a medical emergency and requires immediate medical attention. Whenever a sudden loss of vision occurs, where a previous diagnosis of migraine has not been made, medical attention should always be sought.

Total loss of vision is uncommon and is more likely to be due to many reasons such as: a congenital condition (congenital cataracts may be able to be removed by an eye specialist); congenital small eyes (for which there is no treatment); retinitis pigmentosa (for which there is no treatment), an inherited condition affecting the pigmentation on the back of the retina and resulting in progressive blindness as the person gets older; amblyopia or lazy eye (treated by patching); an infection prior to birth, e.g. German measles.

As people get older, a common reason for reduction in vision is cataracts. Cataracts may be removed to improve vision, providing that there is no significant damage to the macula (the point of maximal vision in the eye) in the form of macular degeneration.

Other causes of loss of vision include stroke; blockage of a vessel supplying the eye (central retinal artery or vein block)—this may be reversed if medical help is sought immediately. Blindness or loss of vision may be caused by infection either in the eye or somewhere in the brain; cancer; direct injury to the eye with a portion of the brain where vision is processed; tumours in the eye (e.g. retinoblastoma, a highly malignant condition and which often requires radiotherapy or removal of the eye. Very rarely this condition occurs in both eyes); retinal detachment (the retina is responsible for transmitting the visual impulses) and a tear in the lining of the back part of the eye—will require surgical repair.

Vision may be affected by glaucoma. Glaucoma is more common in older people and often they will have a family history of glaucoma, but it may also occur in younger people. Treatment of glaucoma involves the use of eye drops and often treatment by an eye specialist using a laser machine to help drain away excess fluid in the eye.

Inflammation may occur in the eye resulting in reduced vision due to optic neuritis (or uveitis) or inflammation of vessels near the eye (temporal arteritis). Both conditions need to be assessed by an eye specialist.

Simple conjunctivitis of the eye does not cause blindness; however, a type of conjunctivitis called trachoma, caused by an organism called chlamydia, may produce blindness and is often associated with clouding of the cornea. This condition occurs due to poor hygiene where infection is transmitted by flies from one person to another. This type of blindness is common in indigenous communities in Australia and in Third World countries.

blisters

See *burns*
See *chickenpox*
See *dermatitis/eczema*
See *genital herpes infection*
See *herpes simplex virus*
See *herpes zoster*

Cause

Blisters on the skin can occur in any location. They may be caused by an infection, a foreign body, an insect bite, dermatitis or a burn.

Infections causing blisters may include chickenpox, shingles oral or genital herpes, impetigo, or clusters of wart-like structures known as molluscum contagiosum.

Symptoms

The blisters may commonly be sore, itchy, red and have watery tops or crusting associated with them. Because of the itching, children commonly scratch them, thus causing secondary infection and redness.

Treatment

Treatment for blisters will depend on the clinical diagnosis. A swab of the blister will be taken and sent to pathology. However, since it may be several days before the results are received, simple solutions such as avoiding scratching, calamine lotion, bathing using Pinetarsol and pain relief should be employed. Antiviral agents may help if it is thought to be chickenpox.

Chickenpox is a viral infection for which only symptomatic treatment is recommended. A vaccination is recommended for children at 18 months to help prevent them from contracting chickenpox. The virus which causes chickenpox is the same virus which causes shingles. Shingles may occur in children but is more common in adults and is characterised by a segmental cluster of blisters on one half of the body. When shingles occurs on the face, it may be accompanied by severe pain and visual disturbance. Post-shingles pain may be very intense and require strong analgesics.

Oral and genital herpes are caused by the herpes virus. Oral herpes may start with a tingling sensation on or around the lips followed by a burning sensation and the appearance of blisters. Genital herpes may start as a burning sensation situated anywhere from the buttocks to the inner thighs, genital area and pubic region. Often men will complain of less severe symptoms with a genital herpes infection than women, who may complain of pain on urination or pain on intercourse.

Treatment for genital herpes is available in the form of treatment for an acute episode or suppression treatment for a long-term treatment.

Impetigo is a form of bacterial infection resulting from bacterium called staphylococcus or, less commonly, streptococcus and is easily treated with antibiotic medication. This medication may include amoxicillin and a cream to insert inside the nose, the most common site of origin of the staphylococcus.

Treatment for molluscum contagiosum is simple but effective. Simple abrasion to the surfaces of the molluscum contagiosum lesions will result in their spontaneous regression.

Preparations used for the treatment for common plantar or palmar warts will also effectively treat the lesions.

Treatment for insect bites consists of simple symptomatic treatment. Stingoes will relieve the lesions. Sometimes application of a mild steroid cream will be necessary to relieve the ongoing itching.

Treatment of burns includes applying cold water immediately to the area affected.

blood disorders

See *anaemia*
See *bleeding*
See *Hodgkin's disease*
See *leukaemia*
See *platelet dysfunction abnormalities*
See *spleen disorders*

blood in the urine

See *bladder cancer*
See *haematuria*
See *prostate cancer*
See *urinary tract infection*

blood pressure

See *atherosclerosis*
See *heart attack*
See *hypertension*
See *hypotension*

Blood pressure is generated during a cycle of contraction and relaxation of the heart. When the heart contracts, the pressure which is generated in the cardiovascular system is termed systolic pressure. When the heart relaxes, the pressure which is generated is referred to as diastolic pressure or lower value. Abnormalities of blood pressure may be defined as either an increase in the normal reading known as hypertension or a decrease in the normal reading known as hypotension, respectively.

body odour

Cause

Body odour is commonly caused by excessive amounts of perspiration associated with skin bacteria and poor body hygiene. Some body odours may be attributable to bad breath, ingestion of certain food types (e.g. garlic, curry, onions), smoking and infections such as tonsillitis, vaginitis and incontinence. The most common sites for body odour are under the arms and in the groin.

Treatment

Treatment includes adequate attention to body hygiene, including the provision and use of antiperspirants and deodorant preparations, shaving axillary hair, washing clothes, and reducing caffeine intake. Injection of axillary sweat glands with Botox can control excessive sweating, as can wedge resection of axillary sweat glands. Treatment with Botox is temporary, of limited effectiveness and expensive.

Surgical excision of sweat glands may be of benefit to some patients with excessive underarm odour and perspiration.

boils

Cause

Boils are the result of a severe localised deep infection of the skin.

Symptoms

The symptoms associated with boils are tenderness, redness of the skin and a localised lump.

Treatment

Treatment of boils includes administration of oral antibiotics, or intramuscular injection of antibiotics or incision using local anaesthetic and packing the cavity of the boil with a dressing material. Dressing the area will need to continue until the cavity has reduced in size. Antibiotics may include amoxicillin, cilicaine intramuscularly or erythromycin. Often application of a cream inside the nose is also recommended. If boils are a recurrent problem, investigation to exclude diabetes may be warranted.

bowel motions, black

See *stomach cancer*
See *colon cancer*

bowel obstruction, large

See *colon cancer*

Cause

The most common cause of a large bowel obstruction would be due to a mass, most often malignant tumour or cancer of the colon. Other causes may include obstruction by a polyp or by faecal impaction.

Symptoms

Symptoms of a large bowel obstruction may include pain accompanied by abdominal distension or an inability to pass bowel motions. Other symptoms may include blood in the bowel motions.

Treatment

Treatment is aimed at determining the cause of the obstruction and then relieving it either by physical means, in the case of faecal impaction or by surgical means in the case of malignant tumours.

bowel obstruction, small

Cause

Obstruction of the small bowel may occur due to tumour, cancer, a polyp or twisting of the bowel, resulting in intermittent abdominal pain or colic as the bowel contracts in order to relieve the obstruction. Obstruction of the small bowel may also come about because of adhesions from previous surgery, previous infection or severe endometriosis.

Symptoms

Abdominal pain is the most common symptom and the severity will depend on the degree of the obstruction of the bowel. Sometimes patients with small bowel obstruction will present with vomiting.

Treatment

Treatment of a small bowel obstruction is to relieve the obstruction, whatever the cause.

brain tumours

Primary brain tumours are divided into six classes:

1. Tumours of the skull

2. Tumours of the meninges (coverings to the brain)

3. Tumours of the cranial nerves

4. Tumours of the support tissue of the brain, called gliomas

5. Pituitary tumours

6. Congenital tumours which include craniopharyngioma, chordoma, germinoma, teratoma, dermoid cyst, angioma, haemangioblastoma.

Secondary brain tumours may occur as a result of spread from other cancers in the body, e.g. breast cancer, melanoma and lung cancer.

Cause

The cause of brain tumours is unknown.

Symptoms

Symptoms from brain tumours result from the effects of the increase in the size of the tumour and increasing intracranial pressure and include headache, vomiting and problems of muscle coordination. Symptoms of changes in temperature, pulse or respiratory rate may occur, as well as drowsiness, lethargy, impaired mental functioning and personality changes. Patients with pituitary tumours may present with headaches, visual field defects, over- or under-secretion of one or more pituitary hormones. Patients may also present with absence of periods (amenorrhoea), regression of secondary sexual characteristics and infertility. In men, pituitary tumours may result in impotence, testicular atrophy, infertility and regression of secondary sexual characteristics.

Treatment

Treatment will depend on the nature of the tumour, the position and type of pathology. Surgical excision, radiotherapy and/or chemotherapy are used depending on the diagnosis. Malignant tumours may require all three modalities of treatment and in most cases of malignant brain tumours, a favourable prognosis cannot be guaranteed. Surgical excision of benign tumours should result in cure. Treatment for pituitary tumours includes ablative radiation therapy or surgery, which is usually done via the approach through the nose and into the cranial cavity, through the sphenoid bone of the skull behind the nasal bones. Following surgical excision, radiotherapy and/or chemotherapy, replacement hormone therapy will need to be evaluated and monitored.

breast cancer

See *prostate cancer*

Cause

Breast cancer most often appears in the form of a lump which may be detected by the woman herself, the general practitioner, on mammogram or ultrasound. No lump, however, should be regarded as trivial until proven otherwise. Breast cancer is uncommon in women under the age of 30. It may also occur in men, but it is also uncommon. The most significant risk is increasing age. The cause of breast cancer is unknown. Some famlies carry BRCA gene 1 or 2, which is associated with breast cancer in women as well as prostate cancer in men.

Symptoms

The majority of patients with breast cancer present for lump which the patient has detected. Most lumps are painless, but are hard and irregular in shape. Other symptoms may include breast pain or breast tenderness, nipple discharge, disparity in size between right and left breast or puckering of the skin, called *peau d'orange* because it resembles the skin appearance of an orange. Uncommonly, breast cancer may present with symptoms of weight loss, tiredness, bone pain and shortness of breath. There are times when no symptoms may be present at all.

Treatment

There are various forms of treatment for breast cancer. Breast cancer management plans involve either removal of the lump or removal of the breast with or without the glands under the arm, chemotherapy, radiotherapy, breast reconstruction and the possibility of ongoing hormonal replacement.

Treatment can include lumpectomy where the lump alone is removed. This may be followed up with a combination of chemotherapy and radiotherapy.

Mastectomy is also a method of treating breast cancer, where the whole of the breast is removed, with or without the glands under the arm. Radical mastectomy means removing the breast and some of the underlying muscles. Some families have a much greater incidence of breast cancer than others and in these families gene testing may be available at major public hospitals. In some instances where a woman has been identified as being a high risk of developing breast cancer, mastectomy is considered as a means of preventing the onset of breast cancer.

Survival rates for breast cancer depend on early detection. In Australia, any woman over the age of 40 is eligible for free mammogram screening. The key to early detection of breast cancer is a self-examination and regular mammogram investigations.

breast cysts and lumps

See *pituitary gland abnormalities*

Cause

A cyst may appear as a lump in the breast. Not every lump which appears in a breast may be regarded as serious; however every lump needs to be investigated. About one lump in 10 may be regarded as a malignant lump; the rest may be regarded as cystic structures of varying histological appearance.

Cysts are often caused by the nature of the breast tissue and may be influenced by the presence of female hormones and as such may vary in size depending on the timing in the menstrual cycle.

Symptoms

Cysts and lumps may present with or without pain and may vary in size during the menstrual cycle.

Treatment

Treatment of breast cysts involves the doctor taking a history relating to this cyst, examination of the cyst by palpation and often by radiological assessment. Sometimes it may be necessary to perform a procedure called fine needle aspiration, where the needle is inserted into the cyst and some of the contents removed for examination under the microscope. This will give a histological diagnosis and this will then determine the next course of action.

breast discharge

Cause

Discharge from the breast may include milk production or abnormal clear discharge which needs to be investigated. Milk is a normal discharge from the breast following delivery of a child. If milk discharge occurs at times other than this, it is abnormal and may be due to an abnormality in the ducts of the breast or due to some medication such as antidepressants. Milk production may also occur under the influence of increased amounts of prolactin hormone from the pituitary gland. Discharge from the breast may be clear or coloured yellow, green or grey or bloodstained. Yellow, green or grey discolouration may indicate the presence of either an abscess or overgrowth of cells lining the ducts of the breast. Bloodstained discharge may indicate the presence of a malignancy.

Symptoms

Breast discharge may be accompanied by pain, tenderness, breast lump, fever, aches and pains and feeling unwell.

Investigations

Investigations for breast discharge include mammography, ultrasound, MRI (magnetic resonance imaging), a swab for infection, cytology for looking at cells. If abnormal milk production is present, estimation of prolactin hormone should be undertaken and an X-ray of the pituitary gland in the head should be undertaken. Fine needle aspiration may also be done to extract some of the cells from an identifiable lump for examination under the microscope. The surgeon may be able to perform an open biopsy, if a lump is present, in the operating theatre.

Treatment

Treatment for breast discharge will depend on establishing a diagnosis of the discharge.

breastfeeding

See *breast infections*

Cause

Milk is produced by the breast following the delivery of a baby. In the first few days this milk is call colostrum and may appear thin and watery. After a few days, however, the milk supply 'comes in' and the mother is able to breastfeed normally.

Symptoms

Sometimes mothers may experience difficulty in breastfeeding for a number of reasons. The most common reason for difficulty in being able to breastfeed is that of emotional or physical stress. Mothers are encouraged to consume greater amounts of fluids during times of breast-feeding and to ensure a healthy diet.

Sometimes there are problems with babies attaching to the nipple, making breastfeeding difficult or impossible. This may occur if there is a problem of retraction of the nipple, where the nipple is unable to become erect to allow the baby to attach to the nipple. Cracked nipples may also be a problem preventing effective breastfeeding.

Treatment

Most breastfeeding problems will improve with perseverance by the mother, who may sometimes require the assistance of a lactation consultant, advice from her doctor, support from other mothers or attendance at a child health clinic. Mothers may experience sore nipples during breastfeeding, which may be improved by adjusting the infant's position and ensuring correct attachment of a baby to the nipple. After feeding has been completed on each side, mothers may ease the child's mouth from the nipple by inserting her finger into the child's mouth, thus breaking the suction effect. If breastfeeding is causing significant problems for mother and baby, she may be advised to complement feed the baby until such time as breastfeeding is established. If this does not occur, she may well decide to cease breastfeeding and commence bottle feeding.

The cessation of breastfeeding can sometimes prove difficult. The woman is advised to restrict fluids, wear a firm-fitting bra both day and night, take pain relief and not to express milk from the breasts. After a couple of days' rest, production of milk will be greatly reduced. It is not recommended that hormone medication be prescribed in order to speed up this process

breast infection and abscess *(mastitis)*

Cause

The most common cause of infection in the breast occurs during lactation and is called mastitis. This is often due to engorgement of the breast and a blockage of the ducts. Mastitis may occur at other times in breastfeeding mothers and is due to bacterial infection. This may progress to an abscess which will need to be drained.

Symptoms

A breast infection or abscess may present as a lump or as soreness in the breast followed by a localised area of redness and tenderness, fever, feeling unwell and muscle aches and pains.

Treatment

The treatment of mastitis includes provision of antibiotics, analgesia for the pain and increased fluid intake. If mastitis occurs in a breastfeeding mother, she will need to ensure that the baby feeds from the side which is tender in preference to the other side in order to ensure that evacuation of the contents of the breast takes place effectively.

If mastitis occurs in someone who is not breastfeeding, investigations with ultrasound may be required and if the infection does not respond to antibiotics, referral to a surgeon may be required.

If an abscess develops, weaning from breastfeeding may be advised.

breast pain and tenderness

Cause

Pain and tenderness of the breast may be caused by even minor trauma. Tenderness of the breast is common in the days prior to the beginning of the menstrual cycle. Not uncommonly, ill-fitting or underwire bras may also produce pain and tenderness in the areas out towards the underarms. Correct fitting of bras is essential. Breast tenderness may also be one of the early symptoms of pregnancy. If a lump is present and the woman is experiencing pain of the breast, investigations should be undertaken to eliminate the possibility of cancer.

Mastitis might present with pain and tenderness. When women present for regular Pap smears, they should receive information regarding self-examination of the breast. This involves using a flat hand to examine the breast, not the tips of the fingers, as the latter technique will cause more pain and tenderness.

Treatment

Treatment for breast tenderness is to correct any underlying problem, e.g. infection, an ill-fitting bra or premenstrual symptoms with oral anti-inflammatory preparations or paracetamol.

Breast pains or mastalgia may sometimes persist despite the above treatment. A more serious cause must be excluded. Independent of the age of the patient, an ultrasound investigation should be carried out, with or without mammography. Mammography is indicated in women over the age of 40. Before the age of 40, mammography is difficult to interpret because of the dense appearance of the breast on the X-ray.

breath holding

See *children, common problems*

Cause

Breath holding may be caused by tantrums in young children or by simple fainting of children and adolescents. Breath holding associated with tantrums is most common in young children between the ages of two and four years of age and is brought on by emotional stress. Commonly, children do not have breath-holding attacks in the absence of an adult presence.

Symptoms

The child may cry in response to some event, then become pale and blue and even lose consciousness, at which time breathing will recommence.

Treatment

Parents should be reassured that breath-holding attacks are not harmful and are not due to a serious medical condition. They should be reassured and advised not to fuss over the child excessively during an event and that the breath-holding events will disappear with time.

bronchiectasis

Cause

Bronchiectasis is a lung disease caused by chronic infection and inflammation which result in the dilatation and destruction of large bronchial passages. Cystic fibrosis is the most commonly occurring condition resulting in bronchiectasis.

Infections which predispose to bronchiectasis include Pseudomonas, Haemophilus, klebsiella, staphylococcus aureus, histoplasma, non-tuberculosis mycobacteria, adenovirus, measles, whooping cough, influenza and human immunodeficiency virus. Patients on immunosuppressive drug regimes or with aspirated foreign bodies; endobronchial malignancy; connective tissue disease, e.g. rheumatoid arthritis; or toxic inhalation from ammonia, chlorine or nitrogen dioxide are prone to development of bronchiectasis. Patients with inflammatory bowel disease or who have undergone organ transplantation are also more at risk of developing bronchiectasis.

Symptoms

The primary symptom of bronchiectasis is a chronic cough, with large volumes of thick respiratory secretions, associated with shortness of breath and wheezing. Coughing up of blood is not uncommon and fever may be associated with exacerbations of the condition. Chronic bronchitis may mimic bronchiectasis and is distinguished from it by the amount of respiratory secretions which are produced.

The diagnosis of bronchiectasis is based on the patient's medical history and physical examination of the patient's chest, chest X-ray results and sputum results.

Treatment

Treatment for bronchiectasis includes prevention of acute exacerbations of the condition, treating the underlying cause and aggressively managing acute flare-ups. Prophylactic oral antibiotics, e.g. ciprofloxin in patients with cystic fibrosis in particular, are worthwhile considering. Frequent postural drainage of the patient's chest is considered desirable, along with intermittent chest physiotherapy and breathing exercises. Additional treatment depends on the underlying cause of the bronchiectasis.

bronchiolitis

Cause

Bronchiolitis occurs in children and is caused by a viral illness called respiratory syncytial virus, or RSV.

Symptoms

Bronchiolitis occurs in young children, most commonly at two weeks to 12 months of age. They present with coughing, wheezing, some difficulty breathing, rapid respiratory rate and noisy breathing. An audible wheeze is common.

Treatment

The child requires careful observation. This may occur either at home or in hospital depending on how sick the child may be. Observation of the child's colour, pulse and respiratory rate and fluid intake are important. The child may require prescription of a variable dose of oral steroid depending on the child's age, weight and the severity of their illness. Antibiotics are not indicated. If the child remains at home, he or she will usually recover in a few days; otherwise, admission to hospital may be necessary.

bronchitis

See *cystic fibrosis*

Cause

Bronchitis may be defined as infection in the bronchial passages in the lungs.

Symptoms

Bronchitis may be acute or chronic, and may be caused by either a viral or bacterial infection. It is accompanied by a cough, shortness of breath, wheezing, fever and the production of sputum or phlegm, which may be either white, yellow, green or brown in colour, sometimes mixed with blood.

Treatment

If bronchitis is thought to be due to a viral infection, the sputum is more likely to be white in colour or clear and symptomatic treatment is often all that is required. If bronchitis is due to a bacterial infection, antibiotics may be required, e.g. amoxicillin or erythromycin. If bronchitis is felt to be chronic, more active treatment may be indicated. Chronic bronchitis is common in people who smoke. Quitting smoking is recommended.

brucellosis

Cause

Brucellosis is an illness of meat workers and farmers with animals, particularly cattle. It is caused by Brucella abortus (cattle) and Brucella melitensis (sheep and goats). Brucellosis is associated with direct contact with infected animals and with the ingestion of the milk of infected cows. Incubation period is five days to several months.

Symptoms

The condition is diagnosed by a history of relapsing fever. Acute symptoms include fevers, headache, aches and pains, malaise and diarrhoea. If diagnosis is delayed, ongoing symptoms include irritability, headache, weakness, insomnia, anorexia, weight loss, abdominal pains, joint pains and severe depression.

Treatment

Combination therapy with doxycycline, streptomycin and prednisone is recommended.

bruising

Cause

Bruising may present as large or small areas. When bruising presents as a smallish pinpoint area, it is referred to as petechiae or ecchymoses which are congregations of lots of lesions on the body, most commonly on the lower extremities. Inflammation of blood vessels may also produce this characteristic appearance. When bruising occurs as large areas, it is often the result of abnormal bleeding due to the presence of platelet dysfunction or abnormalities of coagulation. Bruising may be the first sign of a disease resulting from bone marrow disease, e.g. leukaemia and abnormalities such as haemophilia. Bruising in young, active children may also occur from normal activities.

Symptoms

There may be no adverse symptoms associated with the condition from the bruising itself and the bruising represents the presenting symptom.

Investigations

Investigations for bruising may include full blood count, including platelet count and coagulation studies. Sometimes a bone marrow investigation may be required to exclude leukaemias, and even gene testing to exclude conditions such as haemophilia.

burns

Cause

Burns may be classified as being deep or superficial. The most severe form of burn will present as full thickness burns and, if extensive, will require management in hospital. A superficial burn may be caused by excessive sun exposure, hot water or steam from domestic appliances. Full thickness burns often result from exposure to direct flame or inflammatory substances.

Symptoms

Symptoms associated with events include redness of the skin, blistering and pain. In the case of full thickness burns, pain symptoms are somewhat less as the sensory receptors in the skin have been totally destroyed. Full thickness burns appear as white areas of skin associated with the burn.

Treatment

Superficial burns may be treated with an application of silver sulphurdiazine cream and covered with a bandage dressing. The cream should be applied daily until the wound has healed. Full thickness burns may require treatment in a hospital or by skin grafting. The most significant risk in treating burns is that of infection and fluid loss from the body, particularly with extensive burns.

calluses, corns

Cause

Calluses and corns occur on the feet in response to abnormal amounts of pressure in weight-bearing areas, where areas of the toes rub together or produce a localised increase in pressure.

Symptoms

Symptoms of calluses and corns include the presence of hard skin on the feet or toes, redness, irritation and infection.

Treatment

Appropriate footwear is important and regular removal of calluses and corns is essential to prevent secondary infection. In the elderly patient this may require referral to a podiatrist for foot care. Foot care is especially important for people with diabetes, who may also require referral to a podiatrist for regular foot care.

cancer

Cause

Cancer by definition means an unregulated overgrowth of cells. If they invade other tissues they are said to become metastatic. Cancer often has an immunological response in the body, and many cancers detected early have a good prognosis for cure. Genetic mutations are largely responsible for the production of malignant cells.

There are two factors which may contribute to the production of malignant cells which are controlled by either oncogenes (which regulate cell growth) or tumour suppressor genes (which play a role in cell division and cell repair, and are critical in identifying inappropriate growth signals in cells). Cells in the body are constantly replacing and hence opportunity exists for abnormal cells to occur if mutations or abnormal cells result from the division. Chromosomal abnormalities may also result in these abnormal cells.

Cancers associated with chromosomal abnormalities

Cancers caused by chromosomal abnormalities include leukaemia; lymphoma; myelo-proliferative disorders and solid tumours of the colon, meninges (coverings of the brain), salivary glands; adenocarcinomas of the bladder, colon, kidney, ovary, prostate, lung, uterus; Ewing's tumour of bone; tumours of muscle; malignant melanoma; neuroblastoma; retinoblastoma; testicular and ovarian tumours; and Wilms' tumour.

Viruses associated with cancer

Viruses are also associated with an increased risk of developing cancer, e.g. cytomegalovirus has been associated with an increase in Kaposi's sarcoma, Epstein Barr virus has been associated with Burkett's lymphoma, hepatitis B virus has been associated with hepatocellular carcinoma, human immunodeficiency virus or HIV has been associated with Kaposi's sarcoma and human papilloma virus has been associated with cervical cancer.

Cancers associated with chemical carcinogens

Chemicals have also been associated with an increased risk of cancer development. Soot and mineral oil have been associated with an increased risk of skin cancer. Smoking has been associated with lung cancer and skin cancer. Asbestos dust has been associated with lung cancer and mesothelioma. Hair dyes and aromatic amines have been associated with bladder cancer. Benzene has been associated with leukaemia. Nickel has been associated with lung cancer and nasal sinuses cancer. Formaldehyde has been associated with nasal cancer and nasopharyngeal cancer. Vinyl chloride has been associated with hepatic angiosarcoma. Painting materials, pesticides, diesel exhaust and man-made mineral fibres have been associated with lung cancer. Alcohol has been associated with oesophageal cancer and oropharyngeal cancer. Betel nuts have been associated with oropharyngeal cancer. Tobacco has been associated with head and neck cancer, lung cancer, oesophageal cancer and bladder cancer. Diethylstilbestrol has been associated with liver cancer and vaginal cancer in exposed female foetuses.

Cancer may occur in almost any part of the body. There are some known predisposing factors which increase the risk of developing some cancers, e.g. smoking is associated with an increased risk of lung cancer, as well as an increased risk of cancers affecting the pancreas and liver. A diet that is low in fibre and high in animal fat is a predisposing factor to an increase in the development of cancer of the stomach and intestines. Increasing age is a predisposing factor for breast cancer and prostate cancer.

Some cancers may be increased due to genetic factors, e.g. colon cancer and breast cancer. Excessive exposure to radiation may be associated with a variety of cancers, including leukaemia and malignancies of the bone marrow. Exposure to ultraviolet light in sun is a well-known risk factor for developing skin cancer either in the form of basal cell carcinoma, squamous carcinoma or malignant melanoma. Malignant melanoma may occur in any part of the body where cells produce melanin and where pigment is contained in tissue. Melanomas may even occur in pigmented lesions of the coloured part of the eye or in the pigmented skin around the anus and external genital area. Human papilloma virus or HPV in males is a known contributing factor to the development of cancer of the penis.

Some cancers are very silent, i.e. the patient may perceive very few symptoms until the cancer is well advanced. Examples include cancer of the kidney or cancer of the ovary.

Lumps in the abdomen are always of concern and often likely due to a malignancy, that is a cancer. Any organ in the abdominal cavity may present with a malignancy, including the bowel, pancreas, ovary, bladder, uterus, liver, kidney and gall bladder.

Prevention

Prevention plays a major part when it comes to cancer. Quitting smoking or never taking up smoking, eating a diet high in fruit and vegetables and complex carbohydrates, and protection of the body from exposure to radiation are all readily achievable ways of reducing the risk of cancer formation. Screening programs are also available and effective ways of monitoring a person's risk for developing cancer, e.g. Pap screening programs, breast screening programs, prostate screening programs, colonoscopy and endoscopy are readily available for everyone, particularly those who have a positive family history or those who have a known increased factor. Pap smears are recommended for women between the ages of 20 to 70. If a woman is sexually active before the age of 20, a Pap smear should be done within two years of becoming sexually active. A Pap smear should be done every two years or more frequently at the recommendation of the treating doctor, if an abnormal smear is detected. During Pap smear screening, an internal examination is used to assess enlargement of ovaries in order to assess for ovarian cancer. In women, self-examination of the breast is an important prevention strategy and mammograms should be performed every two years after the age of 40. Free mammogram screening programs are available in Australia for women over 40.

For cancer of the testicle, a regular self-examination for men is recommended. If a lump is detected, further investigations are recommended to exclude the possibility of testicular cancer, e.g. an ultrasound is recommended and biopsy of the lump may be performed. If cancer is detected, removal of the testicle is recommended.

Vaccination is now available for prevention of contracting human papilloma virus (HPV). The vaccinations are called Gardasil and Cervarix and contain a number of strains of HPV known to contribute to cancer. Vaccination is recommended for both males and females. It is thought that up to 80 per cent of cervical cancer in future will be prevented by this vaccination. Currently, girls in years 10 to 12 at school are being vaccinated with Gardasil as part of the free immunisation schedule and, in future, girls in year 8 at school will be routinely vaccinated against this condition. Boys may also be vaccinated to help prevent transmission of this infection; however vaccination of boys is not currently funded as part of a national immunisation program.

Prevention is always preferable to treatment.

Symptoms may be absent or minimal or patients may present with abdominal pain. Most cancers, if treated early, have a good prognosis for recovery.

Investigations

Investigations are specific to the area of the body which is being investigated, e.g. kidney, uterus, liver. Investigations include pathology tests and radiographic testing which includes X-rays, ultrasound, CT scan and MRI scan.

Treatment

Treatment for many cancers will often require excision of the lump. Some tumours may also require additional treatment in the form of chemotherapy and/or radiation therapy and, in the case of breast cancer, hormone suppression may be recommended. Some tumours like kidney tumours may not involve either chemotherapy or radiotherapy as they are insensitive to both forms of treatment. The first principle of treatment for cancer is prevention.

cardiomyopathies

Cause

Cardiomyopathy is a general term applied to an abnormality of cardiac muscle function that is not caused by anatomic or valve defect of the heart. This may occur as a result of viral infection, excess alcohol ingestion or for no known or apparent reason.

Symptoms

Symptoms of cardiomyopathy will vary depending on the extent of impairment of the muscle function of the heart. They include shortness of breath, rapid heart rate, swelling of the ankles, tightness in the chest, lack of energy and fatigue.

Investigation

An echocardiography is done to determine how effectively the heart is contracting. This function is expresssed as a percentage of the volume of blood in the heart and is called the ejection fraction. A value of 60 per cent or more is considered normal.

Treatment

Treatment for cardiomyopathies is aimed at maintaining the best cardiac function and includes correction of hypertension, preventing heart attack, improving quality of life of the patient and modification of dietary and lifestyle factors .

cardiopulmonary resuscitation *(CPR)*

Cardiopulmonary resuscitation (CPR) should be able to be performed by any member of the community, even children. Courses are available for people to undertake training, often as part of a first aid certificate.

Anyone who is found to suddenly collapse and fall to the floor, particularly if their colour starts to deteriorate, should be considered in need of CPR.

The hallmarks of CPR are as follows:

D.R.A.B.C.D.

Danger

Remove the patient from danger providing you yourself are not in danger. Call for assistance from any other person around, including calling for an ambulance immediately.

Response

Try to elicit a response from the person who has collapsed.

Airway

Clear the airway of any obstruction.

Breathing

Tilt the patient's head back, grasp their chin between your thumb and index finger and commence mouth-to-mouth breathing.

If there is concern of contamination from secretions from the patient's mouth and if the rescuer does not have access to some form of hygiene control such as a clean handkerchief, vigorous compression of the chest will also provide some oxygenation of the lungs.

Circulation

Commence cardiac compression by placing the heel of your hand on the lower third of the patient's sternum. It is now recommended that a single person administer both the breathing and the cardiac compressions. A rate of 100 cardiac compressions per minute is recommended. Cardiac compression should be continued until such time as an ambulance arrives. The person providing the resuscitation may tire quickly from this activity, so a relief person should be on standby.

Defibrillation

The most common rhythms for a heart during a heart attack is an uncontrolled contraction of the heart called ventricular tachycardia or complete stopping of the heart called asystole. Both of these situations are appropriate for defibrillation by electrical shock to the heart.

Defibrillation will be one of the first things that the ambulance attendants will do on arrival and is regarded as one of the most important actions to be taken when a patient has been observed to collapse suddenly. Some medical surgeries are now equipped with their own defibrillator machine and it is recommended that medical and nursing staff be familiar with the operation of the defibrillator and receive regular updates on its use.

Once the ambulance and ambulance officers arrive, unless the person performing the CPR is trained in CPR, the ambulance officers will take over management of the patient.

cardiovascular system problems

See *blood pressure*
See *cardiomyopathies*
See *chest pain*
See *cholesterol*
See *coronary artery disease and atherosclerosis*
See *endocarditis*
See *heart attack*
See *hypertension*
See *palpitations and arrhythmias*
See *valvular disorders of the heart*

carpal tunnel syndrome

Cause

Carpal tunnel syndrome is caused by entrapment of the nerves to the hand caused by pressure from the surrounding fibrous tissue bands on the front of the wrist.

Symptoms

Symptoms of this condition include pain in the hand or fingers, numbness and weakness of the muscles of the hand. Symptoms are precipitated and exacerbated by occupations involving excessive use of the hands and the need for fine motor control of the hands. The most problematic time of day for patients with carpal tunnel syndrome is often at night when they complain of numbness and tingling in the hands and fingers.

Treatment

Treatment for this condition is successfully achieved by a simple operation releasing the nerves. Anti-inflammatory medications may temporarily improve the symptoms of numbness and paraesthesia. These days, carpal tunnel procedures are also possible by keyhole surgery, consequently reducing the amount of convalescent time and time off work. On some occasions, repeat procedures may be necessary; however this is relatively uncommon.

cataracts

Cause

Cataracts are caused by cloudiness in the lens inside the eye. It is the lens in the eye which allows a person to focus on small print and then look into the distance. The lens changes refractive power in order to do this by becoming fatter (more powerful) or thinner (less powerful), thus allowing the rays of light which entered the eye through the pupil to focus appropriately on the retina. Where a cataract forms, the rays of light become scattered in the lens before reaching the retina, thus forming a blurred image on the retina or blurring of vision.

The most common cause of cataracts is ageing. These are called senile cataracts. Excessive exposure to ultraviolet light from the sun or from a solarium may contribute to the formation of senile cataracts. Cataracts have many other causes. They may be an inherited condition due to in-utero infection, as in the case of a mother who contracts German measles during pregnancy; as a result of injury to the eye; due to diabetes; through lack of oxygen at birth; heavy metals, e.g. lead and mercury; and as a result of prolonged dosages of steroid use, e.g. treatment of severe asthma and some autonomic diseases.

Symptoms

Patients with senile cataracts, i.e. caused by old age, complain of increasing blurring of vision, which usually comes on slowly over a period of time. Patients who are diabetic may also complain of blurred vision due to a changing refractive error of the lens in the eye; however this does not constitute cataract formation necessarily, but is related to fluctuations in blood sugar level associated with diabetes. Patients may also complain of difficulty distinguishing colours, particularly blue, green and yellow. Cataracts may be accompanied by other ageing changes in the eye including macular degeneration, the point in each eye of maximal acuity which affects the ability to read small print. The presence of long-standing cataracts may lead to glaucoma.

Treatment

Cataracts may be removed by an ophthalmologist. These days, it is possible to remove the lens and insert an intra-ocular lens. Variable results follow removal of the cataracts depending on the presence of coexisting eye problems, particularly problems involving the macular area of the eye.

cellulite

See *hypothyroidism*
See *weight management problems*

Cause

Cellulite is just another word for fat deposits commonly found around the hips and thighs, and produces a characteristic marbling of the skin.

Treatment

Treatment of cellulite is weight reduction, increased exercise, low fat intake and a calorie-controlled diet. Liposuction and body sculpturing will improve the appearances of these fat collections, but treatments are costly and have risks. Liposuction requires an anaesthetic and there is a risk of fat embolism, which means that small pieces of fat may become dislodged and travel to the brain, causing the same effects of mini stroke. It is, however, becoming a more commonly performed procedure for those people who are able to afford cosmetic surgery. It is recommended that anyone thinking of cosmetic surgery should research the qualifications of their surgeon and the anaesthetist before committing to the surgery.

cerebral palsy

See *children, common problems*

Cause

Cerebral palsy covers a group of conditions which occur in children either before, during or after birth, up to and including the age of five years. Conditions result from brain damage to one or more parts of the brain. Cerebral palsy may result from prematurity, prenatal infection, placental abnormalities resulting in a reduced amount of oxygen to the brain, cerebral haemorrhage, birth trauma, lack of oxygen during the delivery phase. Cerebral palsy may also arise as a result of severe jaundice of the newborn (kernicterus), infection of the central nervous system (meningitis or encephalitis) or severe systemic sepsis.

Symptoms

Children with cerebral palsy may present with symptoms of increased muscle tone called spastic tone, incoordination of muscles called ataxia or athetosis or mixed forms of the condition may occur. Symptoms may also include delayed developmental milestones; problems with speech, swallowing, vision, hearing; intellectual disability; problems of mobility; and problems with activities of daily living. A diagnosis of cerebral palsy is dependent on a non-progressive state of the condition.

Treatment

Early intervention is important for the treatment of children with cerebral palsy. This may include physiotherapy, occupational therapy, speech therapy and specialist educational input. Depending on the level of intellectual functioning, attendance at educational facilities may include either integration into regular school, special school or schools for the handicapped. In some instances, people may require lifelong assistance in order to maintain as normal a life as possible.

cervical cancer

See *human papilloma virus*

Cause

It is thought that 70 per cent to 80 per cent of cervical cancer is caused by exposure to the human papilloma virus (HPV). This is the most commonly occurring malignancy in women worldwide.

Symptoms

A woman with early stages of cervical cancer may have no symptoms whatsoever. Worldwide screening programs for cervical cancer in the form of the Pap smear are able to detect the earliest forms of abnormalities in cervical cells. Symptoms such as vaginal bleeding, bleeding after intercourse and intermittent spotting may all be symptoms of early cervical cancer.

Prevention

By preventing infection with HPV, 70 per cent to 80 per cent of cervical cancer may be prevented. Vaccination is now available for males and females in order to prevent the spread of infection. This comes in the form of a vaccination called Gardasil which now forms part of the recommended vaccination program. It is a course of three vaccinations over a period of six months. It is recommended that young females be vaccinated soon after starting secondary school.

A Pap smear is recommended for women over the age of 20 or earlier once they have been sexually active for two years and is recommended every two years providing that the results are normal. If an abnormal Pap smear results, more frequent testing is recommended depending on the degree of abnormality. Referral to a gynaecologist may be indicated if a high-grade abnormality is detected.

Treatment

Treatment for abnormal Pap smears may require examination using a colposcopy investigation, diathermy of the cervix, cone biopsy, Lletz procedure or even hysterectomy. For women who have had a hysterectomy because of abnormal cells, ongoing vaginal vault smears will be required for the foreseeable future.

chest pain

Life-threatening

See *abdominal aortic aneurysm*
See *heart attack*
See *angina*
See *lung cancer*
See *palpitations and arrhythmias*
See *pleurisy*
See *pneumothorax*

Cause

Any patient who presents with chest pain immediately thinks that this is related to heart pain (heart attack). There are many causes of chest pain. In looking for a cause for chest pain, important factors include the age of the patient, a history of any recent injury, a history of recent infections with or without coughing, present occupation and any previous history of medical conditions.

Any patient presenting to a general practice surgery complaining of chest pain should immediately be referred to the treatment room of the surgery. These days, most surgeries employ nursing staff who are based in the treatment room and most patients presenting with chest pain will have their blood pressure and pulse taken by a nurse, followed by an ECG (electrocardiogram), except perhaps in cases of children presenting with chest pain.

Life-threatening causes for chest pain include heart attack or angina, pericarditis, problems involving the heart valves, pulmonary embolism (blood clot in the lung, particularly for women on the pill), pleurisy, severe chest infection, lung cancer, aortic aneurysm, rupture of the lung (pneumothorax). Pneumothorax may occur spontaneously or may occur in patients with known respiratory disease.

Symptoms

If a patient presents with pain across the chest which they describe as a crushing pain or a tight band around the chest, sometimes described as an elephant sitting on it, the diagnosis is heart attack until proven otherwise, even if the ECG looks normal. The duration of the pain is also an important factor in this instance, because if the pain has been present only a very short period of time, the ECG may still be normal even in the presence of a heart attack. The patient may complain that the pain is present more commonly down the left arm than the right and, in addition, may be present on either the right or left side of the jaw. This also favours a diagnosis of heart attack.

Treatment

When a patient presents complaining of chest pain, prompt attention should be paid to determining whether this pain is cardiac in origin. If it is decided that a potentially life-threatening condition is present, immediate transfer to the nearest hospital is recommended.

A patient in whom a cardiac origin for pain is suspected, should be placed on oxygen immediately, be given oral soluble aspirin, be given nitrolingual spray (if available) and an ambulance called for transportation to hospital.

Non life-threatening

See *gastro-oesophageal reflux*
See *helicobacter pylori infection*
See *osteoarthritis*
See *osteoporosis*
See *peptic ulcer*
See *shingles*

Cause

Causes of non life-threatening chest pain may include prolapsed vertebral disc or spinal tumour, oesophageal spasm, reflux or severe indigestion, peptic ulcer, helicobacter pylori infection, musculoskeletal injuries or shingles.

The presence of a peptic ulcer or a history of a peptic ulcer, may go from being a non life-threatening situation to a life-threatening situation if the ulcer ruptures. In the presence of a ruptured peptic ulcer, immediate transfer to hospital is necessary.

Symptoms

Local tenderness in the abdomen, on the chest wall front or back, would favour a diagnosis of musculoskeletal origin. A history of recent heavy lifting or strenuous exercise would favour a diagnosis of either musculoskeletal pain or, alternatively, a prolapsed disc. The presence of localised redness or blisters associated with the pain would favour a diagnosis of early onset of shingles or herpes zoster infection. In this instance, the person may also be complaining of feeling feverish with body aches and pains as well as chest pains.

Treatment

If it is decided that a potentially life-threatening condition is not present, a detailed history and examination of the patient will then be undertaken in order to determine the cause of the pain. This may include a chest X-ray to determine the presence of any infection in the lung. Other investigations may be arranged for a later date and include an endoscopy to assess for the presence of reflux, oesophagitis or peptic ulcer.

At the time of endoscopy, it may be found that the patient is suffering from an infection called helicobacter pylori, which is a common cause of peptic ulcers.

Eradication of helicobacter pylori involves triple therapy, in the form of antibiotics and anti-reflux preparations called proton pump inhibitors. Usually a course of this treatment will last for a week, but may need to be repeated again at some later date. After treatment has been completed, a follow-up test is necessary to determine that the infection has been eradicated. This does not involve having a repeat endoscopy, but may be done by a helicobacter breath test at a pathology department. This test needs to be done six weeks after the eradication treatment has been completed. If it is found that eradication is not complete, another course of treatment will be undertaken. Helicobacter pylori is associated with an increased risk of cancer of the stomach, hence the need for eradication.

Treatment for musculoskeletal pains may include an X-ray or CT scan of the back, pain relief, hot packs, rest and possibly physiotherapy.

Treatment for shingles is provided in the form of a prescription for antiviral medication which, if administered within the first 72 hours following the first signs of the pain, is effective in treating the infection of shingles. Sometimes, after the shingles infection has cleared, post-herpetic pain may persist and be severe, even interfering with the person's sleeping at night. Referral to a pain clinic or pain specialist may be required.

Patients presenting with an acute fracture resulting from osteoporosis may receive relief from the pain by injection of the vertebra affected by an osteoporosis crush fracture. This procedure is done by specifically trained radiologists in a hospital setting and usually will give good relief to this acute pain. This procedure is done with the assistance of X-ray guided technology and helps to stabilise the fracture in the bone and provide ongoing support to the bone to prevent further collapse of the vertebral body.

chickenpox

See *immunisation for childhood infectious diseases*

Cause

Chickenpox is a viral illness caused by one of the herpes viruses called varicella zoster virus. It is very infectious and epidemics occur amongst people without immunity.

Symptoms

Symptoms of chickenpox include acute onset of slight fever, runny nose and the general feeling of being unwell, followed by an outbreak of blisters with watery tops anywhere on the body (these are called vesicles). The vesicles are teeming with virus particles and are very infectious. The chickenpox virus is spread by droplet infection from coughing and by direct contact with the blisters. The incubation period for chickenpox is around two weeks. The infectious period lasts from the two days prior to the appearance of the rash until after all blisters have dried up and formed crusts on top. Most people who contract chickenpox suffer only a relatively minor illness; however some people may suffer a more severe reaction to the disease and deaths from chickenpox still occur.

Treatment

Treatment for chickenpox is primarily symptomatic with pain relief, fluid replacement and decongestants used if necessary. Prevention of chickenpox is achieved by immunisation which includes a vaccine which is recommended for administration to children at 18 months of age. The vaccination may be administered to people of any age and up until the age of 13 years, one administration only is required. After the age of 13, two doses of chickenpox vaccination are recommended, to be administered two months apart to give full protection.

child abuse

Cause

Child abuse may present in the form of physical, emotional or sexual abuse or neglect, and there is much written about this topic.

Symptoms

Children who are the subject of child abuse may present with recurrent injuries such as bruises or fractures and come to the notice of either their local doctor, local hospital or teacher. Young children may also present with symptoms of failure to thrive, be withdrawn and be struggling at school.

Treatment

There are many support agencies available to provide assistance to families and provide treatment to children who are subject to child abuse. It is everyone's responsibility to care for the welfare of their children.

If child abuse and neglect is suspected by a medical practitioner, mandatory reporting exists and they must report their suspicions to the authorities.

childhood infectious diseases

See *infections*
See *immunisation for childhood infectious diseases*

Vaccinations available
Chickenpox
Haemophilus influenza B
Tetanus, diphtheria, pertussis (or whooping cough) (Triple Antigen)
Measles, mumps, rubella (or German measles) (MMR)
Meningococcus
Polio
Pneumococcus
Hepatitis B

For older children, adolescents
Human papilloma virus (Gardasil)

Cause

Infectious diseases of childhood are listed above and distinction is made between those infectious diseases for which an immunisation is available and those for which no immunisation is available. The infectious diseases for which an immunisation is available include tetanus, diphtheria, pertussis or whooping cough, measles, mumps, rubella, meningococcus, pneumococcus, chickenpox, haemophilus influenza B, polio, rotavirus, hepatitis B, human papilloma virus. These are all preventable infectious diseases. The National Health and Medical Research Council recommends an immunisation schedule for these diseases commencing at two months of age.

Symptoms

Children with infectious diseases may become quite ill and some of the above infections more than others have a high mortality rate, i.e. children may die if they do not have the protection from immunisation. Many of the above infectious diseases these days are relatively uncommon as a large percentage of the population has antibodies to them so that epidemics do not develop.

Many of the above infections have common symptoms which include temperature, lethargy, not eating or drinking and wanting to sleep. Some of these infections will be accompanied by a rash. These include measles and rubella as well as chickenpox, which produces small watery blisters with the rash.

Treatment for tetanus is twofold: to limit the effects of the tetanus toxin, which produces the lockjaw, and to eliminate the infecting bacteria, by use of antibiotics such as metranidazole or penicillin.

Diphtheria is a life-threatening illness, as is polio (which used to be referred to as infantile paralysis), meningococcal disease (has a characteristic rash), pneumococcal disease and rotavirus (which produces severe diarrhoea in children).

Diphtheria world wide occurred in epidemic proportions as recently as the mid 1950's worldwide and can be rapidly fatal within minutes. Treatment includes antibiotics such as penicillin, erythromycin, rifampin, or clindamycin. Rapid response is essential once the disease is suspected.

Human papilloma virus may be contracted very early after males or females become sexually active and may lead to cancer of the cervix in females, cancer of the penis in males or to genital warts, another form of human papilloma virus and a cause of cervical cancer. See human papilomavirus.

Whooping cough or pertussis has a characteristic cough involving repeated prolonged episodes of coughing followed by a prolonged effort for inspiration. It is the characteristic 'whooping' sound of the inspiration which lends the name to the condition. Whooping cough is treated with erythromycin, clarithromycin, or azithromycin. Non-immune contacts of an infected person should also be treated prophylactically.

Whereas polio is associated with muscle weakness. Treatment for polio may require assisted ventilation to aid breathing, and other symptomatic support until the signs of infection subside. There are no definitive medications to treat the acute disease once it has occurred.

Mumps presents as an inflammation of the parotid glands which are located just below and in front of the ear lobes. There are varying degrees of swelling of the parotid glands. The parotid glands may simply be tender and the patient may not feel significantly unwell.

Meningococcal disease is a serious infection which causes meningitis, and commonly a characteristic generalised rash. By the time that the rash has appeared, particularly in young children, the infection is well under way. The condition progresses rapidly from the time of initial infection and is not infrequently fatal. Young children and adolescents are particularly susceptible in the spring and winter months. Urgent treatment with antibiotics is required, often before investigations confirm the presence of the infection and this is an essential element to successful recovery.

Haemophylus influenzae B can cause meningitis, epiglotitis (swelling of the throat, obstructing the airway), joint infections and pains, and pneumonia. Young children may require treatment in intensive care. Treatment includes administration of potent antibiotics, e.g. third or fourth generation cephalosporins, semi-synthetic penicillin, or chloramphenicol is required for effective treatment.

Pneumococcus is one of the bacteria of the streptococcus family which as a group of bacteria commonly causes respiratory infections. It is a particularly potent bacterium, and shows increasingly resistance to an increasing number of antibiotics, particularly in countries of Europe, and USA. Care is required in treating those infected with Streptococcus pneumoniae to use a drug to which the organism is sensitive, e.g. using penicillin, amoxicillin-clavulanate, cephalosporins, cephtriaxone, and vancomycin.

Chickenpox or (varicella virus) infection has a characteristic rash, with watery blisters on top, that are often itchy. The infection does respond to antiviral agents such as acyclovir which will shorten the duration of the disease, but the products are expensive and not government subsided for this condition, and therefore preclusive economically for most families.

Most of these infections will present some common symptoms which include fever, lethargy or malaise and treatment is mostly symptomatic, i.e. relief of symptoms with pain relief, the occasion to relieve the temperature and aches and pains. There are occasions when people who become quite ill may require admission to hospital; more commonly, this may involve adults but also may include children.

No vaccinations available
Scarlet fever
Molluscum contagiosum
Plantar warts
Hand foot and mouth disease
Glandular fever

Scarlet fever is an infectious disease caused by a streptococcal infection often associated with a sore throat or tonsillitis. It is treated with penicillin.

Molluscum contagiosum are wart-like structures 2 mm to 3 mm in diameter with what seems like a volcano crater in the centre. These are caused by a minor viral infection and may be treated with abrasions to the tops of the craters, painted with treatments which are also used for plantar warts, frozen with liquid nitrogen or burnt with diathermy.

Plantar warts are also caused by a viral infection and may be found on the palms of the hands or the soles of the feet. In the early stages, the person may feel that there is a foreign body under the skin, particularly in the foot. Some people are more prone to contracting plantar warts and may have lots of them. Treatment methods include application of topical wart killer, freezing with liquid nitrogen or diathermy. Plantar warts are commonly contracted by adults using public shower facilities in gymnasiums and public swimming pools.

Hand, foot and mouth disease is caused by a virus where small blisters occur on the hands, feet and in the mouth. This occurs commonly in day-care centres and kindergartens but is a minor infection only. It is infectious, but not cause for excluding the child from day care or kindergarten. Treatment for this condition is symptomatic.

Glandular fever or infectious mononucleosis is caused by a virus called Epstein Barr virus. It may occur at any age; however patients in their late teens, 20s and 30s are more affected by this condition. On occasions patients may require prolonged periods of time off school or work in order to recover. Symptoms include fever, temperature, sensitivity to light, sore throat and tonsillitis, aches and pains, lethargy, nausea, vomiting.

Treatment is symptomatic, i.e. pain relief, adequate fluids, rest. Often patients in their 20s and 30s have increased sensitivity to alcohol, sometimes for periods of up to 12 months to two years. If alcohol is consumed they may feel nauseated or even vomit. This is because during the acute phase of the illness, the virus adversely affects the cells in the liver, making them more sensitive to later consumption of alcohol. In this case abstinence from alcohol consumption is the treatment.

children, common problems

See *adenitis, mesenteric*
See *bad breath*
See *balanitis*
See *bed-wetting*
See *boils*
See *breastfeeding*
See *breath holding*
See *cerebral palsy*
See *child abuse*
See *childhood infectious diseases*
See *convulsions*
See *deafness and hearing loss*
See *immunisation*
See *infections*
See *knock knees*
See *otitis externa*

See *otitis media*
See *pigeon toes*
See *tonsillitis*

chlamydia

Cause

Chlamydia infections may cause not only urinary tract infections but also respiratory infections such as pharyngitis, bronchitis, pneumonia.

Symptoms

Symptoms include fever, cough, sputum production and pneumonia.

Treatment

Treatment involves antibiotics where the drug of choice is tetracycline or erythromycin or azithromycin.

cholera

See *infectious diseases for adults*

Cause

Cholera is an infectious disease caused by a bacterium called Vibrio cholerae and is transmitted in infected water supply.

Symptoms

Symptoms include abdominal pain, watery diarrhoea, muscle cramps, malaise leading to dehydration, poor urine output and circulatory collapse and death if it is not treated urgently.

Treatment

Rapid correction of fluid loss and monitoring of electrolyte loss are urgent priorities. Intravenous fluids may be required in hospital under medical observation.

cholesterol

See *coronary artery disease and atherosclerosis*
See *heart attack*
See *stroke*
See *transient ischaemic attack*

Cholesterol is the name given to a fat measured in the blood during a pathology test. There are a number of different sorts of fats which are called lipids. Another important measurement of fats in the blood is triglyceride and, together with cholesterol, these are important indicators of future potential disease.

Cholesterol is necessary in the body in making cell membranes, steroids which are produced by the body and in the production of bile acids. The types of fats are classified according to the size of the molecules and may be defined as high-density cholesterol or lipoprotein (HDL) or low-density cholesterol or lipoprotein (LDL). Measurement of cholesterol and triglyceride in the body is important because excessive amounts may lead to the production and accumulation of atheroma plaques on the inner surfaces of blood vessels, most importantly arteries. It is the accumulation of atheroma plaques which produces blocked arteries leading to either a heart attack or stroke.

Cause

Increased levels of lipids in the blood may be defined as either primary or secondary causes. Primary causes of increased lipids may be due to the single or multiple genetic problems associated with overproduction of cholesterol and triglyceride in the blood or abnormal clearance of HDL in the blood.

Secondary causes of elevated cholesterol and triglyceride are more common and are related to lifestyle factors and excessive dietary intake of saturated fat, cholesterol and poly-unsaturated fatty acids. Other common secondary causes include diabetes, excessive alcohol, kidney problems, hypothyroidism, administration of some drugs (some diuretics, beta blockers, oestrogen and progesterone).

Symptoms

There may be no symptoms at all associated with an increase in cholesterol and triglyceride in the body but one of the earliest signs of elevated cholesterol or triglyceride may be the onset of high blood pressure. Excessive amounts of cholesterol and triglyceride may lead to acute pancreatitis and fatty liver.

Treatment

Treatment is indicated for all patients with cardiovascular disease and for some patients who have yet to have symptoms. Health authorities have produced specific guidelines for prescribing medication for patients with elevated cholesterol and triglyceride. The guidelines are focused on reducing levels of LDL and triglyceride, raising HDL and treating metabolic syndrome which may lead to diabetes mellitus.

chronic obstructive airway disease (COAD)

See *emphysema*

Cause

Chronic obstructive airway disease or emphysema is most commonly the result of long-term heavy smoking. Other causes may include damage to the lung by heavy air pollution and chronic airways infection. Some families are known to have an enzyme deficiency in the lung which predisposes them to this disease. This enzyme is called alpha1 antitrypsin and patients may be screened for this enzyme to see if they have a predisposing factor to the development of this condition.

Symptoms

COAD is characterised by deterioration in lung function. It is associated with chronic productive cough, sputum production and, as the condition becomes worse, shortness of breath, wheezing and even difficulty talking in sentences without becoming short of breath. Patients may experience increasing tiredness, lethargy, reduced exercise tolerance and problems sleeping at night. An increased frequency of chest infections is also often a problem.

Investigations

Assessment of the severity of chronic obstructive airway disease is based on performing lung function tests. These tests may include spirometry, where the patient is required to expel as much air from the lungs as possible as quickly as possible into a special machine called a spirometer.

Treatment

Treatment for chronic obstructive airway disease is aimed at keeping the lungs as free from infection as possible, preventing further damage to the lungs and maximising effective oxygenation of the blood. Patients may require antibiotic treatment for lung infections, ventolin to maintain the best possible clear airway, administration of the medication called tiotropium. It also helps to maintain the best lung function. Patients may also benefit from administration of inhaled steroid and sometimes by injectable steroid preparations. As the disease progresses and shortness of breath becomes more prominent, patients may also require the provision of home oxygen, which will need to be recommended by a specialist chest physician. Quitting smoking is also highly recommended.

cirrhosis of the liver

Cause

Cirrhosis of the liver is the leading cause of death worldwide. In developed countries the most common cause of cirrhosis of the liver is chronic, long-term alcohol excess or the effects of a hepatitis C viral infection. In many Asian and African countries, cirrhosis of the liver most commonly occurs as a result of chronic infection with hepatitis B. The exact cause of cirrhosis is unknown.

Symptoms

Symptoms associated with cirrhosis of the liver may be very few for many years and often first presenting symptoms are non-specific and may be complaints of weakness, loss of appetite, no energy and weight loss. Signs of malnutrition are commonplace and may be secondary to poor appetite or poor food intake in association with excess alcohol intake. Malabsorption of fats and fat-soluble vitamins are also commonplace in this disease.

Diseases of the pancreas go hand in hand with cirrhosis of the liver and further contribute to malabsorption of ingested food material.

The clinical signs include muscle wasting, enlargement of the parotid glands, reddish appearance to the palms of their hands, increased breast size particularly in men, testicular atrophy and loss of peripheral sensation.

Treatment

Prognosis for cirrhosis of the liver is often unpredictable and treatment is dependent on the cause of the cirrhosis, the severity, the presence of complications and whether the person continues to consume alcohol. In general terms the treatment is symptomatic and includes the withdrawal of factors contributing to liver damage, the provision of adequate nutritional factors including supplementary vitamins and the treatment of underlying causes and complications.

Drugs which are known to be metabolised in the liver should be reduced and wherever possible not prescribed.

clotting disorders

See *coagulation disorders*

coagulation disorders

See *cirrhosis of the liver*
See *factor v Leiden*
See *infection*

Cause

Coagulation disorders are either hereditary or acquired.

The most commonly occurring hereditary coagulation disorder is Haemophilia A (which is caused by a deficiency of clotting factor VIII and Haemophilia B (which is caused by a deficiency of clotting factor IX). Both of these entities are clinically identical. Haemophilia A is more common, accounting for 80 per cent of haemophilia patients.

Acquired coagulation disorders include deficiencies of Vitamin K, liver disease (including liver disease resulting from alcohol abuse) resulting in coagulation problems and disseminated intravascular coagulation (which may occur as a complication of pregnancy or due to the effects of overwheling infection in the body or as a complication following prostatic surgery or following venomous snakebite injury).

Symptoms

Symptoms include bleeding into joint spaces or haemorrhages resulting from minor trauma.

Treatment

Treatment for haemophilia requires replacement of the deficient clotting factor. These products are supplied by the Red Cross Transfusion Services.

coeliac disease

Cause

Coeliac disease is a condition relating to a sensitivity to gluten which is contained in many food products.

Symptoms

The symptoms of coeliac disease may include failure to thrive in children, abdominal pain and distension, diarrhoea which may be offensive to smell and lack of appetite,

Investigations

If it is suspected that a patient may have coeliac disease, investigations may include estimation of faecal fat and the biopsy of the duodenal mucosa. Blood tests may be performed but some are less reliable and less sensitive.

Treatment

Treatment of a patient with coeliac disease is to remove gluten from the diet. If the patient follows a gluten-free diet vigorously, symptoms will disappear; however the diet regime is a very rigorous process. More gluten-free products are now appearing in the supermarkets and restaurants are becoming more aware of the dietary restrictions applied to people with coeliac disease.

cold sores

Cause

Cold sores are the result of an infection caused by a virus, herpes simplex. There are two types of herpes simplex: herpes simplex 1 and herpes simplex 2. Herpes simplex 1 is the most commonly occurring herpes infection around the mouth. Herpes simplex 2 more commonly occurs around the genitals.

Symptoms

Cold sores may be found around the mouth, nose and lips. Herpes simplex lesions are very infectious and are easily spread from one person to another; they may also be transferred from one place to another on a single person. It is recommended not to touch a lesion which may occur on the face and then touch another part of the body without washing your hands in between. Herpes simplex virus may also be transferred to the eye and around the eye. When this happens, it becomes a serious infection called a dendritic ulcer of the cornea. Sometimes a patient with such a lesion may be referred to a specialist eye doctor and vision can sometimes be seriously impaired. Herpes simplex infection around the mouth may also be transferred to the person's sexual partner's genital area through oral sex.

Treatment

Once a patient becomes infected with herpes simplex, recurrence of the infection may occur again at any time throughout the rest of the person's life. Cold sore creams are available for treatment around the mouth. These creams need to be applied frequently as soon as symptoms of tingling are felt around the lips or mouth.

Alternatively, the person may apply ice packs to the area of the lip for as long as the tingling persists. Antiviral agents are also available and highly effective in aborting an episode of cold sore outbreak around the mouth and face. These medications are available only on prescription and it is recommended that people who suffer from herpes infection outbreaks on the face have a supply of these medications available for immediate use.

colds and flu or viral upper respiratory tract infection *(URTI)*

Cause

Often called the common cold or flu, these are viral infections and highly contagious.

Symptoms

Symptoms often start with sneezing and a runny nose with a clear discharge, sore throat and cough, sore eyes, body aches and pains, feeling tired and lethargic, no energy and slight fever. Patients often complain of headache. Yellow or green sputum production will be absent except at times when a secondary infection may also the present.

Treatment

The treatment for a viral cold (upper respiratory tract infection or URTI) is symptomatic and includes rest, paracetamol for pain relief, cold and flu tablets, steam inhalations containing eucalyptus or menthol and nose blowing. For young children who are unable to nose blow, a product called Fess is available to assist in clearing the nose. Adequate fluid intake is recommended.

Seasonal flu during the autumn and winter months is common. People who are prone to chest infections or who have chronic medical problems are advised to have a flu injection each year when it becomes available, usually at the beginning of March in Australia. This vaccination gives some protection to some of the flu viruses which are thought to be present in the coming months; however it does not confer 100 per cent immunity for any one year.

There is currently no vaccination available for bird flu which authorities say will lead to widespread, severe infections if it does spread into the community.

colic, baby

Cause

Pain associated with constricted movement of the gut is called colic. Colic is a common symptom in children under the age of three to four months. In this age group, it is due to the fact that the child's gut has not yet developed coordinated contractile movement of food passing through its intestines. Colic may also result from excessive amounts of air which the baby may swallow during times of feeding. This will improve with time and perseverance.

Symptoms

Infantile colic occurs in babies between two and 16 weeks of age, and is characterised by prolonged crying, sometimes for hours on end. Crying commonly occurs in the late afternoon and early evening, in association with irritability. If the baby is ingesting large amounts of air during times of feeding, the ingested air will need to pass through the gut and be expelled as flatulence or wind.

Treatment

Given time, infant colic will settle with improved coordinated movements of the baby's intestines. Parents at this time will require reassurance and explanation by the treating medical practitioner. Medications are also available to treat this condition. In the meantime, preparations such as Infants' Friend, paracetamol for babies and good feeding technique will improve the symptoms.

colon cancer

See *anaemia*

Cause

Colon cancer may commence with the presence of polyps in the bowel which progress to become malignant lesions. These may be detected during colonoscopy examination. Colon cancer may also be related to a low-fibre diet, high in animal protein.

Symptoms

A change in bowel habit may be the first sign of colon cancer. This may also be accompanied by bleeding from the bowel occasionally or with each bowel motion. The bleeding is likely to be bright red in colour as opposed to being dark or black in colour which usually indicates that the bleeding is coming from higher up in the gastro-intestinal tract, e.g. stomach.

If constipation is present and recent in onset, a diagnosis of colon cancer must firstly be considered, particularly in adults.

Investigations

Colon cancer is investigated by colonoscopy. Prior to colonoscopy, a CT scan or an ultrasound of the abdomen may detect the presence of a lump in the bowel, and proceeding to a colonoscopy is then mandatory.

Treatment

If detected early treatment of colon cancer will lead to a satisfactory outcome. Sometimes, however, the symptoms are few and the condition is well advanced before a diagnosis is made. Anyone who has a family history of bowel cancer should be advised to have regular colonoscopy screenings to exclude the possibility of bowel cancer. Testing for small amounts of blood in the faeces is another way to detect early bowel cancer. These kits are available from general practitioners and pathology services. Prior to using the kit, patients are advised to have a diet excluding meat products for a period of time to avoid a false positive reading.

Once the diagnosis of colon cancer has been made, a recommendation will usually be made for surgery to remove a portion of bowel affected by the cancer. This will be done by a specialist surgeon. Following recovery from surgery, additional treatment with chemotherapy may also be recommended. Repeat colonoscopies will then be required on a regular basis to exclude the possibility of recurrence of the condition.

colonic polyps

See *anaemia*
See *colon cancer*

Cause

Colonic polyps and colon cancer are related as cause and effect. A polyp is any mass of tissue which protrudes into the cavity of the bowel. Polyps may be flat or on a stalk-like formation. In many instances there is a positive family history of both. The main concern is that what may start as a polyp, may develop into a malignancy. The aim is to identify a patient with colonic polyps prior to the development of colon cancer.

Symptoms

Abdominal cramps, abdominal pain or distension may occur in the presence of a large polyp or a polyp which has developed into cancer.

Colonic and rectal polyps may not present any symptoms until such time as a malignancy has formed. On occasions polyps may produce rectal bleeding in microscopic amounts. Some patients with colonic polyps may even present with anaemia where it is presumed the patient is losing significant amounts of blood or they detect significant amounts of bleeding from the bowel.

Investigations and Treatment

Test kits for detecting small amounts of rectal bleeding are available for the patient to perform at home and then present to the pathology department for analysis. These test kits detect small amounts of blood in the bowel motion. A diagnosis of polyps and even colon cancer may be made by colonoscopy or CT study. Colonoscopy is the investigation of choice, as the polyp may be able to be removed at the time of the investigation. Polyps may also be multiple.

colon problems

See *abdominal pain*
See *cholera*
See *Crohn's disease*
See *coeliac disease*
See *colon cancer, colonic polyps*
See *constipation*
See *cystic fibrosis*
See *diarrhoea*
See *diverticular disease*
See *gastroenteritis*
See *haemorrhoids*
See *inflammatory bowel disease*
See *irritable colon/bowel*
See *ischaemic colitis*
See *typhoid*

coma

Cause

Coma may be defined as a state of severe altered mental alertness, where the person is unresponsive either to verbal command or to other stimulation, including pain. A state of coma may be produced by stroke, head injury, fracture of the skull, brain tumour (including secondary malignant deposits), meningitis, encephalitis, epilepsy, drug overdose organ failure (heart, kidney or liver), diabetes coma or terminal illness. Coma may be induced to treat severe and uncontrolled epilepsy or severe asthma.

Treatment

Coma is managed in a way which is dependent on the cause and is aimed at sustaining life until recovery is possible, or until such time as the disease process progresses and life becomes extinct.

confusion

Cause

Confusion may be defined as a state of altered mental alertness.

Symptoms

This may be due to head injury, dementia (including Alzheimer's disease), transient ischaemic attack, stroke, following an epileptic fit, during acute illness with fever, depression, schizophrenia, post-traumatic stress condition, hypothyroidism or anaemia.

Treatment

Treatment for a confusional state will depend on the medical cause.

congenital dislocation of the hip *(CDH)*

See *hip pain*

conjunctivitis

See *eyes*

Cause

Conjunctivitis may be caused by a bacterial or viral infection. Conjunctivitis due to viral or bacterial sources is very infectious and is easily spread from one person to another in families and particularly where groups of children congregate as in kindergartens and day-care centres. Allergic conjunctivitis also occurs. Chlamydia infection also causes eye infections, particularly in indigenous communities, causing trachoma, but it may also occurs in newborn babies in the first couple of weeks of life. Conjunctivitis in the newborn may occur as a result of gonorrhea infection, where the mother is infected with the condition and the baby becomes infected during the birth process.

Symptoms

Bacterial conjunctivitis presents with sore red eyes which are often stuck together in the mornings due to discharge in the night, discharge from the eyes, swollen lids and tearing of the eyes. Viral conjunctivitis presents with watery discharge from both eyes, whereas a herpes infection usually occurs only in one eye. These symptoms may or may not be associated with an upper respiratory infection with nasal discharge, coughing, sputum, sore throat. These symptoms are however not usually present with a herpes infection of the eye.

Allergic conjunctivitis is usually associated with spring and autumn, hay fever and a past history of allergy. Symptoms of chlamydia conjunctivitis, if present for long enough, will produce cloudiness of the cornea and loss of sight.

Treatment

Treatment of bacterial conjunctivitis includes frequent washing of the eyes with warm water, administration of antibiotic eye drops and, on occasions, administration of oral antibiotics for severe conjunctivitis, particularly in the presence of an upper respiratory infection. Either a warm or cool face washer applied as a compress to the eyes will also relieve the symptoms of the condition. Warm compresses to the eyes will relieve the symptoms of allergic conjunctivitis. Viral conjunctivitis does not require antibiotic treatment.

Treatment for herpes simplex of the eye includes administration of an antiviral agent called acyclovir. This should be administered five times a day for two weeks. This condition will usually warrant referral to an eye specialist. Treatment for chlamydia infections include erythromycin antibiotics and sometimes surgical intervention by an ophthalmologist, particularly in Third World countries and indigenous populations. Antibiotic treatment for neonatal gonorrhoea infection of the eyes is recommended.

constipation

Cause

By definition, constipation means difficulty in passing bowel motions which are hard in consistency. Constipation may be sudden onset or chronic in nature. If constipation is recent in onset, a diagnosis of colon cancer must firstly be considered, particularly in adults. If constipation is chronic, attention should be directed towards eating habits, use of laxatives, fluid intake and a history of similar problems in other members of the family. Sometimes patients will describe periods of constipation following diarrhoea. This may indicate the presence of irritable bowel syndrome or may be simply due to the fact that following an episode of diarrhoea there is insufficient faeces accumulating in the bowel to pass in the next couple of days. This by definition does not constitute constipation.

Similarly, if people are in the habit of taking laxatives in order to achieve a bowel motion, the muscle in the wall of the bowel becomes dependent on the laxatives and spontaneous bowel motions become more difficult to achieve. If this practice is current, the presence of an eating disorder should be considered.

Eating regular meals which contain a balance between carbohydrates, protein, small amounts of fat, fruit, vegetables and wholegrains are essential for the production of normal bowel motions. Constipation is also caused by dehydration and commonly occurs during periods of prolonged travel, especially air travel, when fluid intake is not adequate. Individuals are also sensitive to changed lifestyle factors such as living situations, e.g. sharing a flat, sharing a house with relatives or the presence of visitors in the house, where access to toilet facilities may become congested. Some people are also reluctant to use toilet facilities at work or school to produce bowel motions, either because of lack of privacy or because the toilet facilities are suboptimal.

Constipation in children can sometimes be behavioural in nature. An inherited condition in children called Hirschsprung's disease, a congenital absence of nerve fibres in the muscle of the bowel, should be excluded with a referral to a paediatrician, particularly if the child has a history of constipation.

Constipation may occur during pregnancy either due to the taking of iron tablets, or because of the effects of the pressure of the foetal head pressing on the bowel in the pelvis.

Symptoms

Constipation is defined as a difficulty passing bowel motions, hard bowel motions that may look like small pebbles or not passing bowel motions on a daily basis. Constipation may or may not be accompanied by some rectal bleeding either from a small anal tear or fissure caused from the strain of trying to pass a hard bowel motion or from the presence of coexistent haemorrhoids, which may accompany chronic constipation.

Treatment

Treatment is directed towards identifying the cause of the constipation, most commonly analysing the person's diet and fluid intake. Elderly people in particular may become so constipated that manual removal of large amounts of faeces becomes necessary, even requiring administration of a light anaesthetic in order to do so. Sometimes administration of rectal suppositories and enemas are required in order to relieve a hard plug of faeces in the lower part of the bowel. Colonoscopy may be indicated to exclude the possibility of colon cancer. Colonoscopy is particularly important for older patients and patients who have a positive family history of colon cancer.

In order to diagnose Hirschsprung's disease, children may require an anaesthetic, colonoscopy and biopsy of the bowel.

contraception

See *amenorrhoea*
See *contraception, emergency*
See *pregnancy*
See *oral contraceptives*

There are a number of methods of contraception to choose from and it may require a couple to try different methods to decide the right one for them.

The oral contraceptive pill (OC) was first used in the late 1950s and is still the most common form of contraception. It comes in two forms: the combined pill—which contains oestrogen and progesterone (there are many different products available)—and the progesterone only pill. The mini-pill is used during breastfeeding. The oral contraceptive pill is around 98 per cent safe in preventing unwanted pregnancy. Some women may experience nausea with the oral contraceptive pill and some weight gain; however this is less with the progesterone pill than for most other pills. Some pills are used specifically for the problem of acne but also act as effective contraceptive agents.

Failure of contraceptive methods may require emergency contraception or may result in pregnancy or termination of pregnancy.

Injectable forms of contraception include the three-monthly progesterone intramuscular injection and the implanon device, a two-inch device inserted under the skin of the upper arm which is active for three years. Some women experience no period for the duration of the use of the device and some women may have unpredictable irregular bleeding, but each person is different and may need to try the device to know if they are likely to have unwanted side effects. In most cases the irregular bleeding will settle within a couple of months following insertion of the device.

An intrauterine contraceptive device (IUCD) called Mirena is a relatively new device and suitable for women who have had a child and want ongoing contraception, and is the device of choice for women around the menopause. It is a locally acting progesterone device which lasts for up to five years. The IUCD is fitted inside the uterine cavity and may stay in place for a number of years without being removed. The IUCD must be fitted by an experienced person either at a family planning clinic, by a gynaecologist or a general practitioner who is trained to fit these devices.

The male condom is still one of the most common devices used besides the oral contraceptive pill. To be most effective, it should be used with a spermicidal cream or gel. Some of the condoms will also have an anti-HIV (nanoxynol 9) agent to help protect from infection with human immunodeficiency virus, but these are not usually freely available from local pharmacies. Safe sex should be practised until a couple decide that they will make a firm permanent commitment to each other.

The female condom is a disposable device which is placed inside the vagina prior to intercourse and acts as a barrier to prevent sexually transmitted diseases and pregnancy. They are less commonly used than male condoms and some would say more difficult to master.

The diaphragm is a rubber dome-shaped cap which is used inside the vagina during intercourse and needs to be retained inside the vagina for at least six to eight hours after intercourse. A diaphragm must be fitted to the individual size of each woman.

The rhythm method and the withdrawal method of contraception are the least reliable methods of prevention of pregnancy. The rhythm method relies on abstinence of sexual intercourse during the period of time in the middle of the woman's cycle when fertility is at its maximum. The withdrawal method requires a great deal of communication between the two parties involved in the sexual activity and also a great deal of coordination and timing of the event. Pregnancy rates for both these methods are the highest of any of the methods of contraception.

Lactation and suppression of ovulation is a method of contraception used by mothers who are breastfeeding their babies in the first six to 12 months following delivery. This may be accompanied by the use of the mini-pill to further promote contraceptive reliability. Lactation itself acts as a contraceptive mechanism, particularly while the child is being fully breastfed.

Tubal ligation for women and vasectomy for men are permanent methods of contraception, which are not designed to be reversible. If at a later date reversal of either of these procedures is desired, micro-surgical technique is necessary by skilled trained surgeons. Even then, the risk of ectopic pregnancy for the woman is increased. An alternative to reversal of a vasectomy for men is testicular aspiration of sperm.

Emergency contraception means provision of the morning-after pill which, if taken within 72 hours of unprotected intercourse, will result in contraceptive measures. Most effectively, emergency contraception should be taken within 24 hours following unprotected sex. The morning-after pill consists of taking two tablets 12 hours apart and this will result in a period within the next four to six days.

Safe sex

The choice of contraception is a personal one, dependent on affordability, reliability, effectiveness, ease-of-use and convenience, which is often dependent upon lifestyle factors, knowledge of alternatives and a preference for one method versus another.

contraception, emergency— morning-after pill

See *oral contraceptives*
See *genital herpes, herpes simplex infection*

Cause

Emergency contraception is often required when intercourse occurs in the absence of any form of contraception or if intercourse occurs and a condom breaks or inadvertently comes off.

Treatment

The morning-after pill is now available in the form of two tablets which are taken 12 hours apart as emergency contraception. The pills should be taken within 72 hours after the unprotected intercourse, but preferably within 24 hours. Often the patient will report that emergency contraception is needed as the condom broke during intercourse the previous night. It is recommended that the morning-after pill be taken if unprotected intercourse occurs in the middle of a menstrual cycle when the woman is not on the contraceptive pill.

The middle of the cycle is the time most likely to produce a pregnancy and termed the fertile period of the cycle. The morning-after pill acts to prevent fertilisation of the ovum and prevents implantation of any embryo which may result from unprotected intercourse. Bleeding as a result of taking the morning-after pill will take place within the next four to six days following taking the pills. The morning-after pill may sometimes produce nausea which may be treated with anti-emetic medication, e.g. anti-nausea medications.

It is recommended that if the woman is to continue with sexual activity, that ongoing contraceptive precautions are taken in order to prevent future unwanted pregnancy and to prevent the need for further emergency contraception. If condoms are the method of contraception, correct use and application of the condoms also needs to be reviewed. Practising safe sex is emphasised.

Safe sex means the suppression of ovulation with one of the methods of hormonal suppression, in addition to using condoms for protection from sexually transmitted diseases. Couples often feel that it is not necessary to continue with the use of condoms once the relationship has become steady; however, indiscretions do occur without the other party being aware until some other emergency occurs, such as the contraction of a sexually transmitted disease such as genital herpes. If genital herpes does occur, the person will carry the infection indefinitely, may experience outbreak of further episodes of infection, and pass the infection on to any future sexual partner. There is treatment and suppression for genital herpes, but no effective cure for the disease, i.e. no means of eradicating all signs of it entirely from the body once infection has taken place.

convulsions

See *epilepsy*
See *pregnancy, associated problems*

Cause

Febrile convulsions are caused by increasing temperature in some susceptible children but convulsions may also occur as a result of epilepsy in either adults or children. Febrile convulsions may be associated with the onset of an upper respiratory infection or ear infection or even fever associated with gastroenteritis. Convulsions might also be caused by the onset of epilepsy, head injury, meningitis or encephalitis, severe dehydration, severe hypoglycaemia (low blood sugar) and electrolyte imbalances in the blood, severe temper tantrums in children or hysteria associated with fear or anxiety, stroke, tumours of the brain, liver or kidney disease, migraine, hydrocephalus (excess fluid and pressure around the brain), high blood pressure including that associated with pregnancy (pre-eclamptic toxaemia), some inherited neurological conditions, and injuries to the brain sustained during pregnancy or delivery.

Investigations

Investigation for determining the cause of a fit is aimed at making a diagnosis. Investigations may include performing a lumbar puncture in order to exclude the presence of serious infection, e.g. meningitis and performing brain wave tracing or electroencephalogram (EEG).

Treatment

The onset of epilepsy for the first time in children, either with or without the presence of fever or in adults, should be investigated.

If it is known that the person is a diabetic, attempts should be made to administer glucose either in the form of an injectable emergency kit, which diabetics should carry with them as a precaution for such emergencies or if the person is sufficiently awake, administration of a sweet drink. Assistance should be sought by calling the ambulance and taking the patient to hospital.

If adults experience an epileptic fit, certain restrictions will be placed on the individual regarding driving until such time as the convulsions (or epilepsy) are stabilised.

Treatment for febrile convulsions firstly involves managing the convulsion itself, by ensuring a clear airway, attempting to reduce the fever by application of wet towels to the child and removing the child from any source of potential danger. Administration of paracetamol is recommended to reduce the fever. The child should then be transported to hospital for further observation and investigation as necessary.

In the case of an epileptic fit occurring in a pregnant woman, stabilisation of the patient is required, followed by serious and urgent consideration of delivery of a baby under strict, controlled medical supervision.

coordination

See *damage to the spinal chord*
See *demetia*
See *epilepsy*
See *hydrocephalus*
See *hypothyroidism*
See *intoxication with alcohol*
See *motor neurone disease*
See *mutiple sclerosis*
See *Parkinson's disease*
See *stroke*

Cause

Problems of coordination include cerebral ischaemia resulting in transient ischaemic attacks or stroke; Parkinson's disease; dementia; hypothyroidism; damage to the spinal cord following injury; tumour; or birth injury; epilepsy; multiple sclerosis; hydrocephalus; motor neurone disease; and intoxication with alcohol. Problems of coordination or clumsiness in children should be investigated to determine the cause. This is often done by specialist paediatricians or by a paediatric neurologists.

Symptoms

Coexistent symptoms in the patient are important in determining the likelihood of one or other of the above diagnoses. Patients who are older are more likely to be suffering from the effects of transient ischaemic attacks as a result of impaired blood flow to the brain, Parkinson's disease or dementia, motor neurone disease or intoxication with alcohol. Clumsiness or poor coordination in younger patients is more likely the result of an inherited neurological condition or the result of an injury to the brain resulting during pregnancy or delivery. Sometimes determining the cause may remain a diagnostic dilemma.

Treatment

Treatment for coordination problems is also difficult. Where diagnosis has been made in children, physical therapy, e.g. physiotherapy or occupational therapy, may help to improve the child's functional capacity. If the child presents with the coexistent problem of seizures or epilepsy, treatment of the epilepsy may also improve overall coordination ability.

Treatment for coordination problems in the elderly is aimed at improving the functional cerebral blood flow, minimising as much as possible the effects of dementia and attempts to stabilise the patient's gait with walking aids as required by the patient.

corneal ulcer

Cause

Corneal ulcers may be caused by excessive wearing of contact lenses, which results in a localised infection. A foreign body on the cornea may produce a corneal ulcer, and conjunctivitis may result in multiple small corneal ulcers, which may be bacterial or viral in origin. Herpes simplex virus may cause severe ulcer of the eye. Persistent rubbing of the eyes because they are itchy and sore may result in a superficial corneal ulcer. The presence of an entropion (turning in of eyelids) of one or both eyes may result in constant rubbing of the lower eyelashes on the conjunctiva, resulting in a corneal ulcer. Ectropion (turning out of eyelids) occurs when the lower lid becomes very droopy and loses contact with the surface of the eye, often exposing a small portion of the inner surface of the conjunctiva of the lower lid. This may also lead to dry eye, watering of the eye and exposure or drying out of the cornea.

Symptoms

Symptoms of a corneal ulcer may include redness of the eye, watering of the eye, pain in the eye, irritation of the eye and sensitivity to the light and may at times involve impairment of visual acuity depending on the severity and position of the ulcer, and the amount of inflammation caused.

Treatment

Treatment of corneal ulcers is aimed at relieving the irritation and treating the infection. Relieving the irritation may involve removing a foreign body, suspending wearing contact lenses for a period of time, removing eyelashes which are rubbing on the cornea, or application of additional artificial tears to the eye in the case of dry eyes. Treatment for entropion might at times require an operation to relieve the irritation on the eye. Treatment for ectropion may include frequent administration of artificial tears or a lubricating gel to the eye to prevent drying out of the cornea and often will include surgical correction.

coronary artery disease and atherosclerosis

See *angina*
See *heart attack*
See *heart failure*
See *hypertension*
See *stroke*

Cause

Coronary artery disease involves an impediment of blood to the coronary arteries due to a blockage caused by a build-up of atheroma or cholesterol deposits. Coronary symptoms may also be due to spasm in the coronary arteries.

Symptoms

Coronary artery disease and atherosclerosis in the coronary arteries may be due to ischaemic heart disease, angina, heart attack or sudden death. If coronary artery disease and hypertension are left untreated, cardiac failure or heart failure may result.

Treatment

Prevention of coronary artery disease involves reducing the risk factors, e.g. quitting smoking, weight loss, a healthy diet, regular exercise, control of cholesterol, control of blood pressure and active management of diabetes. Surgical treatment may include coronary artery bypass graft operation and/or stenting of the coronary arteries to correct stenosis or blockage.

coronary syndrome

See *angina*
See *atherosclerosis*
See *cardiomyopathies*
See *chest pain*
See *cholesterol*
See *heart attack*

cough

See *asthma*
See *bronchiectasis*
See *bronchitis*
See *brucellosis*
See *cardiovascular system*
See *cystic fibrosis*
See *emphysema*
See *heart failure*
See *infections*
See *lung abscess*
See *lung cancer*
See *pneumonia*
See *Q fever*
See *smoking*
See *tuberculosis*
See *upper respiratory tract infection*
See *whooping cough*

Cause

Coughing is a symptom which most people have experienced at some point in time. It may be associated with an acute upper respiratory tract infection, bronchitis, post-nasal drip, smoking or, in the case of children, a possible inhaled foreign body in the lungs. Coughing may also be a prominent symptom in asthma.

Coughing may produce sputum which is either clear, yellow, green or bloodstained. Not uncommonly, sputum produced by smokers may be brownish in colour due to a combination of the effects of small amounts of blood mixed with the products contained in cigarette smoke. There are many other causes associated with coughing which may indicate the presence of a more sinister complaint. Most upper respiratory tract infections and chest infections will produce some degree of coughing. In the vast majority of cases, coughing is associated with viral upper respiratory tract infections.

Sometimes coughing may be associated with coughing up blood. More sinister causes may include heart failure, lung cancer, severe lung infections including pneumonia, tuberculosis, lung abscess, bronchiectasis, cystic fibrosis, emphysema, inhaled foreign body, pulmonary embolism (or blood clot on the lung), whooping cough (an infectious childhood disease), Q fever (associated with meat workers and people farming cattle), legionnaire's disease, brucellosis (also associated with meat workers and cattle farmers), sarcoidosis (an uncommon and difficult condition to diagnose) and congestive heart failure.

Symptoms

Coughing may be associated with increased temperature or fever, body aches and pains, sputum production, night sweats, recurrent bouts of respiratory infection and in some children failure to thrive. In children, recurrent episodes of respiratory infection and failure to thrive may be the first signs that the child may have cystic fibrosis.

Investigations

In most cases, if coughing is a predominant symptom, no initial investigations may be indicated. If, however, the patient complains of copious amounts of yellow, green or bloodstained sputum, a chest X-ray, CT of the chest and sinuses or bronchoscopy—for serious cases. The chest X-ray may at this stage also reveal the presence of other pathology including heart failure, lung cancer, pneumonia, bronchiectasis or cystic fibrosis The patient might also need a full blood count, including white cell count, sputum culture looking for infective organisms, serology of blood or the presence of antibodies to infectious diseases, e.g. whooping cough, Q fever, brucellosis, tuberculosis, to determine the extent of their infection.

Treatment

The treatment for viral upper respiratory tract infection includes symptomatic relief such as paracetamol for fever, aches and pains; nasal inhalation; and perhaps an antihistamine to help dry up the nasal secretions. The duration of the illness will last for four to five days, after which time symptoms should start to improve. If symptoms do not improve and progress to a point where sputum becomes yellow, green or bloodstained in colour, the patient should be reviewed by the doctor and an antibiotic added to the regime to avoid a secondary bacterial infection. If a condition other than viral or bacterial respiratory infection is detected, other specific treatment options will be required. Bronchodilators may be indicated if the person is experiencing wheezing or if the person with an infection is also asthmatic.

coughing blood *(haemoptysis)*

See *bronchiectasis*
See *bronchitis*
See *cystic fibrosis*
See *lung cancer*
See *pneumonia*
See *tuberculosis*

Coughing up blood is called haemoptysis. It is a serious condition and requires immediate medical attention.

cramps

Cause

People are prone to feeling cramps, particularly at night. This occurs most commonly in the lower legs and calf muscles. Sometimes this may be related to a relative degree of physical activity, abnormalities in the electrolytes in the blood and sometimes to the presence of diabetes.

Investigations

People complaining of cramps should be investigated with full blood count, electrolyte levels and screening for diabetes.

Treatment

Nocturnal cramps in the absence of other pathology may be treated with massage to the calf muscle, a hot-water bottle and stretching of the muscle.

Crohn's disease

See *bleeding*
See *colon problems*

Cause

Crohn's disease is caused by an inflammation of the wall of the gut.

Symptoms

Crohn's disease is an inflammation of the small or large intestines and is associated with abdominal pain and change in bowel habits. It frequently involves the passing of dark blood in the faeces and the presence of bloody diarrhoea. Episodes may be intermittent or continuous.

Treatment

Various medications are available in the treatment of Crohn's disease. This may involve indications such as anti-inflammatory medication or prednisone, which may be in the form of oral or rectal administration. It is an uncommon condition but if severe, it may require the removal of affected portions of the gut or even at times the entire large gut.

Investigations

A colonoscopy and biopsy will confirm the diagnosis.

croup

Cause

Croup is caused by a viral infection, most commonly caused by the Para influenza virus, which results in swelling of the mucous membranes lining in the lungs, causing a characteristic cough associated with the onset of croup. It is a respiratory disease of children usually six years or younger. It can be very frightening for parent and child.

Symptoms

Croup has a characteristic cough which sounds like that of the seal barking—the general practitioner who hears a child in the waiting room with this cough may be able to make the diagnosis before even seeing the child.

Croup is most common in children from the ages of six months to six years. As children get older, the likelihood of croup occurring becomes less. Most commonly, the onset of croup occurs during the night, often waking the child and parents simultaneously. It tends to occur more during the winter months.

Children who present with croup will often do so firstly in the middle of the night. It is often a concerning symptom for parents experiencing this illness for the first time. Steam inhalation will help such as running a hot shower so the child can inhale the steam.

Treatment

Mild croup only requires symptomatic treatment with paracetamol and steam inhalation. Treatment for more severe croup includes administration of oral steroids for two days, depending on the age and weight of the child. It is recommended that this treatment continue twice a day for four doses after which time the child should be reviewed by the local doctor. The child would usually recover on this regime.

The child's room should be kept warm and paracetamol may be administered. If the parents are concerned and the child is significantly distressed, the parents should be advised to take the child to hospital where additional appropriate treatment will be administered. This will usually be in the form of oxygen and perhaps an injection of subcutaneous adrenaline.

crying baby

See *baby, problems*

Cause

Crying is a baby's way of communicating certain needs. A baby will cry when it is hungry, needs changing, is feeling sick or unwell and when it wants attention. Parents will learn that there are different characteristics to crying depending on the baby's needs. It is of concern if the baby cries and the basic needs of hunger, change of clothing or need for attention have been provided. Ongoing crying may indicate that the baby is unwell.

Symptoms

The baby may have a temperature, abdominal pain, reflux, constipation or diarrhoea, sore ears or sore throat. Older babies may be teething or have a fever. Some babies with developmental abnormalities may cry as a result of cerebral irritation, with or without a fever or may have an injury to some part of the body due to either birth trauma, subsequent injury including a fall or underlying congenital abnormality.

Treatment

If the basic needs of the baby are attended to and crying continues, medical assistance should be sought to determine the cause of the crying and to formulate a management plan.

cryptosporidium

Cause

Cryptosporidium is an organism which causes diarrhoea and is transferred from one person to another by the oral/ faecal route.

Symptoms

The symptoms associated with cryptosporidium infection include watery diarrhoea, abdominal cramps, fever, nausea and vomiting which may last up to two weeks. Loss of appetite is also common and, in association with diarrhoea, may lead to weight loss. The means of transmission of cryptosporidium include the ingestion of contaminated water, including small amounts from contaminated swimming pools, contaminated food and from animals.

Treatment

Treatment for cryptosporidium includes symptomatic treatment only as there is no effective treatment to combat the organism. When infection has taken place in common user areas, e.g. community swimming pools, closure of the area is necessary and the area must be treated, such as draining the pool and ensuring filtration is adequate, before it is safe for the community. It is important that parents monitor children with diarrhoea to ensure that they do not participate in swimming activities or other activities where the infection can spread.

Cushing's syndrome

See *adrenal gland*

Cause

Cushing's syndrome or Cushing's disease, results from an excess of production of cortisol from the adrenal cortex or as a result of tumours arising in the pituitary gland. Cushing's syndrome may also result from administration of corticosteroids, adrenal adenomas or carcinoma of the adrenal glands.

Symptoms

Symptoms of Cushing's syndrome include truncal obesity, hypertension, weakness and fatigue, amenorrhoea, hirsutism, oedema, osteoporosis and sugar in the urine.

Treatment

Patients with pituitary tumours should be treated with surgical removal of the tumour. If an adrenal tumour is diagnosed following investigations, adrenal cortical tumours should be removed surgically. Following surgery, patients will receive cortisol treatment.

cystic fibrosis

Gut symptoms

Cause

Cystic fibrosis is a condition inherited in an autosomal recessive pattern of inheritance. Inherited medical conditions are carried on genetic material called genes, which are portions of chromosomes. This means that each parent carries a gene for cystic fibrosis. Couples with these genes have a one in four chance of a pregnancy resulting in a child with cystic fibrosis. They have a two in four chance of having a child who is a carrier for the condition and a one in four chance for a child of the same couple to have a child who is neither a carrier nor affected by the condition.

Cystic fibrosis may affect the lungs and the gastrointestinal tract. Cystic fibrosis is relatively common in the community and accounts for approximately 1 in 2500 live births. The lifespan of a person with cystic fibrosis is often reduced.

Symptoms

The condition may present in infancy with a failure to pass the first bowel motion, called meconium. Children may present with recurrent chest infections, failure to thrive and malabsorption. In addition to respiratory problems, they will experience a deficiency of digestive juices from the pancreas which processes and digests food.

Investigations

In order to determine a diagnosis of cystic fibrosis, gene testing will be carried out. If the child is experiencing recurrent respiratory infections and failure to thrive, there is sufficient indication to undertake gene testing. Gene testing and sweat chloride tests are used for diagnosis.

Treatment

There is no cure for cystic fibrosis, yet gene therapy appears hopeful. Treatment is determined by the presence of symptoms.

Cystic fibrosis may require treatment for both the lung component and gastrointestinal component of the disease. The latter comprises provision of supplementary pancreatic enzymes to prevent malabsorption and assist with digestion of food. Some patients with cystic fibrosis may receive organ transplantation, most commonly lungs. Good nutrition and supplementary pancreatic enzymes improve gut function and minimse symptoms of malabsorption.

Respiratory symptoms

Cause

Cystic fibrosis is a condition inherited in an autosomal recessive pattern of inheritance. Inherited medical conditions are carried on genetic material called genes, which together form chromosomes. This means that parents of people with cystic fibrosis each contain a gene which, when combined, produce a child with the condition.

Symptoms

Children who are born with cystic fibrosis may experience recurrent respiratory tract infections; coughing; sputum production; wheezy; noisy breathing at times; respiratory distress; slowness in gaining weight and may be small for their age. This is called failure to thrive.

Investigations

In order to determine a diagnosis of cystic fibrosis, gene testing is carried out. If the child is experiencing recurrent respiratory infections and failure to thrive, there is sufficient indication to undertake investigation by gene testing. Other testing is done in the form of a sweat chloride test.

Treatment

There is no cure for cystic fibrosis. Treatment will be determined by the presence of respiratory symptoms. In some instances organ transplantation may be considered, although this in itself does not represent a cure.

Early treatment of chest infections using appropriate antibiotics is essential. Life expectancy and quality of life for the patient with cystic fibrosis have improved with the advent of treatment methods.

cytomegalovirus

Cause

Cytomegalovirus is one of the herpes viruses.

Symptoms

An infection with cytomegalovirus is manifested by fever, hepatitis, pneumonia and in neonates, may cause still birth. If contracted in utero, this infection may cause brain damage, hearing and vision impairment and intellectual disability.

The virus may be excreted in the urine for up to 12 months following infection.

Treatment

Treatment is symptomatic only and includes pain relief and paracetamol for regulation and reduction of fever.

dandruff

See *dermatitis/eczema*

Cause

Dandruff is a common problem for many people and is caused by the flaking of the skin of the scalp. Excessive amounts of flaking of the skin of the scalp is abnormal and may be caused by dermatitis or by psoriasis.

Excessive shampooing or excessively stringent hair products, either shampooing or colouring products, may cause flaking of the scalp.

Symptoms

Wherever there is skin on the body, loss of the outer layers of skin will take place. This occurs on a daily basis and the outer skin is replaced with fresh skin from the lower layers which are being produced all the time.

Dermatitis may appear at other sites on the body in conjunction with the scalp.

Psoriasis is a skin condition associated with redness and patchy areas of flaky skin anywhere on the body. It is not itchy.

Treatment

Simple remedies should always be tried before reaching for more complicated solutions. Simple dandruff may be treated by modifying or changing shampoo or other hair products to suit the individual or modifying the frequency of application of any hair products. Medicated shampoos are available. If symptoms persist, application of a once-weekly corticosteroid solution to the scalp, applied to well towel-dried hair, may improve the symptoms.

deafness and hearing loss

See *ear infections*

Deafness is defined as a hearing impairment which may be temporary or permanent, static (non-progressive) or progressive. It may be classified as conductive hearing impairment or sensori-neural hearing impairment.

Hearing responses are measured in decibels and when a hearing test or pure tone audiogram is done, responses up to 20 decibels (DB) are regarded as normal.

Hearing may be tested using a pure tone audiometry and may be used with children as young as four to five years of age. Other measures will be necessary for children younger than four years.

Cause

Temporary

Temporary hearing impairment is more likely to be conductive and may occur in children or adults in association with an upper respiratory and middle ear infection, which may be accompanied by fluid in the middle ear or Eustachian tube dysfunction, sinus infection or excessive wax in the ear canal. Once the infection or wax or foreign body, has been cleared, the hearing should return to normal.

Exposure to loud noises, which may include industrial noise or loud music, may result in loss of hearing. If exposure to loud noise continues over a period of time, gradually hearing loss will result which will be permanent. If a person is exposed to a sudden loud noise, they may experience a 'ringing' in the ears for a variable amount of time. If this sort of exposure is an infrequent event, more than likely the hearing will recover.

Wax production in the ears is a normal function of cleaning the canal of debris. Some ears are more efficient in this cleaning function that others. Pressure trauma and perforation of the eardrum may also result in hearing loss.

Permanent causes of hearing loss include exposure to industrial or ongoing loud noise, some medication (termed ototoxic) and damage to the ear as a result of pressure trauma.

Sensori-neural causes of hearing loss include skull fracture, congenital problems with or without the presence of family history, maternal rubella during pregnancy or Paget's disease. These causes represent a static process where the hearing loss is unlikely to deteriorate further. Progressive sensori-neural hearing loss occurs with otosclerosis, hardening of the bones in the ear which conduct sensory impulses, tumours of the acoustic nerve or tumours in that part of the brain responsible for the sensation of sound, i.e. the temporal lobe.

Permanent

Permanent hearing loss is more likely to be due to sensori-neural causes. Some drugs may damage the acoustic nerve causing permanent damage to transmission of impulses going to the brain, thus hearing loss. Skull fractures may damage the acoustic nerve or may alternatively damage that part of the brain responsible for hearing.

Some families may have a history of inherited hearing loss. Sometimes this may be associated with a chromosomal abnormality.

Maternal infection with German measles during pregnancy results in a condition called the expanded rubella syndrome, which is associated with deafness, vision defects, cataracts and intellectual disability.

Trauma to the ear including barotrauma may result in dislocation of the ear ossicles, which are small bones in the middle ear which are responsible for the conduction of sound vibrations from the exterior to the acoustic nerve and then to the brain.

Paget's disease of the bone produces new bone formation and if this occurs around the nerves which course through the skull bone, damage to any of the nerves which travel in the bone may result in permanent hearing impairment.

Otosclerosis develops as people age, resulting in a stiffening of the joints which connect the ear ossicles or bones so that they are less efficient in conducting sound vibrations from the exterior to the acoustic nerve. This results in increasing hearing loss.

Tumours of the acoustic nerve may damage the nerve by directly invading the nerve tissue substance or the part of the brain responsible for registering hearing as a sense. Alternatively, surgery for removal of the tumour may result in hearing loss.

Damage to the hearing neural paths may also occur following meningitis, either due to the infection itself or sometimes due to medication used to treat the infection.

Symptoms

Hearing problems in children should be suspected if they do not achieve the usual developmental milestones. Often a child who is deaf may start to make sounds, then stops and fails to respond to voice signals. It is important that a child be diagnosed as early as possible with hearing impairment in order to develop speech and communication skills.

With acute infections, the patient may complain of pain in the ear or popping noises, with adults and older children unable to valsalva (i.e. pop your ears by holding your nose tightly and blowing). Being able to valsalva is most important for people who may wish to go diving and this test is part of assessment when undergoing a dive medical examination. Inability to do so may result in barotrauma to the ears if the person continues the diving activity.

The early signs of hearing loss, particularly in the case of industrial exposure or exposure to other forms of loud noise, may be a sensation of ringing in the ears or tinnitus. If the source of the noise continues or is repeated often enough, the ringing will persist after the stimulus has been removed and at some point the tinnitus will become permanent, accompanied by hearing loss.

Treatment

Cleaning the ears of wax may need to be done periodically, either with medication in the form of drops or by syringing the ears out with warm water. People should not try to syringe out their ears at home as damage may be done to the eardrum. Cotton buds should also not be used as the wax is pushed further into the ear canal causing further problems.

If a child has been diagnosed at an early age with hearing impairment, investigation should be undertaken as soon as possible. If there is no temporary cause found for the condition, the child may need early intervention with speech therapy, teaching of sign language and consideration for a cochlear implant.

Hearing aids are available for both children and adults; however wearers often complain of unwanted noise and often find them only of moderate success.

Prevention is the key to industrial hearing loss, by wearing protective ear equipment.

dementia

Cause

Dementia may be classed as static or progressive in nature. Static dementia may occur following a single major event, e.g. head injury, cardiac arrest or stroke. Progressive dementia occurs in conditions such as Huntington's disease, drug and alcohol nutritional deficiency state, brain tumours, Parkinson's disease, multiple sclerosis and amyotrophic lateral sclerosis. Alzheimer's disease is one of the progressive forms of dementia, as is the dementia which may accompany AIDS.

Symptoms

Symptoms of dementia include depression, anxiety, paranoia, changes in personality, forgetfulness, losing or misplacing possessions, short-term memory problems, diffuculty naming simple objects, repeating previous conversations or questions.

Treatment

Treatment of patients with dementia involves treatment of any coexistent illness, withdrawl of any potentially toxic drug, provision of adequate mental stimulation, removal from any potentially harmful situations, good nutrition, keeping the patient's surroundings consistent. Medication may assist in some cases, e.g. donepezil hydrochloride and memantine hydrochloride.

dengue fever

See *tropical diseases*

Cause

Dengue fever is endemic in tropical areas and is caused by a virus called flavivirus, transmitted by the Aedes mosquito. Incubation period is three to15 days.

Symptoms

Symptoms include chills, lethargy, aches and pains particularly in the legs and joints, fever, conjunctivitis, headache, rash particularly on the face, swollen lymph glands and the palms and soles of the feet become swollen and red. Convalescence may take several weeks.

Treatment

Treatment for dengue fever is symptomatic only, with relief of headache, aches and pains.

Aspirin should be avoided. Prevention of the disease may be achieved with the use of mosquito nets in the tropics and insect repellent.

dental problems

See *gastroesophageal reflux*
See *halitosis*

Cause

Dental problems arise due to poor dental hygiene, decay formation or retraction of the gums due to periodontal infection or the onset of menopause.

Symptoms

Dental problems may present with a history of localised pain or more widespread pain if there is significant infection and abscess formation, localised swelling, inability to chew on the affected side, localised sensitivity to hot or cold food in the mouth and pain in the salivary gland when food is placed in the mouth.

Treatment

Treatment for dental problems is oral antibiotics, usually amoxicillin, pain relief and an appointment to see the dentist for treatment. As people age, scale builds up more readily on the teeth and retraction of the gum line occurs, allowing infection in the gum to occur. Significant dental infection is a predisposing factor to the onset of coronary heart disease. Regular flossing and brushing of the teeth is essential to ensure good dental hygiene.

depression

See *anxiety*
See *bipolar disorder*

Cause

It is often difficult to determine the cause of depression. Sometimes depression may result from one or more situational crises being experienced by the patient. This precipitating event or events may vary from one person to another and is often accompanied by anxiety.

Post-natal depression may occur weeks or months following the delivery of a baby. Women not infrequently report that the birth of the baby experience is different from that which they anticipated, particularly if there are problems in some way with the baby, either due to prematurity, illness or behaviour such as feeding difficulty, crying or colic. Sleep deprivation is also a factor in the development of post-natal depression.

Symptoms

Symptoms may include loss of interest in daily activities; a feeling of lack of fulfilment; weight loss or weight gain; loss of appetite; either insomnia or increased hours of sleeping throughout the day and night which is characterised either by an inability to get to sleep, or alternatively, getting to sleep followed by early morning wakening; fatigue; muscular aches and pains; lethargy; loss of energy; lack of self-esteem; difficulty with concentration; poor performance at either school or work; indecisiveness; feelings of helplessness, worthlessness and despair; forgetfulness; unexplained sadness; suicidal thoughts; and preoccupation with thoughts of death. In the elderly patient depression is particularly difficult to recognise and maybe misdiagnosed as dementia. Recognition of depression in children may also be very difficult.

Treatment

Treatment commences the minute the patient enters the office of the medical practitioner. Establishing a good rapport with the patient is most important and listening to what they have to say. The patient may be unaware of any reason for their feeling this way. If thoughts of death and suicide are prominent in the patient's mind, consideration of inpatient treatment in an appropriate facility should be considered. Referral to a psychiatrist or psychologist is also an important consideration. Exclusion of the underlying medical condition is also necessary before a treatment plan can be established.

A full blood count and thyroid function test should be undertaken. Often listening to the patient, which may take a considerable amount of time and patience on the part of the general practitioner, will allow them to formulate an appropriate treatment plan.

Medication may also play an important part in assisting the person to recover from depression. There are many different types of medication to choose from when deciding on a pharmacological agent. It is important to restore the normal sleeping pattern to the patient as quickly as possible. In order to do this a mild sedative or mild sleeping tablet may be necessary before the patient retires at night. In addition, provision of antidepressants may be necessary.

Selecting the right agent for the individual patient is sometimes more challenging. Review of the patient's progress on a regular basis is very important; this includes reviewing the lifestyle factors of the patient as well.

dermatitis/eczema

See *skin problems*

Cause

Dermatitis and eczema go hand in hand and indicate a sensitivity of the skin.

Symptoms

Symptoms of dermatitis and eczema include acute or chronic skin rash accompanied by redness, crusting and scaling of the skin, itchiness. It may also include skin which is weeping and oozing. Patients may have a family history of similar problems and may also have a history of other allergies, asthma and hay fever. Dermatitis may occur in any position on the body, but eczema is more commonly seen on the face, around the neck, on the scalp and in the creases of the body, i.e. elbows, behind the knees and in the groin area.

Treatment

Careful explanation to the patient or to the parent of the child regarding the condition is important. Patients are advised to avoid the usual soaps and instead use a sorbolene-based bath lotion, using warm but not hot water. Patients should be encouraged not to rub or scratch affected areas and to try to avoid becoming overheated. Application of a moisturising agent such as sorbolene is recommended and on occasions the addition of hydrocortisone cream may be required. If dermatitis is particularly severe, e.g. on the arms or legs, occlusive wet dressings may be indicated. Some patients will also require the use of oral steroids in order to control the symptoms. Referral to a dermatologist may also be required.

diabetes

See *obesity*
See *smoking*
See *weight management problems*

Cause

Diabetes is a disease of glucose metabolism and is subdivided into Type 1 diabetes (previously called juvenile onset diabetes or insulin dependent diabetes) and Type 2 diabetes. Diabetes mellitus Type 1 is a condition which more commonly arises in childhood, adolescence or early adulthood where the cells in the pancreas stop producing insulin in quantities required by the body. This is thought to be an autoimmune disease which may be the result of a viral infection.

Diabetes mellitus Type 2 is defined as impaired insulin secretion with variable degrees of peripheral insulin resistance leading to hyperglycaemia or elevated blood sugar. Type 2 diabetes mellitus is more commonly found in adults who are overweight.

Symptoms

Hypoglycaemia may occur at times in conjunction with the administration of medication for diabetes as a result of lack of food intake in the case of Type 1 or insulin dependent diabetes. Hypoglycaemia may occur at times with Type 2 diabetes if administration of medication and meal times are not coordinated appropriately.

Early symptoms of diabetes included hyperglycaemia or high blood sugar and later include polydypsia (drinking a lot of fluids), polyphagia (requiring eating more frequently) and polyuria (passing a lot of urine).

Patients with Type 1 diabetes are usually young whereas patients with Type 2 diabetes will present later in life, often in their 40s, 50s, 60s or later. Mature-onset diabetes is often accompanied by obesity, high blood pressure, elevated cholesterol, sedentary lifestyle, poor eating habits with a diet high in saturated fat and sugar (or more correctly high in compounds called carbohydrates which are converted into glucose in the body). Later complications of diabetes include vascular disease of the heart, brain, kidneys and vessels in the legs and feet, peripheral neuropathy or altered sensations in the extremities (most importantly in the legs and feet) and an increasing predisposition to infections anywhere in the body. When an infection occurs, control of blood sugar becomes more difficult, thus producing an escalating set of events which calls for intervention by the treating practitioner to regain control of the blood sugar.

Specific attention should be paid to the care of feet in diabetics, as minor infections can spread rapidly leading to major problems and even amputation of toes and portions of the lower limbs. Diabetics also require regular monitoring of their retina or back of the eye. Diabetic retinopathy sometimes requires laser therapy by an ophthamologist in order to preserve sight.

Investigation

The diagnosis of diabetes mellitus is made by performing a glucose tolerance test. A glucose tolerance test is performed by taking blood from a patient who has fasted from nine o'clock the previous evening, administering a standard known amount of a substance containing glucose, then measuring the blood glucose again in two hours' time. A glucose reading of 11mmol/litre is diagnostic of diabetes.

Treatment

Treatment for Type 1 diabetes includes the provision of injectable insulin in order to control the blood sugar level. There are many different types of insulin on the market and the choice of product will be determined by the treating physician and the needs of the patient.

Treatment for Type 2 diabetes includes diet management, weight reduction, exercise, blood sugar level monitoring, control of cholesterol levels and blood pressure. The aim of treatment is to return the blood sugar levels to normal reading. If this cannot be achieved using the previously stated parameters, the addition of oral hypoglycaemic agents may be required. If normal blood sugar levels remain elevated and are not controlled using oral hypoglycaemic agents, even the Type 2 diabetic may need supplementary insulin in order to control the blood sugar readings.

Treatment for an acute episode of hypoglycaemia is to administer to the patient a sweet drink or lolly or alternatively, to administer some fruit, e.g. banana.

Complications associated with either Type 1 or Type 2 diabetes are multiple and lead to primary vascular complications that may affect large and small blood vessels alike. Micro vascular disease is the basis to the common and most devastating complications of diabetes and include diabetic retinopathy (disease of the retina in the eye, which may lead to significant visual impairment), nephropathy (disease of the kidney, which may lead to renal failure) and neuropathy (disease of peripheral nerves, which may lead to impairment of sensation particularly in the lower limbs, rendering them more susceptible to injury and ulcer formation). Micro vascular disease also dramatically impairs the healing of skin, leading to the possibility of deep ulceration which may easily become infected.

Intensive control of blood sugar levels may improve diabetes control and therefore lessen the degree of complications which a patient may sustain; however once damage to eyes, kidneys and peripheral nerves have taken place, the damage to these organs is irreversible.

Education of the patient is a vital ingredient in helping them to understand their disease, as well as assisting them in preventing the complications of diabetes. Regular surveillance of the diabetic patient as well as the involvement of diabetic educators, podiatrists, eye specialists and dietitians form the basis to providing ongoing care for any diabetic patient and a working relationship between all the professions is essential.

dialysis

Dialysis is a treatment for patients with renal failure. Dialysis occurs as either peritoneal or haemodialysis and is used as a means of controlling electrolyte and fluid balance in the body. This may continue either short or long term, depending on the nature of the condition causing the renal failure. Some patients may go on to require kidney transplantation.

In haemodialysis, the patient's blood is pumped into a dialysis machine and in a series of complex exchanges, reduction in urea, creatinine and fluid takes place and the blood is then returned to the patient. In-home dialysis machines are available, but are extremely costly. Patients often need to have dialysis several times per week, so it has a big impact on the patient and the family in terms of time, cost, time off work if the patient is working and large costs to the community.

diarrhoea

See *bleeding*
See *coeliac disease*
See *colon cancer*
See *colon problems*
See *Crohn's disease*
See *gastroenteritis*
See *tropical diseases*

Cause

Diarrhoea is defined as frequent passage of a loose bowel motion which is unformed and often watery. Most commonly, acute diarrhoea will be the result of an infective process, e.g. viral gastroenteritis, salmonella, staphylococcus (food poisoning), enteropathic organisms and rotavirus in children.

In some patients, stressful situations may also result in diarrhoea. Some patients may experience diarrhoea due to certain foods, overeating rich food and some medication, in particular antibiotics. Diarrhoea may also result from inflammatory and ischaemic processes in the gut.

Symptoms

Diarrhoea may be accompanied by abdominal pain, which is cramping or colicky in nature, a feeling of being unwell, fever and loss of appetite. On occasions diarrhoea may also contain blood.

Treatment

Most cases of diarrhoea are treated symptomatically as they constitute a viral infection. Symptomatic treatment includes fluid replacement, pain relief and relief for vomiting and diarrhoea. If diarrhoea, particularly bloody diarrhoea, is a recurring problem, referral to a gastroenterologist is recommended. A stool culture may show the presence of specific gut infections; however in the case of viral gastroenteritis, a stool culture is often negative.

diphtheria

See *immunisation for childhood infectious diseases*

Cause

Diphtheria is caused by an organism called corynebacterium diphtheria.

Symptoms

Diphtheria is a potentially life-threatening condition which involves an infection in the upper airways in both adults and children, which can lead to obstruction of the respiratory passages causing sudden onset of breathing difficulties. As a result of immunisation programs, diphtheria is now an uncommon infectious disease in childhood.

Treatment

Treatment for diphtheria remains prevention by vaccination of infants at two, four and six months, a booster at four years and subsequent boosters for adolescents at 15 years. If diphtheria is diagnosed in a patient, admission to hospital is mandatory.

disturbed patients

See *alcohol abuse*
See *depression*
See *smoking*

Cause

Disturbed patients may present as a result of substance abuse either from alcohol, marihuana or other recreational drugs, onset of dementia or from severe depression.

Symptoms

Patients who display disturbed symptoms may present with suicidal thoughts, an acute episode of psychosis (schizophrenia) or bipolar disorder (with mood swings from euphoria to severe depression). Patients may appear agitated, confused, paranoid and display memory problems, hallucinations (auditory or visual), cloudy thinking, abnormal thought processes and have difficulty articulating their symptoms. Patients with bipolar disorder may present in an episode of acute euphoria when family or friends note excessive non-purposeful activity and may be accompanied by reports of not sleeping, excessive spending, alcohol or drug use or may even be described as the 'life of the party'.

Treatment

There is a need to exclude a physical cause for the behaviour from thyroid, anaemia and acute brain syndrome (due to ischaemic problems).

If suicidal, patients should be referred to an acute facility for assessment and treatment. Dementia patients will need assessment from a psychogeratrician and medication is available which will improve the symptoms to some extent, but often the results may be disappointing. With an acutely disturbed patient, there is a need to ensure the safety of the patient and the household. Patients with an acute psychotic episode need urgent assessment and treatment either as an outpatient (provided there is no risk of self-harming and social support is available from family of friends) or in-patient in an acute facility. If symptoms are due to drug use, this will need to be addressed at some point, often not at the time of the episode if the patient is disturbed and not able to process the advice. Detox centres are available for this purpose also. Patients with bipolar disorder may require hospitalisation to manage an acute episode, then continue with oral medication, antipsychotic medication and mood stabilisers, e.g. Haloperidol, Risperidone or Olanzapine, with or without lithium.

diverticular disease

Cause

Diverticular disease is a condition affecting the colon due to long-term consumption of a low-fibre diet. Diverticulae (or outpocketings in the gut wall) may occur anywhere in the large bowel and is caused by increased pressure inside the lumen of the gut. The condition is uncommon before 40 years; however with increasing age the condition becomes more common. Diverticular disease may sometimes result in inflammation of the bowel associated with severe pain, peritonitis, perforation of the gut and even abscess formation. This is termed diverticulitis.

Symptoms

Most people with diverticular disease report no symptoms; however if diverticulae become inflamed, pain may result, sometimes bleeding. In the case of diverticulitis, patients will often experience severe abdominal pain, tenderness in the abdomen on the left lower side or even pain in the left upper leg. Sometimes perforation of the gut may result in a communication between the gut and the vagina in women, i.e. a fistula, which results in vaginal discharge containing faeces.

Investigations

The diverticulae may be an incidental finding when patients complain of abdominal pain and rectal bleeding as a result of a colonoscopy investigation.

Treatment

Treatment of diverticular disease is aimed at reducing the spasm in the gut which is often responsible for the pain. Also, patients will be advised to increase the fibre content of their diet. Anti-spasmodic medication may improve the spasm and therefore the pain; however most people with diverticular disease will not require more complex treatment or intervention. Some patients may become extremely ill and require hospitalisation. Where diverticulitis occurs and results in perforation of the gut, surgical intervention will be required. For a patient with diverticulitis who is not very ill, home treatment with a liquid diet oral antibiotics, e.g. penicillin and metronidazole, may be all that is required.

diverticulitis

See *colon problems*
See *diverticular disease*

Cause

Acute diverticulitis occurs in less than 10 per cent of patients with diverticular disease. The term diverticulum refers to small bubble-like pockets in the wall of the large bowel. These occur commonly in all adults over the age of 50 years of age and are seen readily on barium enema studies and on colonoscopy.

Symptoms

Acute diverticulitis presents with symptoms of abdominal pain and may be associated with symptoms of chronic constipation over a prolonged period of time.

Investigations

Investigations for acute diverticulitis include estimation of the white cell count, the presence of pus and blood in the stools. In addition, an abdominal ultrasound and CT scan is often performed.

Treatment

The treatment of acute diverticulitis includes intravenous antibiotics, e.g. amoxicillin, gentamicin and/or metronidazole (flagyl), analgesia for pain, either intravenously or intramuscularly and no food or fluids by mouth until the gut recovers. There may be occasions where surgery is required for complications of acute diverticulitis, e.g. an abscess formation or a perforation of the gut.

dizziness

See *alcohol abuse*
See *anxiety*
See *ear infections*
See *ear wax*
See *hypotension*
See *heart attack*
See *Meniere's disease*
See *palpitations and arrhythmias*
See *Parkinson's disease*
See *stroke*
See *transient ischaemic attacks*

Cause

Dizziness is a term used to describe a state of feeling unsteady on the feet. A distinction between dizziness and vertigo lies in the fact that in vertigo, the patient describes a sensation of movement of the body or the surroundings.

Some drugs may cause the feeling of dizziness in particular antibiotics, anticonvulsant medication and aspirin. Other causes may include problems with the cervical spine. Conditions of the ear and central nervous system may also contribute to a feeling of dizziness—these include labrynthitis (a viral infection affecting the balance mechanism of the ear), anxiety, fainting episodes, ear infections, motion sickness, head injury, tumours of the acoustic nerve and central nervous system, intracerebral infection, wax in the ears, alcohol use, Parkinson's disease and Meniere's disease. Conditions of the cardiovascular system may also contribute to a feeling of dizziness, e.g. postural hypotension, heart attack, irregularities of the heart rhythm, problems with the heart valves, blockage in the arteries supplying the brain, stroke or transient ischaemic attacks.

Investigations

Persistent dizziness is a complaint which should be investigated to eliminate or identify a cause.

Treatment

Symptomatic treatment of dizziness may include removal of wax from the ears, rest, reassurance and medication, e.g. prochlorperazine, to minimise the effects.

domestic violence

See *child abuse*

Cause

Causes of domestic violence are complex and often multifactorial and it is difficult to pinpoint causative agents. Some degree of domestic violence may be culturally based and is minimised by society, but Western culture determines that domestic violence in any form is unacceptable.

Domestic violence may take the form of any physical, sexual, emotional maltreatment of another member of the household. Most commonly, domestic violence is committed by male members of the household and is directed towards female members, of any age.

Symptoms

Symptoms of domestic violence in a household may take the form of other members of the household presenting with evidence of injuries to various parts of the body. Law enforcement authorities report that with most violent crime, the perpetrator is a person known to the victim. Violence may be precipitated by the effects of alcohol, drug addiction or psychiatric conditions. The cycle of domestic violence is well documented, where an explosive episode of violent abuse is followed by remorse, repentant phase, followed by tension build-up and precipitating event, which may be trivial, followed by another violent outburst.

Treatment

Treatment is twofold, with the aim of reducing explosive episodes of the perpetrator on each occasion and increasing the coping skills of the victims. Sometimes this may only be achieved by separation.

dry hair

See *hypothyroidism*

Cause

Dry hair may be caused by excessive hair washing and overuse of hair products which are unsuitable, including shampoos, colours and other hair treatments. Dry hair may also be caused by hypothyroidism. Some medication may result in changes in the quantity and quality of hair growth. Post-natally some women may experience dry hair or hair loss.

Treatment

Treatment of any underlying medical condition is important. Appropriate treatment of hair is important and may include use of appropriate shampoo; use of conditioners at the time of washing hair; avoiding heating products in hair such as hot rollers, curling wands and heat driers which are set on a hot setting. People who swim frequently need to pay special attention to their hair, such as using a swimming cap, to prevent the effects of chlorine.

dry skin

See *dermatitus/eczema*
See *hypothyroidism*
See *psoriasis*

Cause

Dry skin may be caused by dermatitis, eczema, ageing skin, psoriasis and keratosis pilaris. Hypothyroidism may also produce dryness of skin. Dry skin may also be produced by taking regular excessively hot showers.

Symptoms

Dry flaking skin, including dandruff, may be presenting problems.

Treatment

Reducing the temperature of the water when bathing will improve dry skin, as well as bathing with a sorbolene soap substitute and soaking in a tepid bath versus showering. The addition to the bathwater of bath oil is also recommended. After showering or bathing has been completed, applying body moisturiser is recommended. Bath oil will help remove the plug of keratin which blocks the opening of the hair follicle, producing inflammation in skin.

dysmenorrhoea *(painful periods)*

See *periods, painful*

dysuria *(pain on passing urine)*

See *urinary tract infections*

Cause

Urinary tract infections are relatively common for women during their reproductive life, more so than men. Dysuria is the term applied to the painful passing of urine. The most common cause of dysuria is a bladder infection, irritable bladder syndrome, the presence of a foreign body, e.g. a tampon which may have been present for some time, trauma which may occur during intercourse or associated with sporting activity. Vaginitis may also present with the painful passage of urine in women of any age and atrophic vaginitis in women who are post-menopausal.

Symptoms

The symptom of pain on passing urine is explained by the fact that when the tissue is infected, inflammation occurs and pain is felt when the bladder contracts during micturition.

Treatment

Treatment for a urinary tract infection includes good history-taking, provision of a specimen to pathology to identify a bacterial cause and the provision of antibiotic therapy. Education of the patient regarding hygiene precautions is also advised, particularly for women who are sexually active and post-menopausal. Women who are post-menopausal may require the provision of some topical oestrogen, in order to minimise the effects of urinary tract infection, in addition to an antibiotic.

ear diseases

See *otitis media*
See *otitis externa*
See *deafness and hearing loss*
See *Meniere's disease,*
See *rubella*

ear infections

See *deafness and hearing loss*
See *otitis externa*
See *otitis media*
See *tropical ear*

ear lobes, infected *(perichondrititis)*

Infected ear lobes and perichondrititis have common causes, symptoms and treatment.

Cause

Perichondrititis is an infection of the cartilage or gristle part of the ear lobe. It may become infected with the insertion of earrings which pierce the cartilage of the ear.

Symptoms

Symptoms may include pain, localised swelling, redness and tenderness. On occasions an abscess may form, which may require drainage.

Treatment

Treatment of perichondrititis involves the prescription of oral antibiotics, most commonly penicillin. Any abscess will need draining and earrings may need to be removed.

ear pain

See *deafness and hearing loss*
See *ear lobes, infected*
See *mastoiditis*
See *otitis externa*
See *otitis media*
See *perichondritis*
See *temporomandibular joint*

ear wax

See *deafness and hearing loss*

ears, pressure problems

See *deafness and hearing loss*

eating disorders *(anorexia, bulimia)*

See *adolescent health, problems*

Cause

Eating disorders are thought to arise because of a disturbance in body image. More commonly these disorders arise in the teenage years, but may persist into adult life.

Symptoms

Symptoms may include preoccupation with being thin, exercising excessively, being overly conscious of all food intake, not eating regularly, taking laxatives or diuretics to reduce weight, constant weighing, regurgitation of food, hiding food or taking food away from the family meal to eat elsewhere and discarding it and amenorrhoea.

Treatment

Treatment often requires specialist psychiatric intervention and at times in-patient management on an IV drip, with nasogastric feeding. Medication may be necessary to prevent regurgitation of food, such as Prochlorperazine or Metoclopramide.

ectopic pregnancy

Cause

A pregnancy which implants in the fallopian tube is called an ectopic pregnancy. Ectopic pregnancies are never viable because as the pregnancy increases in size, it will rupture the fallopian tube.

Symptoms

A pregnancy test will be positive and around six to eight weeks into the pregnancy, a woman may start to experience some vaginal spotting, amenorrhoea, vaginal bleeding and lower abdominal cramping pain on the left or right side. The severity of the pain will increase the larger the ectopic pregnancy becomes. If the ectopic pregnancy ruptures, the woman may suddenly experience a sudden drop in blood pressure and feel faint.

Investigations

The presence of an ectopic pregnancy may be determined with the use of a pelvic ultrasound, which will find an ectopic pregnancy in the fallopian tube. When a vaginal ultrasound is performed at five to six weeks into the pregnancy, it will be found that the uterus is empty and contains no embryonic sac. Instead, it may be evident at that time that a pregnancy has occurred in the fallopian tube.

Treatment

Treatment for an ectopic pregnancy includes laparoscopic removal of the gestational sac. If the ectopic pregnancy ruptures prior to diagnosis, large blood loss may result requiring urgent surgical intervention.

ectropion

See *eyes, red, bilateral*

Cause

Ectropion is caused by a laxity of the eyelid.

Symptoms

Symptoms of ectropion include watery eyes, dry eyes and, on occasions, exposure of the cornea, particularly during sleep.

Treatment

Treatment for ectropion includes supplementary drops for the eye to prevent drying and surgical correction of the deformity in the eyelid.

eczema

See *dermatitis/eczema*

emphysema

See *chronic obstructive airway disease (COAD)*
See *respiratory symptoms*
See *smoking*

Cause

Chronic obstructive airway disease, known as emphysema, is most commonly a result of long-term heavy smoking. Other causes may include damage to the lung by heavy air pollution and chronic airways infection. Some families are known to have an enzyme deficiency, alpha 1 antitrypsin, in the lung which predisposes them to this disease. Patients may be screened for this enzyme to see if they have predisposing factor to the development of this condition.

Symptoms

Chronic obstructive airway disease is characterised by deterioration in lung function. It is associated with chronic productive cough, with sputum production and as the condition becomes worse, patients will experience increasing shortness of breath, wheezing and even difficulty talking in sentences without becoming short of breath. It is possible that in the worst cases, shortness of breath may become so severe that the patient is unable to generate enough respiratory effort to blow out a candle held in front of the face. Patients may experience increasing tiredness, lethargy, reduced exercise tolerance and problems sleeping at night. Increased frequency of chest infections is often also a problem.

Investigations

Assessment of the severity of chronic obstructive airway disease is based on performing lung function tests. These tests may include spirometry, where the patient is required to expel as much air from the lungs as possible as quickly as possible into a special machine called a spirometer. Most general practitioners will have a computerised spirometry machine which will calculate, among other things, the forced expiratory volume of air from the lungs in the first second of the maneuver. This is called the forced expiratory volume or FEV1. The test will also calculate forced vital capacity of the lung or FVC.

The ratio of the FEV1 divided by the FVC will be reduced for people with chronic obstructive airway disease and, unlike patients with asthma, minimal improvement in these calculations will be seen in response to ventolin administration. Monitoring of lung function may be able to be done using a peak flow meter, which the patient is able to do at home and bring to the surgery at times of consultation to assess the progress of the disease, as well as progress of treatment.

A peak flow meter is a graduated hollow tube where the patient blows vigorously into one end and an indicator inside the tube records the amount of air expelled by the lungs. This device is also used to assess treatment for asthma.

Treatment

Treatment for chronic obstructive airway disease is aimed at keeping the lungs as free from infection as possible, preventing further damage to the lungs and maximising effective oxygenation of blood. Salbutamol is prescribed to maintain the best possible clear airway or administration of the medication tiotropium bromide, which also helps to maintain the best lung function. Patients may also benefit from administration of inhaled steroid preparations and sometimes by injectable steroid preparations. Patients may require antibiotic treatment for lung infections. As the disease progresses and shortness of breath becomes more prominent, patients may also require the provision of home oxygen, which will need to be recommended by a specialist chest physician. Quitting smoking is also highly recommended.

Some patients may benefit from lung reduction surgical procedures or in cases with severe symptoms, a lung transplantation may be considered.

endocarditis

Cause

Endocarditis is a serious and potentially life-threatening condition that involves infection inside the heart, commonly involving a heart valve. The infection is usually bacterial, most commonly due to streptococcal or staphylococcus infection. Endocarditis may occur more frequently with intravenous drug users and patients who have low immunity.

Symptoms

The patient may present with few localising symptoms that may indicate the presence of endocarditis. Symptoms such as increasing shortness of breath, unexplained fever, a heart murmur, tiredness, unexplained patches of small bruising called petechiae on the skin. Discolorations under the fingernails, called splinter haemorrhages, may be present. Endocarditis may result in rupture of the valves of the heart and even abscess formation inside the heart.

Treatment

In order to diagnose endocarditis, it is necessary to demonstrate the presence of infection in the heart either by culturing bacteria in the blood, a CT scan, MRI of the heart or by an ECG. Treatment consists of repairing any damage to the valves concerned, which may require surgery, treating localised infection inside the heart and then ongoing prolonged antibiotic treatment to ensure that the infection has been eradicated and does not return.

endometriosis

See *periods, painful*

Cause

Endometriosis is when the cells which line the uterus, which are under the influence of the female hormones and subject to bleeding with the menstrual cycle, may be located in other parts of the pelvis apart from inside the uterus.

Symptoms

The symptoms of endometriosis will depend on the location of the abnormally placed endometrial cells. Symptoms may include painful periods, pain on intercourse, infertility, pain on urinating and on passing bowel motions.

Investigations

Diagnosis of endometriosis can only be made by direct vision of the lesions concerned using a laparoscope.

Treatment

Treatment for endometriosis includes the provision of anti-inflammatory medications, the oral contraceptive pill in order to suppress ovulation and the growth of endometrial tissue, surgical removal of ectopic endometrial cells; ultimately, in severe cases, patients may require hysterectomy by a gynaecologist.

entropion

See *eyes, red, bilateral*
See *corneal ulcer*

Cause

Entropion is caused by the eyelashes rubbing on the cornea of the eye.

Symptoms

Symptoms resulting from an entropion include sore, red, irritated eyes which result from the constant rubbing of the eyelashes on the cornea or conjunctiva.

Treatment

Treatment for entropion includes plucking the lashes from the eyelids or surgical correction of the eyelid inversion.

enuresis

See *bed-wetting*

epilepsy

Cause

There are various classifications in describing epilepsy; however in general terms seizures may be regarded as generalised or partial. Generalised seizures may be grand mal, tonic/clonic, petit mal, absences or myoclonic. Partial seizures may include local twitching of a hand, limb or eyes or unusual behaviour.

Symptoms

Generalised seizures present with the commonly thought-of seizure of a person who falls to the ground, stiffens and undergoes a series of vigorous convulsions. Petit mal seizures more commonly involve children, in particular children who may also be suffering from cerebral palsy, where the child undergoes a series of behaviours which may include staring into space, ceasing the activity which they were previously doing, lip smacking or chewing. These sometimes lead to a generalised grand mal seizure.

Treatment

Any person presenting with epileptic seizure needs investigation with an electro-encephalogram (EEG), CT scan and basic pathology testing. Usually referral to a neurologist is prudent. Medication is also available to control the fitting.

On occasions, the patient may experience prolonged episodes of grand mal epilepsy, called status epilepticus. This is said to occur when a person's epileptic seizure persists for greater than five to 10 minutes or where the patient experiences more than two seizures and does not fully regain consciousness between these episodes. This constitutes a medical emergency and requires hospitalisation. The usual routine cardiopulmonary resuscitation should be put in place using the D.R.A.B.C.D. procedure—see Cardiopulmonary Resuscitation (CPR).

It is important to ensure the safety of the patient and to ensure an adequate airway until such time as the patient is placed in the care of the ambulance officers and transported to hospital. Once the patient has reached the hospital, there may be occasions when the patient may be required to be sedated heavily using anaesthetic agents which will suppress the epileptic activity. Neurosurgical procedures are now able to ablate local areas in the brain responsible for some types of epilepsy.

epistaxis *(bleeding nose)*

Cause

Bleeding from the nose may occur because a small vessel has been ruptured inside the nostril. This may be related to dry secretions inside the nose, the person picking their nose, chronic nasal congestion, an injury or trauma to the nose. It may be a sign of a bleeding disorder and in adults may be related to high blood pressure.

Treatment

Stopping a nose bleed may be done by direct pressure to the nose using the thumb and index finger, applying ice or diathermy to the inside of the nose under local anaesthetic. Sometimes packing of the nose may also be required. Diathermy will usually require referral to an ear, nose and throat specialist. If the bleeding does not subside, referral to hospital may be required.

erectile dysfunction or impotence

See *diabetes.*
See *prostate cancer*
See *prostate infection or prostatitis and prostate abcess*
See *prostatiic hyperplasia, benign*

Cause

Impotence or erectile dysfunction is one of four causes of male sexual dysfunction. Other problems include altered libido, ejaculation problems and problems with orgasm.

Symptoms

Erectile dysfunctions may be termed either primary or secondary. Primary erectile dysfunction occurs when a man has never been able to achieve a sustained erection. This may occur, however, due to psychological factors associated with severe anxiety and depression, fear of intimacy and anatomical abnormalities. Most erectile dysfunctions arise from secondary causes, i.e. having been able to achieve an erection at some point in time. Around 80 per cent of secondary erectile dysfunction is due to an organic basis, i.e. related to organic disease.

Erectile dysfunction occurs as a result of a complex of neural physiological reflexes and processes. The penis is filled with sinus spaces that connect arteries and veins within the corpus cavernosum and when blood passes into the sinuses compressing the venules, thus blocking the outflow of blood from the penis, an erection results. Many factors affect the ability to achieve and maintain an erection, including psychological disturbance; drugs (for high blood pressure, diabetes, anxiety and depression); alcohol and smoking; medical problems including high blood pressure, diabetes, stroke, epilepsy, multiple sclerosis, peripheral and autonomic neuropathy, physical abnormalities of the penis, e.g. Peyronie's disease, spinal cord injuries, endocrine disorders, hypogonadism and following prostate surgery. Difficulty obtaining erections also increases with age.

Treatment

Underlying organic disease needs to be treated appropriately and, if it is felt that existing medication is contributing to the erectile dysfunction, changes to medication need to be considered and altered as necessary. Treatment methods for organic erectile dysfunction include mechanical agents and drug therapy.

Mechanical agents include the use of a constriction ring which is placed around the penis once an erection has been achieved in order to prevent venous drainage, thereby maintaining an erection. Vacuum devices are available in order to engorge the penis, thereby achieving an erection. Penile implants are also available. They require surgical implantation by appropriate specialists.

A number of medications are available in order to achieve or improve the quality of an erection. These medications include injections in the form of Alprostadil, which is inserted by very fine needle into the corpus cavernosum of the penile muscle and oral medication including Tadalafil, Vardenafil and Sildenafil.

There is some risk to men who have problems with coronary heart disease using any of the above medications. If chest pain or angina is experienced with mild to moderate exertion, the use of the above medications is to be adminstered with extreme caution and only under the direction of the treating medical practitioner. Frequency of use of these medications should also be limited for patients experiencing chest or angina pain on exertion.

Some practitioners in men's health clinics are recommending a trial of regular use of this oral medication with the aim of re-establishing a neural pathway for achieving more spontaneous erections when desired.

Ewing's tumour

See *leg pains*

eye inflammation

Cause
The eye is composed of many different layers of cells which have different functions. Inflammation of the various layers of the eye may lead to a red painful eye, e.g. episcleritis, for which no identifiable cause may be found. Conditions such as iritis and optic neuritis may be autoimmune in nature.

Symptoms
Episcleritis, optic neuritis and iritis of the eye may be associated with either rheumatoid arthritis or alternatively, may be associated with multiple sclerosis.

Treatment
Treatment of these symptoms may require the administrations of topical steroid drops to the eye. In the case of iritis, which is an inflammation of the coloured part of the eye, drops may be necessary to dilate the pupil in order to prevent the iris or coloured part of the eye, from adhering to the underlying lens of the eye. If adhesions occur, an irregular shaped pupil may

result and the defect may be permanent. Dilating of the pupil of the eye should be done with caution as it may produce an episode of acute angle closure glaucoma.

eye or eyelid infection

Cause

Infection in the form of conjunctivitis or blepharitis may start as an infection in one eye and then progress to the other eye. Infection around the eye or eyelids may result from conjunctivitis, blepharitis (a local infection of the area surrounding the eyelashes), a blocked tear duct or meibomian cyst (a localised infection which may present initially as a tender lump on either the upper or lower eyelid). Shingles or herpes zoster may be such a severe infection around the eye and temple area, that on occasions patients may require admission to hospital for management of the infection, of inflammation in the eye and for pain management.

Styes are localised infections involving the base of an eyelash. These infections may come in cluster formation.

Symptoms

All of these infections will have common symptoms of red eye, pain in the eye, headache and, in the case of shingles or herpes zoster, fever, severe body aches and pains, malaise and feeling unwell.

Treatment

Treatment for conjunctivitis, blepharitis and meibomian cyst, consists of administration of topical antibiotics, either in the form of drops or cream. They may also require administration of oral antibiotics. On occasions a meibomian cyst may require incision in order to drain the pus from the lesion. This is a simple process to do.

Treatment for shingles involves prescription of an antiviral agent called acyclovir, pain management and monitoring the vision of the eye.

eye trauma

Cause

Eye trauma may be caused by a blow to the head, particularly around the area of the eye or orbit (the part of the skull which houses the eye). This may result in bleeding into the eye, called hyphaema. A direct injury to the eye from a squash ball may produce a hyphaema as well as a fracture to the wall of the orbit. This is called a blowout fracture.

Tradesmen who may be hammering may feel that something has hit their eye, most often a metal foreign body, which will be visible on X-ray. In this instance, the eye may not even present as being significantly painful. On occasions, use of a nail gun or staple gun has been known to cause a penetrating eye injury.

Symptoms

Symptoms will depend on the nature of the trauma to the eye and the force of the injury. If a hyphaema is present and the patient is sat upright, accumulation of blood may be visible in front of the coloured part of the eye.

Treatment

A patient presenting with a hyphaema needs to be referred to an emergency department of a hospital, for further assessment by an ophthalmologist. The patient may require admission to hospital, because secondary bleeding into the eye may occur in the next few days following the injury.

eyes

See *flashes and floaters (in the eyes)*

eyes, pressure in

See *glaucoma*

eyes, red, bilateral (both eyes)

Cause

Conjunctivitis, blepharitis, entropion, ectropion are all conditions that may present with symptoms in both eyes. Flash burns result when tradesmen are using welding apparatus. Sub-conjunctival haemorrhage may result from a simple knock to an eye, chemical splashes or from something as simple as pulling up the blankets in bed. Trachoma of the eyelids is an infection caused by chlamydia and is more common in indigenous communities and Third World countries. It may result in blindness, with the constant repeated infection around the eyes, usually from the presence of flies.

Symptoms

A common presentation resulting in a diagnosis of flash burns is that the tradesman has been using welding equipment earlier in the day and will often present in the evening or even after he had gone to bed and has been woken up by severe pain in the eyes. Both eyes are red, watery, sensitive to light and extremely painful.

Sub-conjunctival haemorrhage may have a dramatic presentation. Blood may be clearly visible where the white of the eye would normally be, i.e. the white sclera, however in most cases this represents an external injury to the eye which is only minor.

The presence of a foreign body in the eye will present with a red eye, watering of the eye, sensitivity to light and often the patient may be able to see a spot on the cornea.

Treatment

In order to examine the eyes, it is often necessary to apply a topical local anaesthetic agent. Whilst this may sting initially, it offers immediate relief from the pain. It is, however, never recommended that continuing application of anaesthetic drops is given to the patient to take home. Instead, analgesics in the form of paracetamol, panadeine or codeine is sufficient to relieve the pain. It may be necessary to apply some topical antibiotic ointment to the eyes, more as a lubricant, then cover both eyes with patching and allow the patient to return home.

Removal of a foreign body from the cornea requires administration of a topical local anaesthetic and lifting off of the foreign body and any rust ring which may be present. The eye should then be patched and topical antibiotic drops applied three times a day for the next five days. No treatment is required for a sub-conjunctival haemorrhage.

eyes, red, unilateral (one eye)

Cause

Causes of unilateral red eye include corneal ulcer, eye inflammation, increased pressure in the eye, glaucoma, eye or eyelid infection or eye trauma.

Causes of corneal ulcer include dry eyes, wearing of contact lenses for prolonged periods of time, a foreign body in the eye, herpes simplex infection of the eye, entropion and ectropion. Causes of eye inflammation include episcleritis, iritis, optic neuritis.

Infection in the eyelid may result from conjunctivitis, blepharitis, meibomian cyst, shingles, or a sty.

facial pain

See *headache*

factor V Leiden

See *coagulation disorders*
See *leg pains*

Cause

Factor V Leiden is the most commonly occurring coagulation (blood clotting) abnormality. It occurs as a result of the mutation of the coagulation factors which results in an increased risk of venous thrombosis (blood clotting).

The presence of factor V Leiden disorder is most often diagnosed following an unexplained deep venous thrombosis (DVT). Those with a family history of DVT are at a much greater risk of developing a deep venous thrombosis than a person in the average population. Patients with this condition are more at risk during periods of immobilisation, particularly during travel by any mode of transport which requires seating for more than a couple of hours at a time.

Symptoms

Symptoms of factor V Leiden are pain, most commonly in a lower limb, which may or may not be accompanied by swelling, redness and tenderness over an affected area.

Treatment

Patients with this condition are advised to take precautions during travel and to move around at frequent intervals either by moving around the cabin during plane flight or by frequent breaks in their journey if travelling by car or other forms of road transport.

Patients in whom a deep venous thrombosis has been diagnosed require anticoagulant therapy until such time as the deep venous thrombosis has been resolved. They may also require treatment with injectable anticoagulants until such time as the oral anticoagulants have stabilised the condition. In extreme cases, patients may require admission to hospital until this is achieved. Patients travelling long distances may be required to be treated with prophylactic injectable anticoagulants while travelling.

female reproductive system

Breasts

See *breast cancer*
See *breast discharge*
See *breastfeeding*
See *breast infection and abscess*
See *breast pain and tenderness*
See *retracted nipples*

Menstruation or periods

See *amenorrhoea*
See *periods, painful*
See *menorrhagia*
See *polycystic ovary syndrome*

Ovaries

See *cancer*
See *ovarian cyst, acute torsion*
See *ovarian follicles*

Vagina

See *atrophic vaginitis*
See *bacterial infections*
See *sexually transmitted diseases*
See *thrush*

fever

See *infections*
See *infectious diseases of adults*
See *immune response*
See *immunisation for childhood infectious diseases*

Cause

Fever is a hallmark of an infective process. Fever may also occur in the presence of inflammation, malignancy and immunological disorders. Body temperature is regulated by the part of the brain called the hypothalamus and fever is brought about by a process of conservation of body heat. Metabolic changes are then set up in the hypothalamus which initiates a reflex to increase the body temperature, causing the hypothalamus to increase the body temperature.

A reflex is brought into play where blood vessels constrict at the peripheries and blood is redirected away from the peripheries to the body core, thus trapping heat and raising the body's temperature.

Fevers and temperatures may occur not only in children but also in adults and indicate an infection. The source of the infection may not always be apparent. The most common sources of infection include upper respiratory tract infections, lower respiratory tract infections, i.e. bronchitis, pneumonia, bronchiectasis, sinus infections, ear nose and throat infections, urinary tract infections (with or without the presence of kidney stones), viral infections which may include glandular fever, human immunodeficiency virus or HIV, tuberculosis, infections of the gall bladder, osteomyelitis, endocarditis, malaria, infections associated with malignancy, e.g. leukaemia, cancer of the kidney, liver or lung. Fevers and temperatures may also occur with conditions such as Crohn's disease, inflammatory bowel disease and diverticulitis.

Symptoms

Symptoms of fever include shivering, the body's way of increasing temperature by muscular contractile activity.

In the presence of an infective process, the body may produce more white blood cells in order to combat the infection and in so doing may not be able to keep up with demand as white blood cells are consumed more quickly than they are able to be replaced. Under these conditions, the body may then start to release more immature white cells in order to combat the infection. Initially the number of white blood cells may increase reflecting an increasing demand for body defence cells. If the infection is overwhelming, the number of white blood cells may actually then fall as the body cannot keep up with the demand.

In the presence of infection and fever a tachycardia usually results (except in the presence of typhoid fever, brucellosis and dengue fever which produce a slowing of the pulse). Increased respiratory rate may also occur.

Treatment

Fever should be controlled by the administration of anti-pyretic medication, paracetamol, simple anti-inflammatory preparations for adults and children and the underlying reason for the fever determined and treated.

fevers in children

See *children, common problems*
See *convulsions*
See *fever*

flashes and floaters *(in the eyes)*

Cause

Visual flashes may be associated with the aura before a migraine or may indicate that there is some tension on the periphery of the retina.

Symptoms

Flashes may be experienced as 'sparks' which appear before a migraine headache or may be seen without the headache when the person is in a darkened room. Sparks which are seen with no headache may indicate a posterior vitreous detachment.

Treatment

There is a possibility that if flashes are seen in conjunction with a decrease in vision, referral to an ophthalmologist should be made as this may indicate a retinal detachment, which will need surgical intervention to relieve the tension on the retina and re-attach the retina to the back of the eye.

flatulence *(passing wind)*

See *anxiety*
See *belching, bloating*
See *colon problems*
See *Crohn's disease*
See *helicobacter pylori infection*
See *irritable colon/bowel*

Cause

Flatulence, farting or passing of wind results from the ingestion of air which then must pass through the gastrointestinal tract. Air may be swallowed during meals and with drinks, particularly fizzy drinks, which may result in either bloating, burping or flatulence. Flatulence in association with a feeling of being bloated may be symptoms of an infection in the gut known as helicobacter pylori, an organism associated with cancer of the stomach. Helicobacter pylori infection may be associated with the presence of bad breath or halitosis.

Investigations

Investigation for helicobacter pylori is done by urea breath testing at pathology or alternatively, at the time of endoscopy.

Treatment

Treatment for flatulence is symptomatic. Treatment for helicobacter pylori is by triple therapy in the form of antibiotic therapy and proton pump inhibitor. This treatment is usually taken for a week, then six weeks later the helicobacter pylori breath test is repeated in order to confirm that the infection has been eradicated. Following infection with helicobacter pylori, patients may experience some degree of ongoing bloating and abdominal distension which may be treated with intermittent use of proton pump inhibitor medication.

floppy baby

Cause

To some extent, all newborn babies are floppy, with poor head control. However some newborn babies and even older babies feel as though they may slip through your hands when you pick them up under the arms. If this sign is recognised by the mother, the paediatrician or the general practitioner or child health nurse attending the child in the neonatal period, a diagnosis of floppy baby may be applied. The reason for the floppy feel of the baby is due to low muscle tone and there are a number of reasons for this occurring.

The child may have a form of an inherited low muscle tone, which may improve as the child gets older. Floppy baby may be a sign of cerebral palsy due to birth trauma or an event which has happened during the course of the pregnancy, due to either infection or poor blood supply to the brain of the foetus. Low muscle tone is also a feature of babies with Down syndrome and other neurological conditions, e.g. Duchene muscular dystrophy, an inherited condition of males only, Prader-Willi syndrome, a chromosomal disorder which results in obesity and Ehlers-Danlos syndrome, a condition of increased flexibility of the joints and laxity of the skin.

Treatment

Children who have been diagnosed as floppy babies may often require early intervention with physical treatment, e.g. physiotherapy, occupational therapy and speech therapy.

flu

See *influenza*

folliculitis

Cause

Folliculitis is a term applied to a skin infection due to staphylococcus and pseudomonas infections of the skin.

Symptoms

The symptoms of folliculitis include a rash on the skin which may be red, raised, inflamed and even pustular. It may start as a localised area anywhere of the body, but most commonly on buttocks, thigh or trunk and may spread rapidly to other parts of the body.

Treatment

Treatment is in the form of chlorhexidine wash oral antibiotics or topical cream.

foot odour

Cause

Foot odour is caused by the presence of bacteria on the feet which give off a characteristic odour. Some people are more prone to foot odour than others.

Symptoms

Patients with severe foot odour may present with obvious infection, either bacterial or a mixture of bacterial and fungal (tinea), redness and localised swelling, pain and discomfort.

Treatment

Treatment of foot odour includes frequent washing of the feet and socks, the use of shoe liners which can be frequently changed or washed and rotating footwear so that footwear is not in constant use.

foot pain

See *arthritis*
See *calluses, corns*
See *diabetes*
See *foot strain*
See *smoking*
See *weight management problems*

Cause

The feet are the weight-bearing agents of the body and foot pain may result from a variety of conditions such as vascular disease, diabetes, overweight, arthritis, the effects of smoking, ill-fitting footwear, foreign bodies, ingrown toenails, underheel spurs and plantar warts.

Foot pain may also be caused by chronic crowding of the feet and the nerves supplying the toes, resulting in an overgrowth of tissue around the digital nerves, called a Morton's neuroma. Abnormal sensation associated with peripheral neuropathy may also result in foot pain. Peripheral neuropathy may also be a manifestation of diabetes.

Symptoms

Painful feet may be the result of microvascular disease in the arteries supplying the feet. The pain is caused by a lack of oxygenation to the tissues of the foot which may appear abnormal in colour. Pain may be accompanied by sensory changes, pressure areas resulting in breaks in the skin and even ulcer formation, numbness of the feet, sleep disturbance. Foot pain is common in people with diabetes due to the association of microvascular disease in diabetes.

Treatment

The pain associated with microvascular disease is difficult to treat and treatment measures are aimed at the causative agent, e.g. improving diabetes management, quitting smoking, weight reduction, massage to the feet and paracetamol.

An X-ray of the feet may demonstrate the presence of arthritis. Arthritis is not likely to be localised only to the area of the foot, so that treatment is for generalised arthritis with paracetamol, anti-inflammatory preparations, in association with weight reduction and improved lifestyle factors.

Pain from foreign bodies, bony tumour and plantar warts will be improved by removal of the object. Treatment of ingrown toenails includes good hygiene of the feet, trimming the nails correctly, appropriate use of good footwear and sometimes antibiotic medication to reduce infection, bathing in warm salty water or betadine solution and keeping the feet dry.

Orthotic splints worn in the shoes may help to improve symptoms. These can be made and fitted by a podiatrist or physiotherapist.

foot strain

Cause

Metatarsalgia or stress fracture, may be caused by unusual or excessive amounts of unaccustomed use of the feet, recent commencement of a new physical activity often involving a change of footwear.

Diagnosis

Achieving a diagnosis for pain in the feet from foot strain involves careful history taking and examination of the feet, observation of the patient's gait and may involve recommending an X-ray, CT scan or even MRI of the feet to determine the presence of a stress fracture.

Treatment

Treatment for metatarsalgia includes provision of correct footwear, arch supports for the feet, education of the patient, the application of hot and cold packs, massage and simple analgesic or anti-inflammatory preparations. Treatment for a stress fracture may require splinting of the foot until the pain subsides.

gall bladder problems

See *abdomonal pain*

Cause

The most common condition affecting the gall bladder is that of gallstones. Gallstones may result in biliary colic or an obstruction to the biliary duct system, but biliary colic can sometimes occur in the absence of gallstones, particularly in women. The presence of microscopic stones may be responsible for the pain and abnormal gall bladder motility or an oversensitive biliary tract.

Cholecystitis is caused by an infection in the gall bladder, often in the presence of gallstones. Cholecystitis may occur as a result of an obstruction to the duct by gallstones. Tumours of the bile ducts are usually rare and risk factors include increasing age or an infestation of liver flukes. Cancers of the gall bladder occur most commonly in South American and Asian countries.

Symptoms

Symptoms of biliary colic or infection of the gall bladder may include severe abdominal pain which may radiate to the back, nausea, vomiting. Eighty per cent of gallstones are asymptomatic. Patients with tumours of the gall bladder and biliary duct system present with itchy skin and frequently with jaundice—yellowing of the skin. Patients may present with an abdominal mass, increase in the size of the gall bladder, loss of appetite, weight loss and abdominal pain which resembles that of biliary colic.

Treatment

Treatment for biliary colic includes pain relief and adequate hydration. Most people diagnosed with gallstones will at some stage require removal of the gall bladder, called cholecystectomy. This may be undertaken during an acute phase of an episode of biliary colic or electively at some later date. The operation may be performed by keyhole surgery, thus limiting recovery time, hospital stay and inconvenience to the patient so that the patient is able to return to work promptly, usually within a couple of weeks following surgery.

Ultrasound examination is the best way of detecting the presence of gallstones. Removal of the gall bladder is effective in treating abnormalities; however sometimes patients may experience ongoing sensitivity to rich and fatty food.

To diagnose the possibility of a tumour of the biliary duct system, an ERCP or endoscopic retrograde cholangiopancreatogram, may be required. This procedure requires considerable skill and is limited to a few gastroenterologists who frequently perform the procedure. In some cases, pancreatitis may result from performing the ERCP examination.

Patients who present with an obstruction to the biliary duct system from a malignancy may require bypassing the tumour in the pancreas or in the gastrointestinal system by using a stent or a more extensive procedure called a Whipple's procedure.

ganglion, wrist, forearm

Cause

A ganglion is a lump which most commonly forms at the wrist. It is a collection of fluid, which is responsible for lubrication of the tendons in the wrist. Such ganglion are harmless lumps and unless causing significant problems may be left alone.

Symptoms

The cyst or lump may be accompanied by localised pain and sometimes by restriction of movement of the wrist.

Treatment

Treatment for a ganglion may include observation only, attempt to rupture the cyst or surgical removal. Even after surgical removal sometimes a ganglion in the wrist may recur.

gastro-oesophageal reflux

Cause

Patients with a free flow of stomach contents back into the oesophagus due to poor control of the lower oesophageal sphincter are said to have gastro-oesophageal reflux. Factors which contribute to the presence of gastro-oesophageal reflux or GOR include excessive weight, eating fatty foods, drinking caffeine, carbonated drinks and alcohol, smoking and some drugs, i.e. antihistamines, tricyclic antidepressant drugs, calcium channel blockers, progesterone and nitrates. Severe, ongoing, untreated GOR may lead to a condition known as Barrett's oesophagus, which may in turn lead to cancer of the oesophagus.

Symptoms

The most common symptoms of gastro-oesophageal reflux include heartburn, with or without the presence of reflux, as well as indigestion and inflammation of the oesophagus called oesophagitis. Oesophagitis, if persistent for a long period of time, may produce stricture formation and on occasions may result in the formation of a pre-cancer stage. Common symptoms also include vomiting, loss of appetite and may result in coughing, wheezing and hoarseness of the voice.

Treatment

Treatment for gastro-oesophageal reflux includes elevating the head in bed at night, not eating within three hours of going to bed, avoiding alcohol and coffee before going to bed, as well as avoiding fatty food, chocolate and smoking. Medication is also recommended for people with chronic gastro-oesophageal reflux.

Medications include proton pump inhibitors and H2 antagonists. Surgery is also available to help reduce the effects of GOR. It is most commonly offered to children. Barrett's oesophagus may be treated by surgical removal or by laser therapy. It may or may not regress with medical or surgical intervention so a regular endoscopy is recommended.

gastroenteritis

See *cholera*
See *diarrhoea*
See *typhoid*

gastroenteritis, viral

Cause

Acute gastroenteritis is invariably a self-limiting condition of a few days at the most. Gastroenteritis in children may be associated with fever and diarrhoea and/or vomiting where there is no other identifiable cause. Rotavirus is the most common cause in infants and children and there is now an oral vaccine available for young children, i.e. babies before the age of six months. Other organisms causing gastroenteritis include salmonella, shigella, giardia, entomoeba, cryptosporidium. Dehydration from extreme fluid loss as a result of either watery bowel motions or a combination of diarrhoea and vomiting is a significant cause of death from gastroenteritis, especially in children.

Cholera is an infectious disease characterised by severe, profuse, watery diarrhoea and is highly infectious. The symptoms and treatment for cholera are the same as those for acute gastroenteritis and diarrhoea. Vaccination is available for travellers, particularly those to Third World countries, to prevent infection. Traveller's diarrhoea is thought to be due to a less virulent strain of cholera.

Typhoid is a systemic disease caused by bacteria called salmonella. The diagnosis is made on the clinical symptoms and also by culture of the faeces. The condition is caused by inadequate hygiene precautions after bowel motions.

Symptoms

Symptoms of gastroenteritis include crying in children, refusing breastfeeding or bottle feeding, vomiting, diarrhoea, loss of appetite, fever, nausea.

Treatment

Treatment is aimed at maintaining normal hydration, which may be assessed by the amount of urine output in children and adults and the colour or concentration of the urine.

In children, anti-diarrhoea and anti-nausea medication should be avoided. Instead oral rehydration fluid, which is available from chemists, should be provided frequently. Not uncommonly, children dislike the taste of these preparations, although new preparations on the market are much more pleasing to the taste. As an alternative, lemonade may be diluted with one part lemonade to four parts water for rehydration. If dehydration is severe, as evident by the fact the child may be listless, have poor urine output and be refusing all fluids, admission to hospital may be recommended.

genital herpes, herpes simplex infection

Cause

Genital herpes is caused by the herpes simplex virus, usually Type 2. Genital herpes refers to the presence of herpes simplex infection in the genital area and may be spread from person to person by direct contact with the genital area or by oral sex.

Symptoms

Symptoms of genital herpes include the presence of redness and irritation, localised pain and tenderness, the presence of blister-like lesions called vesicles, feeling unwell, fever and pain on intercourse. These symptoms classically recur in the same area if no treatment is administered.

Treatment

If the presence of genital herpes is thought to be a new infection, it needs to be confirmed by taking a swab, after which time commencement with a normal anti-viral agent is recommended. Acyclovir is the antiviral agent of choice for both treatment of an acute episode and treatment for suppression of the virus.

genital warts

See *human papilloma virus*

Cause

Genital warts are caused by an infection called human papilloma virus (HPV). There are a number of different strains of HPV that occur and are thought to be responsible for producing abnormalities of the cervix in Pap smears. The species of HPV which causes genital warts is thought to be different to the species of human papilloma virus HPV which causes abnormalities on Pap smears.

Symptoms

Genital warts may produce very little in the way of symptoms apart from local irritation and roughening of the surface of the skin around the genital area and inside the vagina. In men, genital warts may occur on the penis, testicles and scrotum, and around the pubic area.

Treatment

Treatment of genital warts includes topical application of antiviral agents, diathermy and spraying with liquid nitrogen.

giardia

See *diarrhoea*

Cause

Giardia is a flagellated protozoan infection, primarily of the gut, called giardiasis.

Symptoms

Symptoms of giardia range from intermittent flatulence to chronic or acute diarrhoea and chronic malabsorption. The diarrhoea is watery and offensive in odour and associated with abdominal cramps, distension, flatulence, nausea, severe upper abdominal discomfort, bloating and anorexia. Chronic giardia infection may lead to malabsorption of fat and sugars which results in significant weight loss. Giardia infection has been associated with failure to thrive in children. The condition is infectious and, not uncommonly, may infect a whole population of students at preschools and day-care facilities and families. It is more common in underdeveloped countries and in non-sewered areas.

Treatment

Treatment for giardia infection is achieved by administration of metronidazole as an oral preparation.

gingivitis

See *halitosis*

Cause

Gingivitis is an inflammation of the gums. It may be caused by injury to the gums, vitamin deficiency including vitamins C and B and iron deficiency. Cancer of the gums is present as a hard, painful lump on the gums.

Symptoms

Gingivitis may produce bleeding and swelling, redness and change in the normal contour of the gums. It may produce retraction of the gum away from the base of the teeth, resulting in dental pain.

Treatment

The diagnosis of gingivitis is based on observations from a dentist and the treatment involves professional cleaning of the teeth around the margins of the gum line, followed by home dental hygiene.

glandular fever

Cause

Glandular fever or infectious mononucleosis is caused by a virus belonging to the herpes group called Epstein Barr virus (EBV).

Symptoms

Incubation period for glandular fever is between four and eight weeks. The acute phase of the illness is marked by severe headache, fever, pharyngitis and enlargement of the lymph nodes. In patients under 20 years or over 40 years, symptoms of glandular fever may be minimal. In the intervening years, however, patients may present with persistent fever, headache which is unrelieved by paracetamol, nausea, vomiting, sore throat and tonsillitis, anorexia and muscular aches and pains.

In patients aged in their late teens to late 30s, the symptoms may be severe and may last for several months following the initial infection. Severe infections may be accompanied by abnormal liver function tests during the acute phase of the illness. It is for this reason that patients with glandular fever are intolerant of alcohol intake for a period of time, which may be up to 12 to 18 months following initial infection.

Treatment

Identification of EBV by pathology testing confirms a diagnosis. Patients in the 20 to 40 years age group may experience significant symptoms and sometimes be unwell enough to remain away from work for weeks on end. There is no specific treatment to assist a patient's recovery. Symptomatic treatment includes bed rest, pain relief using aspirin or paracetamol, treatment for sore throat and nausea, and abstinence from alcohol and fatty foods.

glaucoma

See *blindness*
See *eyes, red*

Cause

Glaucoma refers to an increase in the intra-ocular pressure of the eye and may result from open angle or closed angle glaucoma. Glaucoma is one of the most common causes of blindness and many people with glaucoma are not aware of the problem. The term open or closed angle refers to the mechanism by which fluid is continually generated and drained from the inside of the eye.

The eye is divided into two separate chambers, an anterior chamber which is filled with a watery fluid called aqueous humour and a posterior chamber which is filled with a jelly-like substance called vitreous humour. The two areas are separated by a complex of structures which include the iris and supporting structures and the lens of the eye. If these structures are pushed forward, decrease in the depth of the anterior chamber will result. This condition is referred to as close angle glaucoma.

Open angle glaucoma will result in progressive decrease in vision and may come on gradually. Whereas in closed angle glaucoma, the anterior chamber of the eye is reduced in depth and the escape route for fluid which is generated in the eye is closed off. An episode of closed angle glaucoma may occur acutely, with onset of symptoms also occurring acutely.

Increased pressure in the eye may also sometimes arise as a result of the presence of a long-standing cataract in the eye.

Symptoms

Many people with glaucoma have no symptoms until the condition is well established and permanent damage in the form of loss of vision has already occurred to the eye. This situation is more commonly the case with the condition of open angle glaucoma.

Visual defects may be detected on specialised examination, on computerised equipment called a perimetry machine, which maps out the patient's response to varying intensities and sizes of point sources of light on a plain white illuminated background. This test is standardised and reproducible in the computer program built into the machine and is a way of documenting the progress of the disease and the effectiveness of the treatment.

In the case of closed angle glaucoma, the patient may present with sudden loss of vision, accompanied by pain in the eye.

Symptoms associated with open angle glaucoma may be minimal, insidious and often present as a gradual reduction in visual acuity and decrease in peripheral vision; however by the time the patient is aware of the reduction in visual acuity the disease is often well-established and may be irreversible. Symptoms associated with closed angle glaucoma include pain, headache, reduction in visual acuity and even nausea.

In either case, glaucoma should be suspected if the intra-ocular pressure on testing is elevated or in the presence of a positive family history of glaucoma. Once optic-nerve damage has occurred, return to normal levels of vision may be limited.

Treatment

The aim of treatment for glaucoma is to restore the intra-ocular pressure (IOP) to normal values either by eye drops, medication, surgery or laser methods. Treatment is generally recommended for patients with an IOP of greater than 30 mm Hg.

When an increase in pressure occurs with closed angle glaucoma, the onset of symptoms may be rapid. Acetazolamide tablets may be used in an acute situation in order to relieve the pressure in the eye. Once the pressure has returned to normal, the ophthalmologist will use a special laser machine in order to burn a hole in the periphery of the iris in order to allow the excess fluid in the eye to be reabsorbed. Following an acute episode or in the case of open angle glaucoma, ongoing drops will be required in order to maintain the pressure of the eye in the normal range.

If an over-mature cataract is present in the eye and an episode of glaucoma arises, removal of the cataract is indicated.

glomerulonephritis

Cause

Causes of glomerulonephritis are idiopathic (a definite cause cannot be identified) and post-infectious, such as streptococcal infection, mycoplasma infection, staphylococcal infection, E. coli, pseudomonas, proteus, klebsiella, clostridium, coxsackievirus, cytomegalovirus, Epstein Barr virus, hepatitis B and hepatitis C virus, herpes zoster, measles, mumps and chickenpox.

Symptoms

A diagnosis of glomerulonephritis will usually be made following a history of infection with one of the above agents in association with blood in the urine.

Treatment

Treatment for glomerulonephritis is the management of electrolytes, through fluid management and management of blood pressure in more severe cases. In most cases dialysis is unnecessary. In some cases glomerulonephritis leads to long-term kidney problems where the diagnosis is again based on history of the condition, urine analysis, pathology blood tests and renal biopsy. If progression to this form of glomerulonephritis occurs, treatment with corticosteroids is often necessary, with or without cyclophosphamide and plasmapheresis (plasma filtering procedure). If untreated this form of glomerulonephritis may lead to end-stage renal disease over a period of weeks to months.

goitre

Cause

Goitre is an enlargement of the thyroid gland, which produces thyroxine, which in turn regulates the metabolic rate of the body. Goitre may result from hyperthyroidisim, hypothyroidism or thyroid cancer.

Symptoms

Symptoms of hyperthyroidism include palpitations, fast pulse rate, sweating, weight loss, agitation, diarrhoea. Symptoms of hypothyroidism include dry skin, depression, weight gain, fatigue, lack of energy and constipation.

Treatment

Treatment for goitre depends on the underlying disease. Treatment for hyperthyroidism includes radioactive iodine, neomercazole or surgical removal of part of or the entire thyroid. Treatment for hypothyroidism includes thyroxine replacement hormone. Treatment for thyroid cancer involves total thyroidectomy with subsequent thyroid replacement hormone treatment and monitoring of thyroid hormones.

gonorrhoea

See *sexually transmitted diseases*
See *vaginal discharge*

Cause

Gonorrhoea is a sexually transmitted disease caused by the bacterium gonococcus.

Symptoms

Patients may notice copious amounts of mucus discharge with the bowel motions and pain on rectal examination. Infection of the urethra, cervix, rectum, pharynx and eyes may result, with discomfort and profuse discharge, urinary frequency and vaginal discharge. The reproductive organs are the most frequently infected. Infection in women may lead to pelvic inflammatory disease and sterility. Rectal gonorrhea is common in homosexual men.

Treatment

Treatment of gonorrhoea is with penicillin, assuming sensitivity of the bacteria to the drug and recommendations today include coexistent treatment with doxycycline for a week.

gout

Cause

Gout is caused by a build-up in uric acid in the blood. Uric acid is a breakdown product of protein, in particular of red meat, shellfish and offal meat. Gout may also result from red wine and cheese intake. When uric acid levels increase, crystal deposits form in joints causing pain, tenderness, swelling and redness. More commonly these joints include the big toe, ankle, knee, but any joint may be involved.

Symptoms

The symptoms of gout include acute pain, tenderness, redness, swelling, sensitivity and a feeling of warmth in the joint. The patient may find it difficult to bear weight on an affected joint and may even find difficulty with the weight of the bed clothes on the foot during the night. Accumulation of urate deposits may also be seen at times on bony prominences, which may require surgical removal.

Treatment

Diagnosis of gout requires the identification of crystals of uric acid in the fluid around the joint. Anti-inflammatory preparations are used to relieve the symptoms of an acute episode of gout. The frequency of attacks may be reduced or prevented by regular administration of anti-inflammatory preparations and/or the inclusion of colchicines or allopurinol medications. Allopurinol is used for prevention of recurring attacks and also for prevention of renal stones and gouty arthritis. Patients with gout are advised to increase fluid intake in order to prevent the possibility of developing renal or kidney stones.

The principles of treatment for gout are the same irrespective of the cause. This includes a balance between rest and exercise; heat packs to painful joints; reducing weight if overweight; gentle exercise; simple analgesics, e.g. paracetamol; non-steroid or anti-inflammatory medications, e.g. ibuprofen. At times referral will be necessary to a specialist orthopaedic surgeon or rheumatologist.

Graves' disease

See *hyperthyroidism*

groin pain

Cause

Groin pain may be caused by hernia formation either spontaneously or due to sudden excess of musculoskeletal straining, common in people who participate in lifting weights in the gym; torsion of the testis; arthritis of the hip; conditions of the pelvic organs, e.g. ovarian cysts or tumours, endometriosis; appendicitis; prostatitis; and pelvic inflammatory disease; but hernia is more common in males than females.

Symptoms

Symptoms of pain may be accompanied by muscular spasms, a palpable lump in the groin, fever, malaise, abnormal vaginal bleeding, pain on intercourse, blood in the semen.

Treatment

Musculoskeletal aches and pains and arthritis may be treated with simple analgesic, nonsteroidal anti-inflammatory preparations, a routine of prescribed exercises and stretches of the muscles in the groin and physiotherapy. A hernia is readily treated by surgical correction.

Ovarian abnormalities, pelvic inflammatory disease and endometriosis may require investigation with pelvic ultrasound. If an infection is detected, suitable antibiotics may be prescribed. Ovarian tumours may require surgical intervention. Treatment for prostatitis involves the use of antibiotics, usually over a period of three to four weeks. Treatment for appendicitis is removal of the appendix.

haematemesis *(vomiting blood)*

See *stomach cancer*

haematemesis and melaena

See *colon cancer*
See *stomach cance*

By definition, haematemesis means vomiting blood, which originates from either the oesophagus or stomach. Melaena means the passage of black bowel motions as a result of bleeding in the digestive (gastrointestinal) tract. Melaena is characteristically black in color and thick and sticky in texture, and results from denatured blood as it passes through the gastric juices.

haematospermia

Cause

Haematospermia is a term applied to blood in the semen. The most common cause is a prostate biopsy. Other causes may also include benign prostatic hyperplasia, infections and disorders of the seminal vesicles. Sometimes the cause of haematospermia is unknown and may occur spontaneously.

Treatment

Treatment for this condition is first of all to identify a possible cause, e.g. infection. A urine culture should be performed specifically to exclude a sexually transmitted disease. Prostate specific antigen (PSA) should be performed for the older patient in order to exclude the possibility of prostate cancer. Patients should be reassured that this is not necessarily a sign of cancer nor will it affect their sexual function.

haematuria *(blood in the urine)*

See *bladder cancer*
See *cancer*

See *endocarditis*
See *kidney cancer*
See *ovarian cancer*
See *prostate cancer*
See *renal stones*
See *urinary tract infections*

Definition

Haematuria is a symptom and is defined as the passage of blood in the urine.

Cause

Haematuria may be caused by a urinary tract infection (UTI), urethritis, prostatitis, a renal stone, anticoagulant therapy, following radiation treatment, endocarditis, cancer of the kidney or bladder, ureter, or trauma to the kidney or ureter.

Symptoms

Blood in the urine may be accompanied by symptoms of pain, fever and burning on passing urine.

Treatment

Investigation regarding the cause of haematuria may include a micro-urine test, lower abdominal and or pelvic ultrasound or CT of the abdomen. Treatment of any infection causing haematuria includes the prescription of antibiotics, increased fluid intake, alkalinising agents of the urine, e.g. Ural. Recurrent urinary infection may indicate the presence of a pelvic mass, e.g. an ovarian tumour, which may be compressing the ureter and bladder, resulting in infection.

haemochromatosis

See *liver problems*

Cause

Haemochromatosis is an inherited iron-storage disease, where excess amounts of iron (used to make red blood cells) are stored in the liver. Gene testing of patients with elevated ferritin (iron) will confirm the diagnosis.

Symptoms

There may not be any symptoms, but sometimes a patient with the condition may complain of being tired, lethargic or may at times present with jaundice if the ferritin level is very high.

Treatment

Treatment for haemochromatosis consists of regular blood tests to monitor the level of ferritin in the blood within the normal range. Blood taking may need to be performed monthly to maintain normal levels and, in the initial stages, may need to be weekly until normal levels of ferritin are achieved.

haemophilus influenza B (HIB)

See *immunisation for childhood infectious diseases*

Cause

Haemophilus is a bacteria that causes meningitis, septic arthritis, pneumonia, tracheobronchitis, otitis media, conjunctivitis, endocarditis, sinusitis and acute epiglotitis in young children. It is transmitted through the respiratory tract from infected to susceptible individuals.

Symptoms

Respiratory symptoms predominate with associated fever, headache, aches and pains in the muscles and localised pains. Acute epiglotitis may become a medical emergency with referral to a hospital for management, as it may result in obstruction of the airway. Diagnosis of haemophilus influenza B (HIB) infection is possible following positive sputum or swab results.

Treatment

Treatment is by intravenous antibiotics, with penicillin the drug of choice. Treatment for haemophilus influenza B forms part of childhood immunisation.

haemorrhoids

Cause

Haemorrhoids are large veins which are located around the anal passage. They result from thrombosis in dilated veins around the anus and are commonly referred to as thrombosed external piles. Haemorrhoids occur in the presence of chronic constipation as a result of increased pressure around the rectum, pelvic floor and anal area and during the latter stages of pregnancy from the pressure effects of the baby's head pressing inside the pelvis.

Symptoms

Haemorrhoids are associated with pain around the anal area, swelling of the veins which are associated with an external lump which the patient can feel. Haemorrhoids are associated with rectal bleeding and anal irritation and sometimes itching of the area. Haemorrhoids may be internal or external.

Treatment

Treatment of haemorrhoids is symptomatic, i.e. relief of the swelling by incision of the thrombosed vein, which is done by injecting some local anaesthetic and making an incision into the area and expelling the thrombus inside the vessel, pain relief, suppositories containing vasoconstricting agents, improved diet and treating the constipation, and delivery of the baby.

If the haemorrhoids are internal, banding of the haemorrhoids will improve the symptoms. On occasions more extensive surgery may be required if the haemorrhoids are extensive.

hand, foot and mouth disease

Cause

Hand, foot and mouth disease is a minor viral infection.

Symptoms

Symptoms of hand, foot and mouth disease include blisters, which occur on the hands and feet and in the mouth. It occurs most commonly among children and as it is a minor infection, it does not warrant exclusion from day care or school.

Treatment

Treatment for hand, foot and mouth disease is symptomatic with either paracetamol or ibuprofen and adequate attention to fluid intake.

hangover

Cause

Hangover is a common user term for the symptoms felt after the intake of excess alcohol.

Symptoms

The most common symptoms include headache, nausea, feeling dehydrated and concentrated urine.

Treatment

Treatment of a hangover includes fluid replacement, preferable isotonic fluid (sports drink diluted one part sport drink to two parts water), vitamin B1 replacement tablets (two thiamine tablets immediately) and pain relief with aspirin or paracetomol.

hay fever *(rhinitis)*

Cause

Hay fever is caused by sensitivity to allergens in susceptible people, e.g. dust mites, pollens, food. Often patients may also have a history of asthma, eczema or dermatitis and usually a family history of the condition.

Symptoms

Sneezing repeatedly first thing in the morning is a common symptom but also often at various times of the day, with an itchy feeling in the nose or throat, which may be accompanied by symptoms of asthma.

Treatment

Antihistamines are recommended, preferably non-sedating. Topical steroid preparations up the nose are also quite beneficial and some patients benefit from a course of desensitisation injections.

head lice

Cause

Head lice are wingless, bloodsucking insects which infect the hair on the head.

Symptoms

Head lice may be obvious to a trained observer and commonly run in epidemics in schools, day-care centres and in families. Head lice are transmitted by direct body contact and may present with itching of the head and scratching.

Treatment

Treatment of head lice includes using preparations such as malathion, permethrin and pyrethroid, which are available at local chemists.

headache

Headache and facial pain

See *aneurysm*
See *blood pressure*
See *cancer*
See *dental problems*
See *eyes*
See *hypertension*
See *migraine headache*
See *sinusitis*
See *stroke*
See *temporal arteritis*
See *temporomandibular joint*
See *tension headache*

Cause

The most frequently occurring causes of headache and facial pain are dental pain, sinus pain, eye-related pain, migraine headache, tension headache (or musculoskeletal headache) which may present as a unilateral headache or pain around one eye, mumps, stone in the salivary gland, aneurysm formation, temporal arteritis, high blood pressure, intracranial haemorrhage or impending stroke and the presence of malignancies around the head and neck.

The line between headache and facial pain can sometimes be blurred and causes of both need to be considered together.

Sometimes the patient may complain specifically of facial pain, but in either case the presence of other coexistent symptoms will lead the medical practitioner to suspect the cause of the pain.

Investigations

Less commonly occurring conditions may need further investigations to confirm a diagnosis. Infections such as mumps and stones in one of the salivary glands are not common, but the history will raise the suspicion of the diagnosis, which may be confirmed with further testing.

Treatment

Symptomatic treatment of the headache with paracetamol or ibuprofen is the first line of treatment.

Some conditions may be best managed by referral to the most appropriate specialist or even to an emergency department. These may include serious cardiovascular conditions around the head and neck including aneurysm formation, temporal arteritis, intracranial haemorrhage or impending stroke and the presence of malignancies around the head and neck such as cancer in the mouth or sinuses or bony secondaries. A CT scan of the head and sinuses, MRI imaging or cerebral angiography may detect serious intracranial causes for headaches.

hearing loss

See *deafness and hearing loss*

heart attack

See *cardiomyopathies*
See *chest pain*
See *cholesterol*

Cause

The function of the heart and cardiovascular system is to act as a pump and a conduction device distributing blood and oxygen to the vital organs and to the peripheries and thus to every cell in the body.

The ability of the heart to pump blood efficiently around the body is dependent on the efficiency of the heart as a pumping agent. Heart attack or acute coronary syndrome results from severe obstruction of one of the coronary arteries. Most coronary artery disease is caused by the presence of atheromatous plaques in the coronary vessels which produce blockage in the flow of blood to the heart muscle. If the flow of blood is restricted, the muscle does not receive adequate amounts of oxygen-carrying blood to supply the metabolism demands of the heart. If the blood supply to the main part of the heart is cut off, the muscle, which depends on the artery for blood, then sustains cellular damage. The result is pain called angina. It is also thought to be due to the accumulation of by-products from cellular metabolism, e.g. lactic acid, which is the same product which builds up in the skeletal muscles of athletes after or during prolonged strenuous exertion, particularly when competing long distance. Complications of angina include heart attack or sudden death.

When atheroma builds up in the coronary vessels, these vessels are prone to clot formation on the surface of the plaques. If this occurs in an already narrow vessel, at some time the vessel may become blocked altogether, causing a heart attack or myocardial infarction. Altered platelet function in the vessels also contributes to the formation of the plaque formation in the coronary arteries.

Blockages may occur in either the right or left main coronary artery or their branches. Most frequently it is the left coronary artery involved in myocardial infarction or heart attack. The left coronary artery has a large branch called the left anterior descending branch (LAD branch) which supplies the majority of the left ventricle.

If the blockage to the vessel is detected and treated early, the effects of the blockage may be reversible, hence the reason for early referral of heart attack patients to hospital for treatment. If the treatment does not occur in a timely manner, permanent damage to the heart may result and the portion of the heart supplied by the occluded vessel may start to undergo permanent pathological changes. The muscle of the heart will be replaced with scar tissue which does not function as well as cardiac muscle.

Symptoms

Symptoms of heart attack depend on the degree of obstruction of the coronary arteries involved and range from mild through to moderate and severe. Symptoms include chest pain, with or without shortness of breath, nausea, pallor, sweating and claminess.

Some patients may experience breathlessness for no apparent reason and symptoms may mimic musculoskeletal pains or gastrointestinal pains followed by sudden cardiac death, i.e. some people 'just drop dead' and attempts to resuscitate them fail.

A diagnosis of sudden cardiac death should only be made after exclusion of other possible causes, e.g. pulmonary emboli, drug-related death, stroke, overwhelming infection, severe liver disease, e.g. cirrhosis or sudden perforation of a gastric ulcer.

Following an acute event, complications with heart function may occur and these include conduction defects of the heart's electrical system, called conduction defects or bundle branch blocks, arrhythmias, abnormal function of the heart muscle, heart failure, ventricular aneurysm, cardiogenic shock, rupture of the wall of the ventricle and abnormal function of the valves of the heart. Electrical dysfunction of the heart may be so significant that large parts of the heart become inactive because of scar tissue.

Investigations

The diagnosis of heart attack is made using one of a number of parameters for measuring heart function. These parameters include electrocardiogram (ECG) and the use of blood tests or serological markers which reflect damage to the heart muscle and are released from the heart muscle in the hours following obstruction of a coronary artery.

Investigations to determine cardiac function also include chest X-ray, echocardiography (CT) scanning, Holter monitor, exercise stress testing, cardiac catheterisation, coronary artery bypass graft, and stenting and angioplasty of coronary arteries.

ECG and chest X-ray are often the first line of investigation in the diagnostic procedure for cardiac complaints. An ECG is essential for determining cardiac arrhythmias and cardiac ischaemia. It may also determine atrial and ventricular enlargement and abnormalities of cardiac conduction. A chest X-ray provides assessment of atrial and ventricular size and outline of the pulmonary vessels; however additional tests are required to provide more detailed information of cardiac function.

An echocardiograph is a technique which uses ultrasound waves to produce an image of the heart and the great vessels to and from the heart. It is also able to assess the fitness of the heart muscle, the movement or contractions of the heart muscle, the blood supply to the heart muscle and the functioning of the heart valves.

Trans-oesophageal echocardiography is used to visualise the heart by placing the transducer at the end of the oesophagus. In this way it can assess cardiac structures, such as the left atrium and the area between the right and left atria, because it is closer to the structures being visualised. Stress echocardiography is also performed which allows visualisation of the motion of the heart wall during exercise.

Cardiac catheterisation is an investigation used to assess and quantify abnormalities in the coronary arteries and the chambers of the heart, the valve structures in the heart and major vessels. It is an invasive procedure where the catheter is inserted into the groin and passed up through the vessels and into the heart. Once in place, cardiac catheterisation may be used to perform angiography, intravascular ultrasonography and measurement of cardiac output and even endocardial biopsy, e.g. in the case of tumours arising inside the heart chambers.

Coronary artery bypass grafting is a technique used for surgically correcting and bypassing significant stenoses or blockages in the coronary artery vessels. This technique uses tissue from the patient (usually a vein from the leg) to provide the grafting material for the heart.

This technique requires cardiopulmonary bypass when the heart is stopped and the patient is maintained on a bypass machine which pumps to provide oxygen to the patient. In order to conserve oxygen consumption of the body, the patient is cooled during the procedure.

The risks of coronary artery bypass grafting include stroke or heart attack either during or following the procedure. Some cardiac surgeons will delay procedures for coronary artery bypass graft operations for patients who continue to smoke, as the benefits of performing an operation of this magnitude are such that smoking will significantly minimise the benefits thereof.

During exercise stress testing, the heart is monitored using an ECG tracing. The patient is asked to increase their normal physical activity, e.g. by walking on a treadmill and increasing their cardiac output and oxygen demand on the heart which may then be monitored. The heart rate is increased by the exercise to 85 per cent of the age predicted maximum, or until the patient reports the development of symptoms such as chest pain, at which time the procedure will be terminated. Stress testing is used for diagnosis of coronary heart disease and monitoring patients with known coronary artery disease. During exercise stress testing, further assessment may be undertaken by using radioactive thallium-201 which is injected during the procedure. The aim is to evaluate reversible perfusion defects in the heart muscle, i.e. localised areas of ischaemia in the heart muscle. This is referred to as a thallium stress test.

CT scanning may be used to assess specific conditions in the heart, such as pericarditis, congenital cardiac disorders (especially abnormal arterovenous shunts between the chambers of the heart) and disorders of the vessels such as aortic aneurysm, dissecting aneurysm of the aorta, heart tumours, pulmonary embolism and the presence of chronic pulmonary embolus formation.

Holter monitoring is a technique of continuous ECG and/or blood pressure monitoring over a period of either 24 or 48 hours. The patient is fitted with a device which measures the ECG tracing, heart rate and, at times, will also measure the blood pressure.

Coronary artery stenting and balloon angioplasty are techniques which are used to dilate and bypass local blockages in coronary arteries and their branches. The stents are tubes which are inserted into areas of blockage in the coronary arteries. Some stents also contain slow-release drugs which are designed to prevent repeat blockage in the artery. Balloon angioplasty is a technique used to increase the diameter of the coronary vessels by using a dilatory device which is removed at the end of the procedure.

Treatment

The aim of treatment in heart attack or acute coronary syndrome is to relieve the obstruction of the vessel supplying the heart as soon as possible in order to prevent damage to the heart muscle. Treatment for heart attack or acute coronary syndrome includes anti-platelet drugs (platelets stick to the walls of abnormal coronary vessels and cause clot formation), anticoagulant drugs, nitrate spray or tablets (to relieve spasm in the coronary arteries), beta blockers (to control heart rate), stenting of blocked coronary arteries, fibrinolytic drugs (which break down the blood clot in coronary vessels) and coronary artery bypass graft surgery.

Pain relief is essential and monitoring of the patient's heart function is also essential and preferably carried out in a coronary care unit, with specialist medical and nursing care.

Medical treatment for an acute heart attack includes urgent medical assessment in the general practitioner's surgery with ECG tracings to monitor the heart, administration of oxygen using a face mask, administration of aspirin orally to help prevent or dissolve clot formation in the coronary arteries. Transfer to a coronary care unit is then warranted where assessment may include further drug therapy, assessment of the patency of the coronary vessels and definitive treatment, including emergency stenting of the coronary vessels to prevent damage to the heart muscle as a consequence of lack of oxygen supply.

The patient will then be placed on a program of convalescence medical therapy, including addressing and minimising the predisposing factors for heart attack.

The best prognostic feature for surviving a heart attack and even sudden cardiac death, is the presence of a defibrillator device, which is now carried in all cardiac (specialist paramedic) ambulances, some medical surgeries and of course in emergency departments. Staff and the general public, including children, should be familiar with the principles of cardiopulmonary resuscitation (CPR) which improves the chances of survival.

Prevention

The most effective prevention of sudden cardiac death and heart attack is elimination of the predisposing factor for developing the condition, i.e. quitting or never commencing smoking, regular exercise, reducing obesity, prevention of diabetes, low fat diet, and controlling cholesterol and hypertension.

heart failure

See *angina*
See *atherosclerosis*
See *cardiomyopathies*
See *heart attack*

Cause

Heart failure occurs when the pumping action of the heart is unable to effectively keep the blood flowing around the body without fluid collecting either inside the heart (cardiomegaly) or in the peripheries (peripheral oedema or swelling), i.e. legs or in the lungs. Heart failure may result from the non-functioning of one of the heart valves.

Heart failure or congestive heart failure, is caused by an abnormality of ventricular function. Cardiomyopathies are a form of heart failure, with low ventricular output and disturbances of movement of the heart muscle, i.e. the muscular wall of the heart contracts poorly resulting in low cardiac output.

Symptoms

Symptoms of left ventricular failure include shortness of breath, fatigue, poor exercise tolerance. Right ventricular failure include accumulation of fluid in the abdomen and in the lower extremities. Heart failure is classified by the New York Heart Association into class one to four and are listed below.

Symptoms of heart failure include fatigue, shortness of breath with exercise or with sitting or lying in bed, swelling of the legs and poor exercise tolerance. Patients may also be on medication for high blood pressure and/or diabetes and have had treatment for coronary artery disease, e.g. stenting of the coronary arteries or a coronary artery bypass graft operation.

The symptoms associated with class one heart failure produce no limitation of physical activity. Class two heart failure produces slight limitations in physical activity, e.g. fatigue, shortness of breath, palpitations and angina. Class three heart failure produces a moderate degree of physical limitations which include discomfort at rest, fatigue with mild physical activity, shortness of breath, palpitations and angina. Class four heart failure produces severe symptoms which may be experienced at rest and with any physical activity.

Investigations

Monitoring of blood pressure is important, as is actively treating high blood pressure and achieving good diabetes control. The efficiency of the functioning of the heart muscle is assessed by an echocardiogram. This will estimate the size of the heart, the functioning of the heart valves and the ejection fraction of the heart, i.e. the amount of blood expelled with each contraction of the heart. A larger heart is not necessarily better as the heart becomes inefficient in its metabolism if the heart muscle is too thick.

Investigations such as coronary angiography are also able to determine heart functions, but this is a more invasive investigation requiring day or overnight admission to hospital and the skill of a procedural cardiologist.

Treatment

Treatment of heart failure is aimed at increasing the efficiency of the pumping action of the heart. This is achieved by administration of a class of medications called angiotensin converting enzyme (ACE) inhibitors which help with the efficient contracting of the heart as well as controlling blood pressure, diuretics to help improve unwanted fluid level in the body by increased excretion by the kidney, as well as prescription of a third group of medications called beta blockers. Patients will usually also be prescribed treatment for controlling cholesterol and platelet function.

For patients who go into acute heart failure, treatment should first involve calling the ambulance for emergency transport to hospital.

heartburn

See *oesophagitis, gastro-oesophageal reflux*

Heartburn, dyspepsia and indigestion are other names for gastro-oesophageal reflux.

heel pain

Cause

Tendo achillis or Achilles heel can be caused by several things ranging from tendonitis, bursitis of the heel, a spur, trauma to the heel and plantar fasciitis, to ill-fitting shoes, excessive amounts of physical exertion, a foreign body in the foot and fallen arches.

Symptoms

The person will feel pain in the sole of the foot associated with weight bearing and stretching of the tendo-achillis tendon. With plantar fasciitis the patient complains of pain in the heel with the first step to the floor in the morning.

Investigations

Investigation of pain in the back of the heel includes an ultrasound of the area, looking for foreign bodies in the foot, signs of tendonitis or tearing of the tendo-achilles tendon. X-rays may show the presence of bony spurs.

Treatment

Treatment for heel pain includes prescription of anti-inflammatory medication, treatment with hot and cold packs, inserts in the shoe to correct arch problems and elevation of the heel with an insert for problems with the tendo-achilles tendon. If on ultrasound investigation it is determined that the tendo-achilles tendon has been partially ruptured, surgical repair may be required.

helicobacter pylori infection

See *chest pain*
See *oesophagitis, gastro-oesophageal reflux*

Cause

Helicobacter pylori are a bacteria which produce an infection in the stomach. It may be related to the consumption of contaminated food or water.

Symptoms

Symptoms of helicobacter pylori infection include indigestion, heartburn, dyspepsia, flatulence, bloating and abdominal discomfort. It may cause gastritis, peptic ulcer disease and cancer of the stomach.

Treatment

Eradication of helicobacter pylori involves triple therapy in the form of antibiotics and anti-reflux preparations called proton pump inhibitors. Usually a course of this treatment will last for a week, but may need to be repeated at some later date. After treatment has been completed, a follow-up test is necessary to determine that the infection has been eradicated. This does not involve having a repeat endoscopy, but may be done by a helicobacter breath test at a pathology department. This test needs to be done four to six weeks after the eradication treatment has been completed. If it is found that eradication is not complete, another course of treatment will be undertaken. Helicobacter pylori is associated with increased risk of cancer of the stomach, hence the need for eradication.

hepatitis

Cause

Hepatitis refers to an infection of the liver and may be caused by various viral agents which have been designated hepatitis A to H. Most commonly referred to hepatitis is that of hepatitis A, B or C. Acute viral hepatitis is a diffuse liver inflammation caused by specific viruses.

Other infections may also cause an inflammatory reaction in the liver, e.g. glandular fever.

Symptoms

Symptoms of acute hepatitis include anorexia, nausea, fever, pain in the right upper side of the abdomen, abdominal distension, jaundice, nausea, vomiting, tiredness, lethargy, clotting disorders resulting in an increase in bruising to the skin. Chronic forms of hepatitis, particularly hepatitis B, may ultimately lead to liver cancer.

A patient with cirrhosis of the liver may present with fever, peritonitis, low blood sugar, a high calcium level, high cholesterol and triglyceride.

Treatment

Treatment for hepatitis in the acute phase is symptomatic and supportive during the course of the illness and convalescent phase. If the acute phase of the illness progresses to become a chronic infection of the liver, other treatment measures may be required in order to minimise the effects of long-term infection or inflammation in the liver. Treatment such as interferon has been used for hepatitis C.

Prevention

A vaccination for the prevention of hepatitis is available but only for the forms of hepatitis A and B.

hernia

Cause

A hernia may occur in the abdomen and present as a lump as a result of tissue from inside the abdomen pushing through a weakness or defect in the abdominal wall to form a lump which can be felt or even seen. A hernia may form as a result of a strain, excessive increase in intra-abdominal pressure or as a result of a breakdown from an abdominal wound following surgery.

Symptoms

Patients with hernia may present with pain or a lump. Adult men more commonly present with groin hernia following excessive straining usually involving heavy lifting. This hernia is called an inguinal hernia present as a lump in the scrotum. Hernia may occur on the abdominal wall around the umbilicus, around pre-existing operation scars, in the groin and internally as hiatus hernia.

The hernia may move in an out of the scrotum and at times may become trapped. If entrapment of the hernia happens, the blood supply to the portion of gut which forms the hernia may be impaired. The hernia is then said to strangulate, which requires surgical intervention to ensure that the portion of gut does not die due to gangrene.

Treatment

The treatment for hernias involves either conservative management, e.g. support by a truss or by surgical repair of the area.

herpes simplex virus *(lips or genital area)*

See *eyes*
See *eye or eyelid infection*

Cause

Herpes simplex infection may be either oral (cold sores) or genital. The two strains of the virus are: Type 1, which may occur either on the peri-oral area or on the genital area (it can be spread to the genital area from infected lips of one sexual partner to the genital area of the other during sex) and Type 2, which almost always occurs on the genital area.

Symptoms

Peri-oral symptoms include tingling, a sensation of burning, followed by the onset of blisters and scab formation. Genital symptoms include tingling and burning, followed by areas of ulceration surrounded by areas of redness.

Treatment

Treatment of herpes simplex, either genital or peri-oral, is by an acyclovir preparation either in the form of cream or tablet. For treatment of oral or genital herpes, a private script pack of tablets is now available for immediate use when the symptoms of tingling and burning commence. It is recommended that if a patient is known to have oral herpes, a spare pack of the tablets should be kept on hand for immediate use as soon as the symptoms are felt. In this way, an acute attack will be averted.

Spread of the virus may also take place by kissing, drinking from the same water bottle, using the same cup or utensils or by sharing the same lip gloss or lipstick of someone who is infected. If infection occurs, potential recurrence is lifelong.

herpes zoster *(shingles)*

Cause

Shingles is caused by another of the herpes viruses called herpes zoster. It is the same virus which causes chickenpox in children.

Symptoms

Shingles may occur anywhere on the skin. The most problematic area for it to occur is on the face or forehead when it is called herpes zoster ophthalmicus. It is manifested on the face and scalp in the distribution of one or more branches of the trigeminal nerve.

Symptoms such as pain in the area of the outbreak may precede the onset of the rash by some days. The rash follows a segmental pattern of the body called the dermatomes of the body, which represent the embryological development of the foetus. The rash of herpes zoster on the trunk of the body will not cross the midline of the body on the front or on the back. Pain may be quite intense and may last for some time following resolution of an infection. Children who are not immune to the chickenpox virus may contract chickenpox as a result from exposure to the shingles virus.

Treatment

Prompt treatment of herpes zoster ophthalmicus is recommended with acyclovir in order to minimise the possible effects of involvement of the eye or cornea. If the eye becomes infected, visual impairment may result. Analgesia is often needed for the acute infection and sometimes ongoing after the infection has cleared. The use of oral steroids are sometimes needed for severe infections. Immunity to the virus is conveyed by vaccination with the chickenpox vaccination, with a course of two vaccinations in adults over the age of 13 years of age.

hip pain

In children

See *arthritis*

In adults

See *osteoarthritis*

Cause

Both children and adults may experience hip pain, but for very different reasons. In children, congenital dislocation of the hip (CDH) is tested for at regular intervals in the time before the child becomes fully mobile (at around 12 to 14 months of age) and is caused by a failure of the development of the acetabulum which is cup-shaped and holds the ball of the head of the femur in the pelvis.

Perthe's disease may occur in a slightly older group of children (aged four to 10 years) and it is more common in males than in females.

A slipped femoral epiphysis may result from a minor trauma or fall, particularly in a child that is overweight.

In the case of septic arthritis, no apparent cause for the infection may ever be found, but should always be suspected if a child presents with unexplained pain in the area of the hip.

In adults, osteoarthritis and fracture of the neck of the femur are the most likely causes of hip pain.

In adults, obesity may increase the wear and tear in the hip joint. Adults who engage in regular long distance running often find that the cartilage on the femoral heads has become worn and may require hip replacement as a result. In elderly adults, osteoporosis accompanied by a fall may result in a hip fracture (which carries with it a significant risk of mortality and morbidity), requiring pinning of the neck of the femur (or hip).

Symptoms

Congenital dislocation of the hip in children presents with a click in the hip as early as the neonatal period and if not corrected as soon as possible, will result in a lifelong disability for the child. Perthe's disease represents a condition where the head of the femur crumples as a result of lack of blood supply. In a slipped femoral epiphysis, the child will complain of pain in the area of the hip and immediate referral to an orthopaedic specialist or emergency department is necessary.

Treatment

All hip pain in children requires referral to an orthopaedic specialist for further investigation and management. A child suffering from congenital hip dislocation (CDH) will be placed in a 'frog' splint as a way of encouraging the acetabulum to develop normally. Double nappies is an option designed to produce maximum separation of the hips.

Progress of the child may be monitored by X-ray. Other treatments for hip pains will be undertaken depending on the cause of the pains.

HIV

See *human immunodeficiency virus*

Hodgkin's disease

Hodgkin's disease, also known as Hodgkin's lymphoma, is a cancer of the lymph nodes, spleen, liver and bone marrow.

Cause

The cause of Hodgkin's disease is unknown but genetic susceptibility and environmental associations play a role. Lymphomas were once thought to be distinct from leukaemia; however better understanding shows that the difference between lymphomas and leukaemia is not distinct.

Symptoms

The first symptom that a patient may have is the detection of a lump or a feeling of being tired, lethargic and lacking in energy.

Investigations

Chest X-ray, lymph node biopsy, CT scan of the chest, renal and liver function tests are generally obtained and sometimes an MRI is done.

Treatment

Many people who are treated for Hodgkin's disease make a full recovery (approximately 75 per cent of people). Treatment involves the administration of radiotherapy and chemotherapy drugs over a period of time to be determined by the treating physician. The stage of the disease will indicate the extent to which the patient is affected by the condition. This is done by assessing if lymph nodes are enlarged in various regions of the body, e.g. neck, underarm, groin and inside the abdominal and thoracic cavities.

HPV *(human papillomavirus)*

See *human papillomavirus*

human immunodeficiency virus *(HIV)*

Cause

Human immunodeficiency virus or HIV is caused by an infection of a retrovirus, which destroys white blood cells and results in impairment of cell-mediated immunity, and increases the risk of infections and cancers in humans.

Transmission of HIV requires contact with body fluids, specifically blood, semen, vagina secretions, breast milk secretions or secretions from wounds. All of these body fluids in an infected person may contain the HIV virus to a varying extent. Transmission of the HIV virus is commonly via sexual contact, sharing of blood-contaminated needles, childbirth, breastfeeding or by medical procedures including accidental injury by needle stick.

Needle-stick injury protocol includes referral and immediate treatment using anti-retroviral medications in order to minimise the risk of infection and replication and sero-conversion in cases where it is known that the needle has been contaminated with HIV. The risk from needle-stick injury seems to be greatest if the wound is deep or if the needle is hollow.

Least likely transmission of HIV is via saliva, sneezing and coughing.

Symptoms

Initial symptoms of HIV infection occur one to four weeks following the infection and last from three to 14 days. They include fever, lethargy, pains in the joints, a rash, swelling of the lymph nodes and sometimes symptoms of meningitis. The symptoms are similar to those experienced with acute viral infections or glandular fever.

Following initial infection, most patients with human immunodeficiency virus will remain relatively asymptomatic for months or even years. Diagnosis of the condition may arise as a result of the presence of acute or chronic enlargement of the lymph glands oral thrush, herpes zoster or shingles, unexplained diarrhoea, fatigue and fever.

As symptoms worsen, the patient may progress to the end stage of HIV infection, known as acquired immunodeficiency syndrome or AIDS. Without treatment, the risk of progression from HIV infection to AIDS is about 1 per cent to 2 per cent for the first two to three years of infection and about 5 per cent to 6 per cent per year thereafter, but eventually AIDS will develop. During this time the body is prone to unusual infections which often result in the patient's death. Kaposi's sarcoma and lymphomas and infections are also common in people with HIV infection prior to the onset of end-stage AIDS.

The risk and severity of infection in AIDS patients is related to the lymphocyte count and the patient's exposure to potentially opportunistic infections, e.g. pneumocystic pneumonia, toxoplasmosis encephalitis, cryptococcal meningitis, mycobacterium avium.

The HIV virus also infects non-T cells in the body including brain cells, heart cells and kidney cells resulting in organ damage to the systems of the body.

Treatment

Treatment for human immunodeficiency virus is based on suppressing the virus which causes the condition. This is done by using drugs which inhibit the enzymes which enable the virus to multiply. Patients diagnosed with HIV are commonly on three to four antiviral agents in order to maintain suppression of virus replication; however administration of antiviral agents is usually deferred while the patient is well and the viral load is low.

human papillomavirus (HPV)

See *cervical cancer*
See *genital warts*

Cause

There are numerous strains of human papilloma virus (HPV). Some cause common warts, some cause genital warts, and others cause abnormalities in cervical cells in women. Human papilloma viruses are thought to be responsible for around 70 per cent of abnormal pap smears.

Treatment

Treatment for common warts is achieved by topical preparations, diathermy, liquid nitrogen or, excision. Treatment for genital warts includes topical preparations, e.g. imiquimod, diathermy, liquid nitrogen, or excision. Vaccination is now available in various strains of HPV which will give protection from the development of abnormal Pap smears in women, and also convey protection in men for carcinoma of the penis which is also thought to arise from the papilloma virus.

hyperpituitarism

Cause

Hyperpituitarism occurs in the presence of excess amounts of production of growth hormone due to the presence of a pituitary adenoma. This produces a condition called gigantism and acromegaly. If excess production of growth hormone occurs before the growing phase in a child is completed, i.e. before the growing plates in the bones have fused, the condition is called gigantism. If the excess production of growth hormone occurs after the growing plates in the bones have fused, i.e in adulthood, the condition is called acromegaly.

Hyperpituitarism may also result in the production of milk from the breasts in both males and females in the presence of a prolactin-secreting pituitary adenoma.

Symptoms

Symptoms of gigantism and acromegaly include increased stature, delayed puberty and hypogonadism which is failure of the production of hormones from the ovaries or testicles.

Symptoms of acromegaly include increased coarse facial features and an increase in the size of hands and feet. Coarse body hair and an increase in skin thickness may occur along with increased function of sweat glands, an increase in the size of the lower jaw and malocclusion of the teeth. The tongue is frequently enlarged and degenerative arthritis is common.

Problems commonly occur with peripheral nerves because of compression of the nerves by adjacent fibrous tissue. Headaches are also common. The internal organs including the heart, liver, kidneys, spleen, thyroid, parathyroid and pancreas are also larger than normal.

Symptoms of prolactin-secreting pituitary adenoma include abnormal milk production in women who are not breastfeeding and in men. Patients with prolactin-secreting pituitary adenoma will have elevated levels of the hormone prolactin.

Treatment

Surgery or radiation is generally the treatments of choice for hyperpituitarism.

Treatment for prolactin-secreting pituitary adenoma is a controversial subject. It is felt that for patients with elevated levels of prolactin hormone, observation may be sufficient. These patients will normally present with small tumours or microadenomas. For patients with macro-adenomas, treatments include administration of dopamine antagonists, surgical removal of the tumour and radiation therapy.

A screening test for diabetes is also done.

hypertension

Hypertension is high blood pressure. Blood pressure is generated as a result of the contraction and relaxation of the heart as it pumps blood around the body. The upper limit considered normal for blood pressure is 140/90 irrespective of age. Blood pressure is measured using a sphygmomanometer. When the heart contracts it generates a reading called systolic pressure (the upper reading) and when the heart relaxes it generates a reading called diastolic pressure (the lower reading) and is due to the amount of flexibility in the walls of the arteries of the body.

Blood pressure varies constantly for an individual throughout the entire day.

Cause

Causes of hypertension include kidney disease, narrowing of the renal artery called renal artery stenosis, coarctation of the aorta where a congenital narrowing of the aorta occurs, connective tissue disorders, abnormalities of the endocrine system, excessive alcohol intake, the use of the oral contraceptive pill, asthma relievers, steroids use, cocaine, licorice. In essential hypertension, no discernible cause for an increase in the blood pressure may be found.

Increased blood pressure may also be the result of stress, anxiety, strenuous exercise, smoking, overweight, some medications, hypertension of pregnancy (pre-eclampsia), a tumour of the adrenal gland which sits on top of the kidney (phaeochromocytoma often produces intermittent elevation in blood pressure and is sometimes difficult to diagnose), diabetes, abnormalities of arteries (e.g. renal artery stenosis), cholesterol deposits in arteries, autoimmune diseases (systemic lupus erythematosus, polyarthritis), medical problems of endocrine glands (e.g. thyroid gland, parathyroid glands, adrenal glands), the contraceptive pill and nonsteroidal anti-inflammatory medications, which are often used for arthritis complaints.

Symptoms

Symptoms will depend on the cause of the hypertension. In most instances, elevated blood pressure may cause no symptoms whatsoever, but symptoms may include dizziness, headache, fatigue, nose bleed, nervousness and feeling flushed in the face. The most commonly occurring symptom associated with hypertension is headache. Other symptoms include palpitations, increased sweating, nausea and vomiting, abdominal pains, blurred vision, concentration problems, problems with speech, transient or permanent blindness, sudden collapse, irritability, shortness of breath, chest pains, feeling tired, weakness of the muscles, sensation of pins and needles and nose bleeds.

Treatment

Treatment of hypertension is essential to maintain blood pressure within a normal, acceptable range (upper limit of normal is accepted at less than 140/90 mm of mercury) in order to prevent the possibility of adverse event, e.g. heart attack or stroke. Treatment of hypertension firstly depends on making a diagnosis of the cause of the increase in blood pressure, where possible. This may include prescription of one or more medications including diuretics, beta blockers, ACE inhibitors, calcium channel blockers, angiotensin II (A2As) receptor blockers.

hyperthyroidism

Other names for hyperthyroidism include thyrotoxicosis, Graves' disease, toxic nodular goitre and toxic diffuse goitre.

Cause

The cause of hyperthyroidism is not entirely understood, but is most likely an autoimmune disease resulting in high thyroxine production.

Symptoms

Symptoms of hyperthyroidism include enlarged thyroid, weight loss, tachycardia, heat intolerance, agitation, restlessness, sweaty hands, hand tremors along with atrial fibrillation, fatigue, increased appetite, insomnia, muscular weakness, diarrhoea, prominent eyes, retraction of the eyelids, pain around the eyes and sensitivity to light. There may be some weakness of the muscles controlling eye movements, which leads to double vision.

Treatment

Treatment of hyperthyroidism is with antithyroid medication which decreases the production of the thyroid hormones. Beta-blocking agents may be used to block the effects of the tachycardia, tremor, heat intolerance and diarrhoea. Radioactive iodine may be used for some patients past their child-bearing years. Surgery also offers good prospects for recovery. There is a risk of becoming hypothyroid following some treatments for hyperthyroidism.

hypopituitarism

Cause

Causes of hypopituitarism include pituitary adenomas, craniopharyngiomas, ischaemia of the pituitary gland, shock (particularly post-partum shock), diabetes, sickle cell anaemia, vascular disorders and aneurysms, inflammation such as meningitis, pituitary abscess, infiltration, e.g. in haemochromatosis, following radiation to the skull, autoimmune dysfunction. These causes are referred to as primary hypopituitarism. Secondary hypopituitarism may be caused by hypothalamic tumours, inflammatory process, e.g. sarcoidosis, trauma, surgical trauma to the gland. All these disorders result from factors affecting the anterior pituitary.

Symptoms

Hypopituitarism involving the posterior pituitary produces diabetes insipidus, which is caused by a deficiency of production of anti-diuretic hormone (vasopressin). Diabetes insipidus is a relatively uncommon condition and should not be confused with diabetes mellitus (which means sugar in the urine). Hypopituitarism may produce symptoms of deficiency in hormones from any of the endocrine glands, e.g. thyroid, parathyroid, adrenal, ovaries or testes.

Treatment

Treatment for pituitary tumours includes ablative radiation therapy or surgery, which is usually done through the nose and the sphenoid bone of the skull.

hypotension

Cause

Hypotension or low blood pressure may occur even in young, fit, healthy people and this alone is not an indication for intervention, although some people may become overly concerned at being told that their blood pressure is low. Blood pressure is at its lowest for people who are active during the day between 2am and 4am, after which blood pressure begins to increase in anticipation of a day's activity.

Hypotension may occur as a result of sudden change in position from lying to sitting or standing (called postural hypotension), as a result of prolonged standing in the one position, a result of sudden fright or because of sudden excessive bleeding. Hypotension may also occur at times of severe acute infection including toxic shock syndrome arising from the use of tampons, anaemia, as a result of heart attack or irregularities in heart rhythm, as a result of dehydration due to excessive sweating or excessive loss of fluids due to gastroenteritis, as a result of medications such as antihypertensive agents, tranquillisers, antidepressants, sleeping tablets. Hypotension may also occur as a result of a blood clot travelling to the lungs or brain.

Hypotension in the presence of heart attack, heart disease, cardiomyopathies or arrhythmias is cause for concern and the patient should be referred for treatment to an emergency department.

Symptoms

Severe hypotension may be accompanied by feelings of nausea and vomiting, lightheadedness, feeling faint and sweaty, dry mouth, blurring of vision, feelings of anxiety.

Treatment

If the cause of the hypotension is a simple faint, also referred to as a vaso-vagal attack, the patient should be laid flat and sweet fluids administered. Other treatment for hypotension may require investigation and even admission to hospital to determine the cause.

hypothyroidism

Cause

Primary hypothyroidism is most likely an autoimmune disorder resulting from Hashimoto's thyroiditis. The second most common cause of hypothyroidism is following radioactive iodine therapy treatment for treatment of hyperthyroidism or thyrotoxicosis. Severe iodine deficiency may result in hypothyroidism.

Secondary hypothyroidism my result from a problem in the interaction between the pituitary and the thyroid glands.

Symptoms

Symptoms of hypothyroidism include tiredness, lethargy, no energy, dry skin, cold intolerance and weight gain despite no change in eating habits. Severe hypothyroidism, called myxoedema, may result in a deep voice, apparent lack of emotions, depression and clouding of mental abilities. There may also be puffiness around the eyes and loss of body hair. The patient may experience a bradycardia or slow pulse rate. Constipation may be a feature and the patient may complain of symptoms of carpal tunnel syndrome. The patient may experience heavy periods and as a result may present with anaemia. The thyroid gland may be enlarged and tender.

Symptoms of secondary hypothyroidism include amenorrhoea (or no periods), enlargement of the tongue, low blood pressure and hypoglycaemia.

Treatment

Treatment for hypothyroidism includes replacement therapy of thyroid hormone.

immune response

See *immunisation*
See *immunisation for childhood infectious diseases*

We share the world with an array of micro-organisms which like to invade our bodies as it provides them with a favourable environment in which they can live and replicate. It might be very nice for the micro-organisms, but we run the risk of disease when germs take up residence within us so the body has defences against these would-be invaders. When micro-organisms do succeed in entering our bodies, despite the natural protection which is offered by our intact skin, mucous membranes lining the respiratory tract and the stomach and a substance called lysosome which is present in tears, saliva and nasal secretions, they are confronted with the body's immune mechanisms.

Because micro-organisms undergo extensive mutation to avoid being killed in the body, a more sophisticated system called the acquired immune response has evolved to help the body fight infection. Some germs are so strong that the body needs further help to overcome these, such as antibiotics.

When micro-organisms enter the body, they encounter special cells called phagocytes. These phagocytes comprise special cells called polymorphonucleocytes and macrophages, which generate powerful chemicals which aid in the killing and digestion of germs. For a germ to be destroyed by a phagocyte, it must first become attached to the phagocytes. Some bacteria produce chemicals which attract neutrophils, but others have developed mechanisms to prevent their being attached to neutrophils. The body has then very cleverly dealt with this obstacle by producing a substance called complement which is a series of blood proteins that enhances phagocytosis or ingestion of micro-organisms.

There are other proteins produced by the body called acute phase proteins which assist in the killing of micro-organisms. These proteins include interferon which inhibits viral replication. Some organisms have learnt to avoid complement, so the body develops another mechanism called the antibody. Antibodies circulate in the blood and deal with germs on the outside of cells. This molecule recognises a point on the micro-organisms and attaches to it and at the same time activates the complement system. These antibodies are made by a special type of white cell—a lymphocyte called B-lymphocyte.

When a lymphocyte encounters an infectious agent or a bacterial product, it produces an antibody response. Antibodies appear several days after infection occurs, but the level of antibodies falls quickly. This is called the primary response to the germ. The next time the germ encounters the antibody, the response is much stronger as the number of lymphocytes capable of producing the antibody has increased. The lymphocyte, which has developed a memory, recruits many other lymphocytes to deal with this germ when it again appears. This acquired memory or immunity is very specific, e.g. immunity to mumps virus does not make the body immune to polio virus.

When the body is vaccinated against a particular disease, it is injected with a killed or much weakened form of the germ, but it still has enough chemical sites to stimulate antibody production. Some micro-organisms enter into cells and live inside cells whereas others live outside cells. To deal with lymphocytes which live inside cells, the proteins which make up micro-organisms, bacteria or germs are taken into the cell by a vesicle (or bubble). This bubble is formed when a thin membrane covering the cell of the body wraps itself around the micro-organism.

The body has various ways of ensuring that its lymphocytes do not attack its own cells. This special process, called negative selection, causes cells which might harm the body to be killed or inactivated. Sometimes, however, this system goes wrong and the body makes antibodies against itself. These are called auto-antibodies and damage the body and there are many autoimmune diseases which can result.

When a decision has been made to transplant a patient with a donor organ, e.g. kidney or liver, it is essential that the two people share the same HLA antigen, otherwise the organ will undergo a very rapid rejection at the time of transplantation. There are some infections, e.g. HIV, which interfere with the body's immune system making it ineffective, so that people who are infected with the HIV virus are prone to unusual infections and more susceptible to the development of cancer.

Some people are born with defective immune systems. Some of the resulting diseases are so severe that the person dies in infancy whilst others live with varying disabilities. Some people who are mildly affected may require regular transfusions with antibodies enabling them to live normal lives.

immunisation

See *immunisation for childhood infectious diseases*

Immunisation to a number of infectious diseases was designed to reduce the morbidity and mortality associated with childhood and infant infectious diseases. Immunisation against infectious diseases has changed the profiles of epidemics. Many of the diseases which were considered infectious diseases of childhood have been eliminated due to the effects of vaccination of the population. An epidemic is only likely to occur when an infectious disease presents itself to a population of people who are not immune and the infectious disease is readily transmitted from one person to another. Smallpox for example, has been officially eradicated worldwide according to the World Health Organization and this has been achieved by vaccination. Diseases such as tetanus, diphtheria and polio are now rarities due to immunisation programs worldwide.

immunisation for childhood infectious diseases

Cause

Immunisation schedules particularly for childhood vary from one country to another, and even individual countries are constantly revising and changing the recommended guidelines for their programs. Documenting a detailed immunisation schedule is fraught with the risk of having the recommendation outdated at short notice.

Adults can of course become infected with any if not all of the diseases commonly referred to as infectious diseases of childhood, if not possessing adequate immunity.

Childhood infectious disease vaccinations schedule is recommended commencing from around 2 months and include:

Tetanus, Polio, Whooping Cough, Diphtheria, Hepatitis B,

Haemophylus influenzae B

Pneumococcus

Meningococcus

Measles, Mumps, Rubella

Chickenpox

Symptoms

Childhood infectious disease poses serious threat to life for young children. Infections may be accompanied by high fevers and not uncommonly signs of various characteristic rashes, of coughing, of weight loss, of respiratory distress, of gastrointestinal symptoms, of general malaise, of dehydration and sometimes death. Infection with tetanus (formerly called lockjaw) is associated with uncontrollable muscle spasms and if untreated is inevitably fatal.

Treatment

Treatment for tetanus is twofold: to limit the effects of the tetanus toxin which produces the lockjaw, and to eliminate the infecting bacteria, by use of antibiotics such as metranidazole or penicillin.

Whereas polio is associated with muscle weakness. Treatment for polio may require assisted ventilation to aid breathing, and other symptomatic support until the signs of infection subside. There are no definitive medications to treat the acute disease once it has occurred.

Whooping cough has a characteristic cough and is treated with erythromycin, clarithromycin, or azithromycin. Non-immune contacts of an infected person should also be treated prophylactic.

Diphtheria occurred in epidemic proportions as recently as the mid 1950's worldwide and can be fatal within minutes. Treatment includes antibiotics such as penicillin, erythromycin, rifampin, or clindamycin. Rapid response is essential once the disease is suspected.

There is no medical treatment for acute Hepatitis B. Prevention of the disease is the main aim. Long term consequences of hepatitis B may include cancer of the liver, cirrhosis, chronic hepatitis (of inflammation of the liver), liver failure, or death.

Haemophylus influenzae B (I lib), can cause meningitis, epiglotitis (swelling of the throat, obstructing the airway), joint infections and pains, and pneumonia. Young children may require treatment in intensive care. Treatment includes administration of potent antibiotics, e.g. third or fourth generation cephalosporins, semi-synthetic penicillin, or chloramphenicol is required for effective treatment.

Pneumococcus is one of the bacteria of the streptococcus family which as a group of bacteria commonly causes respiratory infections. It is a particularly potent bacterium, and shows increasingly resistance to an increasing number of antibiotics, particularly in countries of Europe, and USA. Care is required in treating those infected with Streptococcus pneumoniae to use a drug to which the organism is sensitive, e.g. using penicillin, amoxicillin-clavulanate, cephalosporins, cephtriaxone, and vancomycin.

Attention to adequate fluid requirements and replacement is always a high priority and applies to all children with symptoms of vomiting with or without the accompanying symptom of diarrhoea.

Meningococcal disease is a serious infection which causes meningitis, and commonly a characteristic generalised rash. By the time that the rash has appeared, particularly in young children, the infection is well under way. The condition progresses rapidly from the time of initial infection and is not infrequently fatal. Young children and adolescents are particularly susceptible in the spring and winter months. Urgent treatment with antibiotics is required, often before investigations confirm the presence of the infection and this is an essential element to successful recovery.

Measles, Mumps, Rubella come as a combined vaccination for administration to either children or adults. All health workers and prospective mothers should ensure that their immunity to these diseases is up to date prior to embarking on pregnancy, or commencing work in health roles. There is no medical treatment for these diseases apart from symptomatic relief of the fever, headache, and malaise, and topical treatment for relief of the discomfort of the rashes associated with measles and rubella. Measles infection may progress later in childhood to a degenerative condition of the central nervous system called sub-acute sclerosing panencephalitis which is invariably fatal at approximately aged eight or nine years of age.

Mumps produces the characteristic swelling on either side of the neck, due to infection of the parotid glands.

Chickenpox or (varicella virus) infection has a characteristic rash, with watery blisters on top, that are often itchy. The infection does respond to antiviral agents such as acyclovir which will shorten the duration of the disease, but the products are expensive and not government subsided for this condition, and therefore preclusive economically for most families.

impetigo

See *skin problems*
See *dermatitis/eczema*

Cause

Impetigo is due to an infection of the skin with staphylococcus aureus and/or, less commonly, streptococcus pyogenes. The bacteria which cause impetigo live in the nose and are transferred by the fingernails to other parts of the body. Normally a child with a staphylococcal reservoir in the nose picks his or her nose and then scratches the skin in another location, thus transferring the bacteria, which quickly multiplies and lodges in abraded skin. Not uncommonly, children present with impetigo which the parents say started as a bite. This may well be true as the bite becomes itchy, is scratched constantly and is infected resulting in a lesion of impetigo.

Symptoms

A common place for impetigo to start is on the face. The skin appears red, inflamed and eventually a scab will form at the site or sites of the broken skin. Once one skin lesion has occurred, the bacteria can then be transferred to other places. The skin feels itchy, inflamed and scratching occurs, further inflaming the area. The areas of infection quickly increase in size, on potentially multiple areas of the body.

Treatment

Treatment for impetigo includes oral antibiotics, hygiene measures to the skin with bathing and hand washing and prescription of a cream to use inside the nose. The infection responds rapidly to treatment.

impotence

See *diabetes*
See *erectile dysfunction*
See *hypertension*

Impotence is now referred to as erectile dysfunction and may occur in men at any age; however it is more common with increasing age. For older men sustaining an erection may become more difficult because of the effects of coexistent disease; medication, particularly for depression, hypertension and diabetes; or the presence of psychological factors, which may be temporary or permanent.

incontinence

See *benign prostatic hyperplasia*
See *prostate cancer*
See *urinary incontinence*

Cause

Incontinence may include either urinary or faecal incontinence with loss of control of either urination or defaecation. Sometimes both forms of incontinence may occur.

Faecal incontinence is the loss of voluntary control of bowel movements and may result from diseases of the spinal cord, congenital abnormalities, accidental injuries to the rectum and anus (during childbirth), diabetes, advancing age, dementia, faecal impaction, inflammatory processes, tumours of the rectum.

Symptoms

Incontinence may present in one of four different ways. Urge incontinence (or an urgent irrepressible need to urinate); stress incontinence, which is a leakage of urine due to a sudden increase in intra-abdominal pressure, e.g. from coughing, sneezing, laughing or lifting; overflow incontinence with the dribbling of urine from the bladder; and functional incontinence which is associated with physical impairments, e.g. dementia or following stroke.

Treatment

Improvement in incontinence may be achieved with regular pelvic floor exercises, review of prescribed medications and at times surgical intervention. Some medications will improve bladder tone and reduce urinary incontinence. Some medication in the form of tablets or nasal sprays may be used to reduce bed-wetting in children and are also applicable for use in adults. In the elderly, particularly those in nursing homes or who are bedridden, incontinence devices may be necessary.

infections

See *immunisation*
See *immune response*

Cause

Micro-organisms are everywhere and humans co-exist with them every day. Patients often ask, 'Where did I get this from? I have not been near anyone with this.' The fact is you just do not know from looking at someone if they are carrying an infectious disease at the time. It takes only one sneeze from someone at close range to infect another person with an infectious disease.

Bacteria also live on the skin and in the respiratory tract, gastroenterology or digestive tract and the genital tract and constitute normal flora. Whether an organism is able to invade the human host and cause illness or infection depends on a balance between the properties of the host, the organism and the immunity of the host.

The first defence mechanism is the physical barrier provided by the intact skin and mucous membranes. Micro-abrasions in the skin and mucous membranes allow organisms to invade the body, e.g. with sexual activity, an abrasive activity of skin surfaces rubbing on each other causing microscopic trauma and allowing entry of certain organisms.

Symptoms

Bacterial infection may occur following these micro-abrasions producing vaginitis, thrush and allowing the entry of the human immunodeficiency virus (HIV) or AIDS virus from an infected individual to the uninfected sexual partner.

Burns of the skin allow infection to gain entry and this is one of the most significant risks for burns patients and poses a considerable risk for their survival if large portions of the body are affected by burns.

In the respiratory tract, the passages are lined with cells which have an outer layer of cilia or hairs which beat in a wave-like fashion, not unlike wheat fields waving on the breeze. Its function is to propel foreign material away from the surface and up towards the mouth. It also acts as a barrier to organisms invading the mucous membrane and if this barrier is disturbed, infection in the respiratory tract will occur, e.g. bronchitis.

In the stomach (the food receptacle at the end of the oesophagus and not the region of the body sometimes called 'the stomach') hydrochloric acid is present and helps to sterilise ingested material which acts as a barrier to infection. Infection may still occur resulting in vomiting and diarrhoea, which may be called viral gastroenteritis and food poisoning.

Impetigo is a skin infection which is caused by a staphylococcus and/or less commonly streptococcus which lives in the nose. Despite what we might think, everyone picks their nose at some time of the day, week or year, but at least some time in their life. Children are most frequent offenders and least likely to wash their hands on a regular basis. They are also more likely to scratch, poke, prod or play with other parts of the body and in doing so carry the staphylococcal bacteria which by this time are located under the unwashed fingernails to remote places on the body, abrading the skin and causing infection. The lesions then become irritated and further scratching results, and more spread of the bacteria occurs.

Some bacteria also possess enzymes which enhance their penetration of the barrier, e.g. staphylococcus bacteria. The immune system of the body is called to action by mobilising white blood cells to engulf the invading organism and destroying it. If a patient's immune system is compromised by diseases such as acquired immune deficiency syndrome (AIDS), they are unable to fend off invading organisms and hence the body is swamped by even more organisms which are regarded as normal flora. Symptoms occur in the respiratory tract, skin or central nervous system.

Antibody production is also a defence mechanism of the body and is the basis for using immunisation as a means of presenting infectious diseases. It is also the means by which effective immunity may be measured in the body by measuring the levels of immunoglobulin to specific antigens, e.g. measles, Ross River virus.

Treatment

A range of antibiotics are used for treatment of bacterial infections depending on the causative agent and possible allergies of the patient, e.g. to penicillin. Viral illnesses in the main are treated with symptomatic remedies only, e.g. paracetamol for headache, antihistamines for runny noses associated with viral infections. Some specific antiviral agents are used for the treatment of herpes infections or HIV.

List of Infections

Brucellosis

Chickenpox

Chlamydia

Cholera

Croup

Cryptosporidium

Dengue fever

Diphtheria

Giardia

Glandular fever

Gonorrhoea

Haemophilus (HIB), Haemophilus

Human papilloma virus (HPV)

influenza

Hand, foot and mouth disease

Helicobacter pylori infection

Herpes simplex infection

Hepatitis A, B, C

Herpes zoster (shingles)

Human immunodeficiency virus (HIV)

Influenza

Leptospirosis

Malaria

Mycoplasma pneumonia

Measles

Meningococcal disease

Molluscum contagiosum

Papilloma virus (HPV)

Pneumococcus

Polio

Q fever

Rabies

Rheumatic fever

Ross River virus

Rubella

Scarlet fever

Shingles

Staphylococcus aureus

Syphilis

Typhoid

Yellow fever

Tetanus

Tuberculosis

Whooping cough

infectious diseases of childhood

See *immunisation for childhood infectious diseases*

infectious diseases of adults

See *cervical cancer*

See *glandular fever*

See *human immunodeficiency virus (HIV)*

See *human papilloma virus (HPV)*

See *immunisation for childhood infectious disease*

See *pregnancy*

See *sexually transmitted diseases*

See *travel medicine*

See *tropical diseases*

It is recommended that adolescent males and females receive a booster for hepatitis B, tetanus, whooping cough, diphtheria, and that adolescent girls are vaccinated for HPV or human papilloma virus.

HPV has been shown to cause cervical cancer where the vast proportion of disease is caused by previous HPV infection, sometimes from an infection contracted during sexual activity. The more sexual partners that an individual may have in a lifetime, the greater chance of contracting a sexually transmitted disease. The greater the risk of contracting sexually transmitted infections including HPV, syphilis, gonorrhoea, Chlamydia, and HIV. Currently, there are no vaccinations for syphilis, gonorrhoea, Chlamydia, and HIV

Adult women under the age of 45 years are encouraged to be vaccinated against HPV, and there are currently 2 brands of vaccination on the market.

There is growing acceptance that adolescent males also be vaccinated with HPV vaccine to help prevent the spread of the disease further including genital warts. There are multiple strains of HPV, some strains of which are associated with cervical cancer, some cause genital warts, and some cause the more common plantar warts.

Women of child bearing age should ensure that their immunity to Rubella is sound before embarking on pregnancy, because of the risk of damage to the foetus if maternal infection with rubella occurs during pregnancy. The expanded rubella syndrome is the name given to the problems resulting for the child who is infected with rubella in utero. These problems are enduring and life-long, and may include profound deafness, vision defects, severe mental handicap, developmental and learning problems, and heart defects.

It is also recommended these days that parents of newborns be vaccinated for whooping cough, and that grandparents who may be caring for the child also receive a booster as soon as possible after the baby is born.

Annual vaccination for influenza virus is recommended for persons with known respiratory problems such as asthma, recurrent bronchitis, bronchiectasis, heart problems, or diabetes. You should be guided by your doctor to determine if you fall into a special category of increased risk of contracting annual influenza.

Travelers to foreign countries are also recommended to protect their health by seeking travel vaccinations advice for a range of infectious diseases before leaving home soil.

Adults over the age of 65 are advised to have a pneumococcal vaccination, and a booster for tetanus, whooping cough, and diphtheria. If adults have received regular boosters for tetanus during their lifetime, the WHO recommendations on immunisation suggest that further vaccinations for tetanus are not required.

People entering health professional careers are often required to provide proof of immunity or supplement their vaccination with updates for infectious diseases.

There is now a vaccination available for adults to prevent shingles. Two administrations of the vaccine are recommended to maximise the immunity response. The virus which causes shingles is called varicella zoster and is the same as that which causes childhood chickenpox.

infertility, female

See *amenorrhoea*
See *contraception*
See *hypothyroidism*
See *intercourse, problems*
See *in-vitro fertilisation*
See *pregnancy problems*
See *sexually transmitted diseases*

Cause

Infertility is a problem for males and females and investigation of infertility includes investigations for both the male and female partner. For a pregnancy to result, intercourse must occur between the couple at around the time of ovulation, with healthy sperm capable of producing a pregnancy.

Infertility may be the result of anovulatory cycles (no egg produced) for the woman or ongoing use of contraception, infrequent intercourse at times other than the fertile period in the cycle , poor sexual technique, the development of antibodies in the female partner to the male partner's sperm.

Other causes for infertility may include thyroid problems, problems of the pituitary gland which regulates the production of both male and female hormones, the presence of sexually transmitted diseases (STDs) in either male or female partner, vaginismus in the female partner where sexual technique is a problem for one of a number of reasons including pain associated with the vaginal penetration (due to either infection with one or more STDs, tight vaginal opening, endometriosis), lack of privacy for the couple, previous treatment with chemotherapy or radiotherapy of either male or female partner.

Issues exist with infertility after 40 years of age for the female partner. While pregnancy does occur after 40 years, fertility rates are considered lower, the risk of chromosomal abnormalities are higher and the risk of miscarriage higher. For the male partner, the problems of increasing age are not as great and men in their sixth and seventh decades are capable of producing a pregnancy as the production of sperm is a continuous process whereas females are born with a ready store of eggs which are not replaced.

Treatment

Treatment for infertility starts with identifying a possible medical cause in both the male and female member of the couple. This should involve a comprehensive history taking from both people. If a cause is identified, corrective measures should be undertaken. Sperm count and analysis should always be part of an investigation to determine the cause of infertility, even if it is thought that the infertility is related to the female partner.

Other measures include establishing a temperature chart in association with a cervical mucus chart in order to determine the most likely time during the female cycle for ovulation. The fertile period during the female cycle occurs when the woman's basal temperature suddenly rises by around one degree, usually mid-cycle, in association with change in the character of the cervical mucus from being thick and sticky to being watery. This window of opportunity will last for only about one to two days on either side of the day of ovulation.

If a pregnancy is not achieved through natural methods, the next step is administering hormonal stimulation to the female partner in the first part of the cycle. This takes the form of prescribing clomiphene tablets, usually for five days from day five to day 10 of the cycle. If after two cycles, a pregnancy has still not been achieved, referral to a fertility specialist should be undertaken. The couple may then require assisted fertility in the form of some form of in-vitro fertilisation or IVF.

Provision of sperm is available from sperm banks located within clinics providing fertility services. The provision of donor eggs is possible; however there is often a problem with supply unless a private arrangement can be made and a source of supply of donor eggs is found.

infertility, male

Infertility is a diagnosis applied to a couple. Male infertility may be due to defects in either sperm production or sperm emission and infertility due to male sperm causes accounts for about 35 per cent of infertility in couples.

There is not a specific infertility test as such, but infertility is said to exist if no pregnancy has occurred in the presence of unprotected vaginal intercourse between a male and female for a period of 12 months.

Cause

Spermatogenesis, the production of sperm, is a continuous process in men but may be affected by genetic disorders, abnormalities affecting the Y chromosome and endocrine abnormalities (of the adrenal gland, thyroid gland or due to hypogonadism), heat, drugs (anabolic steroids, oestrogen medication, alcohol, recreational drugs) resulting in low sperm counts. Low sperm emission may be related to retrograde ejaculation of semen into the bladder, neurological problems, following prostate surgery or a vasectomy, due to cystic fibrosis and the presence of sperm antibodies.

Treatment

Assessment for infertility should always include examination of a semen specimen, in order to determine the morphology of the sperm and the percentage of highly motile sperm which are most likely to produce pregnancy.

Providing no other medical abnormality is present, low sperm counts may be treated by administration of clomiphene daily for 25 days in any month. This may stimulate the production and increase sperm counts as it acts as an anti-oestrogen; however it does not improve sperm motility or morphology. If sperm counts are less than 10 million per mls, the most effective treatment would usually be in-vitro fertilisation or IVF with injections of a single sperm into single eggs. Alternatively intra-uterine insemination may occur using washed semen samples at a time which coincides with ovulation. If the pregnancy is still unable to be achieved, donor sperm may need to be considered.

inflammatory bowel disease

See *abdominal pain*
See *colon problems*
See *Crohn's disease*
See *diarrhoea*
See *irritable colon/bowel*

Cause

Inflammatory bowel disease may present either in adults or children. It includes Crohn's disease, also called regional enteritis or granulomatous ileitis. Ulcerative colitis is an inflammatory disease which affects the mucosa of varying parts of the colon. There may be a family history of inflammatory bowel disease.

Symptoms

Symptoms of inflammatory bowel disease may include diarrhoea, abdominal pain, abscess formation inside the abdomen, fistula formation both inside the abdomen and from the inside of the gut to the outside of the body (e.g. fistula into the vagina from the bowel and bowel obstruction may arise). The diarrhoea, which is bloodstained, may occur along with fever, loss of weight, loss of appetite, abdominal tenderness and a palpable abdominal mass.

Investigations

Investigations include abdominal X-ray and/or CT scan, ultrasound which may demonstrate the addition of gynaecological pathology, endoscopy, barium enema X-ray. A sigmoidoscopy and colonoscopies may assist with the diagnosis.

Treatment

Treatment of inflammatory bowel disease may require surgery in the presence of a fistula or perforation of the gut. Corticosteroids will be required to reduce the inflammation in the gut; these may be administered orally, by injection or rectally. In addition, other disease-specific medication may be required in order to reduce the inflammation, i.e. methotrexate, azothiaprine.

influenza *(flu)*

Cause

Influenza or flu as it is commonly called, is a viral illness which is highly infectious and can spread from person to person rapidly.

Symptoms

Runny nose, fever, muscular aches and pains, headache are all symptoms of flu.

Treatment

As it is a viral illness, treatment for flu is limited but some response to antiviral agents occurs if they are used early in the disease, e.g. oseltamivir phosphate.

Treatment is mainly symptomatic, i.e. pain relief, decongestants, steam inhalation, nose blowing and fluids. Not infrequently, what starts out as a viral respiratory infection may be further complicated by bacterial infection with the development of coloured sputum, which may be yellow, green or bloodstained. At this time it is appropriate to intervene with treatment in the form of antibiotics, as the viral infection has now been superseded with a bacterial infection.

ingrown toenails

Cause

Ingrown toenails are caused by an incurving of the growing part of the toenail, most commonly the big toe. Other causes may include tight shoes. Some people have a predisposition to ingrown toenails due to the shape of their toes.

Symptoms

Symptoms may include infection, discharge, pain, redness and swelling of the toes.

Treatment

Treatment includes correcting tight footwear and pedicure technique and attention to foot hygiene. If these measures fail, treatment might also include antibiotics, bathing with a betadine solution and wedge resection of the toenail.

injuries to the ligaments

Bursitis

See *gout*
See *psoriasis*
See *rheumatoid arthritis*

insect bites

Cause

Bites and stings may include bees, wasps ,yellow jackets and hornets.

Symptoms

Insect bites are particularly problematic to the skin and cause immediate burning, pain, swelling and redness of the area which sometimes may last for several days.

Treatment

If stingers are still present they should be removed as quickly as possible without further injecting venom into the skin. This may be done by placing a sharp knife flat on the skin and running it carefully towards the stinger, thus lifting it out of the skin. Ice may be applied to the skin and the patient given antihistamines as required. Some people with known hypersensitivity reactions to certain insects may be required to carry with them an Epipen for possible stinging by certain insects.

insomnia

See *anxiety*

See *depression*

Cause

Insomnia is the inability to achieve sleep or difficulty staying asleep. Causes include inattention to sleep hygiene, psychological factors, e.g. everyday worries, anxiety and depression. Sleep apnoea, circadian rhythm disturbances, sleep disorders are also common to shift workers and travellers crossing time zones.

Other factors which cause insomnia include smoking, drinks containing caffeine, some cold and flu preparations, a noisy environment in the proximity of the bedroom, physical pain and certain prescribed medications.

Treatment

Treating insomnia requires attention to maintaining a regular sleep schedule; restrictions of time in bed, i.e. if the person is unable to sleep for 20 minutes they should get out of bed and return to bed when sleepy; avoid daytime naps; have a regular bedtime routine, e.g. bathing, brushing teeth; making the bedroom conducive to sleeping; attention to a comfortable bed and pillows; climate control in the bedroom; regular exercise but not in the evening before bed; relaxation techniques; avoidance of caffeine and other stimulant type foods, e.g. chocolate; quitting smoking; and bright light exposure during the day.

intercourse, problems

See *atrophic vaginitis*
See *cervical cancer*
See *erectile dysfunction or impotence*
See *menopause problems*
See *premature ejaculation*
See *sexually transmitted diseases*
See *urinary tract infections*
See *vaginal discharge*

Cause

Problems with sexual intercourse, called dyspareunia, may occur as a result of virginity; tight vaginal opening; inexperience of the sexual couple; infection either due to localised infections around the genital area, including herpes simplex virus, bacterial infection, thrush or sexually transmitted diseases (STDs); urinary tract infection; fear of pregnancy; lack of oestrogen in the vagina (which is called atrophic vaginitis and usually occurs in women following the menopause or leading up to menopause); immediately or in the early weeks following the delivery of a child; endometriosis; the presence of fibroids; retroversion of the uterus; cancer of the cervix or uterus or ovaries; or ectopic pregnancy.

Men may also experience problems with intercourse including erectile dysfunction; premature ejaculation; sexual inexperience; or problems due to pain associated with sexually transmitted disease or urinary tract infection. Men may also experience discomfort with trauma to the frenulum of the foreskin due to the effects of friction and microabrasion to the penis during intercourse.

Treatment

Talking to the woman and man separately and talking to them as a couple will often reveal the source of the problem. Examination of both partners is important and treatment will depend on the nature of the problem.

intussusception

Cause

By definition, an intussusception occurs when a piece of gut folds in on itself and proceeds to move along the gut taking another fold of gut with it.

Symptoms

An intussusception invariably leads to an obstruction of the gut, associated with severe intermittent waves of pain. These obstructions may occur in the large or small gut and most commonly occur in children.

Treatment

An intussusception can be relieved by barium enema or colonoscopy if the large bowel is involved, but if other areas of the gut are involved surgery may be required.

in-vitro fertilisation *(IVF)*

See *infertility*
  - *male*
  - *female*

In-vitro fertilisation is a form of assisted fertility and means adding sperm to an ovum in a test tube or at least outside the human body. Sperm and eggs are harvested from the male and from the female partners, added together in the laboratory and inserted back into the uterus under controlled conditions. Various techniques are available to assist fertility including artificial insemination and directly injecting the sperm of the male partner into the egg of the female partner. This latter technique takes a great deal of precision and is done with the assistance of a microscope. It is possible to sample the cells of the embryo at a stage when it consists of only a few cells to test for the presence of inherited genetic defects. This is also a highly skilled procedure and is surrounded by many moral and ethical issues.

iron deficiency

See *colon cancer*

Cause

Iron deficiency is common in infants, adolescent girls and pregnant women and may result from inadequate intake of iron-containing food or blood loss. Women will have greater iron intake needs during pregnancy and breastfeeding. Blood loss may be due to internal bleeding such as haemorrhoids or from consistent small amounts of blood loss due to illnesses such as colon cancer. A common cause of iron deficiency in women is menstrual blood loss.

Symptoms

Iron deficiency anaemia results from lack of iron. The patient may complain of feeling tired, lethargic, run-down and having no energy. They may even complain of breathlessness on exertion. Patients with coexistent morbidities, e.g. heart disease, may find that their symptoms are worse in the presence of iron deficiency and resulting anaemia, as the heart has to work harder to pump enough blood to the tissues for oxygenation.

Treatment

Treatment for minor iron deficiency includes attention to daily diet, dietary supplementation with iron preparations and investigation for blood loss from the body.

irritable colon/bowel

See *abdominal pain*
See *colon cancer*
See *colon problems*
See *inflammatory bowel disease*

Cause

Irritable colon or irritable bowel disease is defined as a clinical history of three months of abdominal pain in association with altered bowel habit without proven abnormality on investigation. Irritable bowel or irritable colon is the disease of exclusion of other conditions.

Symptoms

Symptoms include cramping, lower abdominal pain, frequent passage of bowel motions which may be described as ribbon-like in appearance, the passing of wind and a feeling of needing to pass bowel motions frequently. Symptoms may be precipitated by eating, followed by symptoms of bloating and abdominal distension. Stress for any reason may increase the symptoms.

Treatment

Treatment for irritable bowel is based on controlling the symptoms, i.e. identifying that certain foods may produce symptoms, managing stress-related episodes, careful attention to diet including alcohol and beverage intake, and ceasing smoking. Symptomatic relief may be provided by the use of anti-diarrhoea preparations, e.g. lomotil and consideration should be given to a trial of a mild antidepressant to help control stress symptoms.

ischaemic colitis

See *abdominal pain*

Cause

Ischaemic colitis occurs in elderly patients where an obstruction exists to the artery supplying blood to the gut.

Symptoms

Severe sharp, intermittent abdominal pain may occur sometimes in the presence of blood-stained diarrhoea. The pain may be more common after eating a meal. The pain is situated around the belly button. This may be a very difficult diagnosis to make and sometimes gangrene of the gut may result before diagnosis has been made.

Investigations

Investigation is aimed at demonstrating an obstruction to the artery supplying the gut. This may be done by injecting dye into the artery suspected of being obstructed.

Treatment

Treatment will require relieving the obstruction to the vessel supplying the area of gut.

jaundice

See *liver problems*

Cause

Jaundice is a physical finding, not a diagnosis. Jaundice or yellowing of the skin is caused by excess amounts of bilirubin in the body and comes about either from infection (hepatitis A, B, C; septicaemia; other viral infections, e.g. glandular fever), blockage of the bile ducts (e.g. gallstones or malignancy), excess alcohol causing cirrhosis of the liver, drug reactions, fatty liver, haemochromatosis (which is an abnormality of iron), or malignancy of the liver, gall bladder, pancreas and biliary ducts; and from secondary deposits from e.g. cancer of the bowel.

Neonatal jaundice may occur and every newborn is assessed for this symptom. Prematurity increases the risk of neonatal hyperbilirubinaemia and consequently the risk of neonatal jaundice. Marked neonatal hyperbilirubinaemia can cause kernicterus, which is a syndrome associated with neurological damage in the newborn. Severe kernicterus may occur in babies where there is Rhesus incompatibility between the mother who is Rhesus negative and the baby who is Rhesus positive. Brain damage with severe physical developmental abnormalities and disabilities may occur in these babies and even death as a result of brain damage.

Symptoms

Investigations to determine the cause of the jaundice includes a full blood count, liver function tests, tests for hepatitis A, B, C and an abdominal ultrasound or CT scan.

Patients with gallstones may present with several abdominal pains in the upper right side of the abdomen, in association with nausea, vomiting. If the biliary system is completely obstructed, the patient my have pale, chalky-white bowel motions.

Treatment

Depending on the cause, jaundice should settle with appropriate treatment, e.g. removal of gallstones, ceasing alcohol, withdrawal of drug which may be causing the jaundice, appropriate treatment for malignancy. On some occasions, stenting the obstructed bile duct may be necessary in order to relieve the obstruction causing the jaundice, e.g. in cases of cancer of the biliary system.

Treatment of neonatal hyperbilirubinaemia is done with the use of photo therapy and if the condition is severe, an exchange transfusion may be necessary. Prenatal diagnosis of Rhesus incompatibility improves the outcome for the baby of a mother with Rhesus incompatibility.

jet lag

See *colon problems*
See *travel medicine problems*

Cause

Jet lag is caused by rapid travel across more than two time zones. The body has a natural day/ night pattern of being awake or asleep. If this rhythm is rapidly changed, the traveller will feel sleepy during daylight hours and wakeful at night. The normal pattern of sleep and awake should return within a few days.

Treatment

If possible, travellers should start to modify their awake/sleep pattern prior to travel. Short-acting sleeping tablets are worthwhile for brief periods after arrival at a destination.

jock itch/rash

Cause

Jock itch is caused by an infection and environmental factors, e.g. warm weather and restrictive clothing, obesity and with skin surfaces rubbing together.

Symptoms

Men are commonly more affected than women because of the close approximation of the scrotum and thigh. The area may become red, itchy and infected with bacteria or fungal agents.

Treatment

Treatment for jock itch or rash includes topical antifungal agents, e.g. miconazole, ketoconazole, econazole, for 10 to 14 days.

keloid scar

Cause

Keloid scars are a manifestation of pink overgrowth of fibrous tissue arising in an area of an injury or a surgical scar. Some people are more prone to keloid scar formation than others.

Symptoms

Keloid scars are shiny, smooth and dome-shaped in appearance.

Treatment

Treatment for keloid scars involves the application of long-term pressure to the area involved. Some improvement may be achieved by injection of the area using steroids.

keratoacanthoma

Cause

Keratoacanthoma is a type of skin cancer but it is one of the least harmful types of skin cancer.

Symptoms

This type of skin cancer presents as a round, firm, pinkish coloured nodule, often with a central depression.

Treatment

Sometimes these lesions will regress spontaneously and on occasions they have been known to grow rapidly to form very large lesions which then need excision. Sometimes skin grafting of the area involved is extensive. Patients will often want these lesions removed simply for cosmetic benefit.

keratoses *(skin condition)*

See *seborrhoeic keratoses*
See *solar keratoses*

kidney cancer

Cause

The cause of kidney (or renal cell) cancer is unknown; however risk factors include smoking, exposure to asbestos and cadmium, family history, a high-fat diet and obesity. Men are twice as likely to get renal cell cancer as are women.

Symptoms

Carcinoma of the kidney is a notoriously silent disease. Detection of cancer of the kidney may occur incidentally during investigation of abdominal pain or during investigation for hypertension. Other symptoms may include blood in the urine, pain in the loins, a palpable abdominal mass, an obstruction to the kidney or bladder (which may cause renal failure).

Treatment

Treatment for cancer of the kidney is surgical removal of the kidney. The survival rate is not improved by radiation or chemotherapy. Treatment for bladder cancer includes surgical treatment, inplants to bypass the obstruction and chemotherapy.

kidney disorders

See *glomerulonephritis*

kidney/renal failure

Cause

Renal failure may be defined as an acute or chronic decrease in kidney function which causes a build-up of by-products in the body from metabolism as well as fluid build-up.

Acute renal failure may be caused by a sudden loss of large amounts of body fluid, low cardiac output, problems such as septicaemia, liver failure, antihypertensive agents, increased vascular resistance due to the presence of obstruction of the renal artery, thrombosis of a renal vein. It may also be caused by prolonged ischaemia (or lack of oxygen) in the kidney, acute glomerulonephritis and problems such as leukaemia, lymphoma and sarcoid or sarciodosis.

Other causes include precipitation of material in the tubules either due to tumours or stones, obstruction of the ureter and obstruction to the bladder due to a build-up of pressure in the kidney, e.g. prostatic hyperplasia or cancer, bladder cancer, obstruction to the urethra, e.g. by stricture formation.

Chronic renal failure may be caused by diabetes, post-infectious glomerulonephritis, hereditary conditions, hypertension and obstruction to the kidney.

Glomerulonephritis occurs following an infection, most commonly group A beta-haemolytic streptococcus. The diagnosis is suggested by the history and examination of the urine. The prognosis for recovery is usually excellent and treatment is simply supportive until the kidneys recover.

Other types of glomerular disease exist and are termed nephritic syndrome (or conditions of blood and urinary sediment in association with proteins in the urine, oedema, hypertension, elevated creatinine and small urinary output) or nephrotic syndrome which occurs, for instance, in the presence of diabetes and relates to excretion in the urine of large amounts of proteins on a daily basis.

Diabetic nephropathy is a glomerular abnormality of increasing fibrosis associated with metabolic and haemodynamic changes of diabetes. It is slowly progressive and is associated with an increase in hypertension and an increasing degree of renal failure.

Analgesic nephropathy occurs where damage to the kidneys results from a large intake over a prolonged period of time of certain analgesic compounds.

Toxic changes in the kidneys may result from exposure to various heavy metals, in particular lead, resulting in lead nephropathy. Lead used to be a common component in house paint and breakdown of paint on the exterior of houses mixed with rainwater produces run-off and results in excessive amounts of lead exposure. Lead has now been discontinued as a component to house paint; however in many older homes lead paint can still be evident.

Reflux nephropathy is the scarring of the kidneys resulting from reflux of urine from the bladder into the ureter with a back-up of pressure around the pelvis of the kidney.

Symptoms

Symptoms of renal failure include nausea, vomiting, loss of appetite, alterations of conscious state if the condition is left untreated and alterations in fluid and electrolyte balance in the body.

Treatment

Treatment for renal failure is aimed at the cause and involves careful attention to fluid and electrolyte management of the body and either short- or long-term dialysis either until the kidneys recover or until such time as renal transplantation occurs.

kidney stones

See *renal stones*

knee pain or patello-femoral syndrome

See *knock knees*
See *osteoarthritis*
See *pigeon toes*

Patello-femoral syndrome

Cause

Fractures and dislocations may be caused by osteoarthritis, injuries to the ligaments (including the cruciate ligaments and tears in the capsule of the knee joint, tears to the menisci), bursitis, fractures and dislocations of the knee and patella and patello-femoral syndrome, knock knees and pigeon toes. Pain in the knee may be associated with a more general physical cause, e.g. rheumatoid arthritis, gout, psoriasis. Osgood-Schlatter disease is a condition common in teens which is often made worse with sporting activities.

Symptoms

Pain may be experienced in the front, back or on either side of the knee. Pain on movement, walking or while lying in bed may occur. Pain may be associated with localised swelling and tenderness of the knee, increased temperature of the knee and redness or bruising to the knee. Localised tenderness to the knee may occur with Osgood-Schlatter disease, menisci injuries, bursitis and patella conditions.

Treatment

Treatment for various injuries including injuries to the ligaments, fractures and dislocations may need referral to an orthopaedic surgeon. Pain relief is important and some improvement may be made with non-steroidal anti-inflammatory preparations as well as appropriate physiotherapy to the knee. Treatment for Osgood-Schlatter disease is aimed at reducing the amount of irritation to the knee which may limit the amount of physical activity for a period of time. A combination of heat and cold packs will also help.

knock knees

Cause

Knock knees and pigeon toes are a manifestation of a mechanical variation of the alignment of the lower limbs occurring in childhood.

Symptoms

Symptoms may include pains in the knees and discomfort in the lower limbs. Often the mother will notice their child's legs are not straight or that the child sustains lots of falls or is clumsy.

Treatment

Treatment for knock knees and pigeon toes may be achieved by changing the child's sitting posture when sitting on the floor, from sitting in a position where the legs splayed to the side to a position of sitting cross-legged on the floor. Given time, knock knees and pigeon toes will usually resolve spontaneously. If knock knees are particularly pronounced, some cases may involve correction by orthopaedic surgery with osteotomy and re-alignment of the bones in the lower legs. Alternatively a build-up on the soles of the shoes may help to correct the problem.

laryngitis

Cause

Laryngitis is an inflammation of the larynx caused by either a viral infection or by acute or chronic overuse causing hoarseness of the voice.

Symptoms

Symptoms include hoarseness of the voice, with decreased volume. This may be accompanied by an uncomfortable feeling at the back of the throat and may be accompanied by fever, malaise, pain on swallowing and pain in the throat. If hoarseness of the voice occurs for greater than three weeks, investigation by laryngoscopy is necessary in order to eliminate a more serious cause for the hoarseness.

Treatment

Acute viral laryngitis requires only symptomatic treatment and is a self-limiting conditions involving resting of the vocal cords, i.e. minimisation of speaking, warm drinks and if necessary, pain relief.

leg pains

Cause

Pains in the legs may be caused by musculoskeletal problems, problems relating to inactivity, tumours and vascular problems.

Pains caused by musculoskeletal problems include trauma to the legs, which include fractures and sprains and osteoporosis.

Inflammatory causes include Osgood-Schlatter disease, rheumatoid arthritis, osteoarthritis of the hip and knee, tendonitis, osteoarthritis.

Muscle cramps are a common cause for pains in the legs and there are many causes which may lead to cramps.

Infection such as osteomyelitis and septic arthritis may lead to pain in the legs.

Nerve irritation and compression caused by sciatica may lead to pains in the legs as a result of disease of the intervertebral disc, osteophyte formation, narrowing of the spinal canal.

Tumours such as myeloma which is a malignancy of plasma cells in the blood and Ewing's tumour, may cause pain is the legs. The cause of Ewing's tumour is unknown.

Vascular disease in the form of deep venous thrombosis and arterial blockage cause significant problems with pain in the legs. Deep venous thrombosis presents in the deep veins of the legs, usually in the lower legs and results from impaired venous return of blood from the lower legs and back to the heart. Arterial blockage caused by atherosclerosis in the lower extremities causing ischaemia or poor circulation to the tissues is called claudication and commonly occurs during exercise; the distance a patient can walk may indicate the severity of the blockage.

Symptoms

Pain may be associated with swelling and tenderness which may be localised or widespread or worse on exercise or with rest, or may be constant. Coexistent medical problems will help make the diagnosis as will the history of the pain.

Musculoskeletal causes for pain in the leg such as fractures are often diagnosed with the assistance of a history of trauma and the presence of localised tenderness, swelling and bruising. The presence of a fracture may be determined by performing an X-ray, CT scan or an MRI scan.

Osteoporosis is more common in the older population for both men and women. The risk of osteoporosis increases in postmenopausal women and if present in men tends to be more severe.

Symptoms associated with inflammatory conditions such as rheumatoid arthritis and osteo-arthritis may also be diagnosed partly on the history of the condition, the examination of the joint concerned and X-ray confirmation.

The presence of muscular cramps in a patient may warrant further investigation to eliminate the possibility of vascular blockage, diabetes or electrolyte imbalances. Pathology tests and Doppler studies of the vessels will clarify this diagnosis.

Suspicion of infections such as osteomyelitis or septic arthritis may be made using CT examination.

Sciatica is a condition involving compression of the sciatic nerve and producing pain along the length of the sciatic nerve, in the lower back which causes low back pain, referred pain into the leg and knee.

Myeloma causes symptoms of bone pain, renal insufficiency, anaemia, recurrent infections and an increase in serum calcium.

Ewing's tumours are accompanied by pain and swelling in the affected bone and are more common in the age group of under 20 years and are usually very aggressive tumours.

Deep venous thromboses may be asymptomatic or produce pain and swelling in the affected limb. Deep venous thromboses or DVT are a risk for travellers on long distance travel and for some people with clotting disorders which increase their risk of clotting, e.g. factor V Leiden which is an inherited condition. Patients with arterial blockage are more common in the older age group and patients with other forms of cardiovascular disease, diabetes, high cholesterol and obesity.

Treatment

Fractures whether due to trauma or osteoporosis will be diagnosed with the aid of an X-ray, CT scan, bone scan or MRI and treatment using appropriate splinting.

Treatment for other injuries may be improved by a combination of nonsteroidal anti-inflammatory preparations as well as the non-invasive measures such as ice, rest, elevation, physiotherapy and heat packs at night. Simple analgesia will also improve the symptoms.

Treatment for inflammatory conditions includes analgesia, nonsteroidal anti-inflammatory preparations, heat, rest, physiotherapy.

Treatment for rheumatoid arthritis, osteoarthritis and sciatica pain includes similar physical measures, nonsteroidal anti-inflammatory preparations to reduce symptoms and disease modifying anti-arthritic drugs which slow the progression of the disease.

Treatment for myeloma first involves making the diagnosis which may necessitate a bone marrow biopsy to identify the abnormal cells in the bone marrow. Specific treatment includes chemotherapy in association with corticosteroids and blood stem cell transplantation.

Treatment for Ewing's tumour includes a combination of surgery (often amputation), chemotherapy and radiation therapy and most patients with Ewing's tumour will require more than one form of treatment in order to eradicate the tumour.

Treatment for deep venous thromboses (DVT) includes anticoagulant preparations.

Treatment of peripheral vascular disease or arterial stenosis includes minimisation of risk factors, exercise, anti-platelet drugs. Severe peripheral vascular disease may require surgery in the form of angioplasty in order to open the narrowed arteries or surgical bypass of the stenosis and as a last resort, amputation of a portion of the limb may be required in order to minimise symptoms of pain and the possibility of gangrene.

Treatment for factor V Leiden condition involves being suspicious if patients with the condition present with pain in the lower limbs. They may require anticoagulant medication either by injection or by oral administration. The risk in these people for pulmonary embolism if untreated is high and death could occur.

leptospirosis

Cause

Leptospirosis is caused by an organism called a spirochete. Human infection is acquired by contact with infected animals, both domestic and wild, such as rats in canefields.

Symptoms

The disease is characterised by headache, severe muscular aches and pains, chills, fever, conjunctival irritation, enlargement of the spleen and liver and sometimes signs of meningitis. Jaundice may occur in severe cases of the disease, and blood in the urine may occur.

Treatment

Penicillin or doxycycline is recommended. Isolation is not required.

leukaemia

Cause

Leukaemia is defined as cancer of the white blood cells in the bone marrow. It can be divided into acute (myeloid, lymphoid) and chronic disorders (most commonly myeloid and lymphocytic). Age differences occur amongst the different types of leukaemia, namely children present more commonly with acute lymphocytic leukaemia and adults in middle and old age present with chronic lymphocytic leukaemia.

Acute myeloid leukaemia may present at any age, while chronic myeloid leukaemia is more common in young adulthood. Risk of developing leukaemia increases with a history of exposure to ionising radiation, chemicals, infection with certain viral agents, e.g. Epstein Barr, chromosomal trans-locations, immunodeficiency disorders, myeloma proliferative disorders, Down syndrome and certain X-linked disorders. Leukaemias are classified from two different lines of white blood cells—lymphocytic leukaemia and myeloid leukaemia. Anaemia results from reduced red cell production as white cell production takes over the activity in the bone marrow.

Symptoms

The most commonly presenting symptoms in leukaemia include anaemia, infection, easy bruising and bleeding. Other symptoms include fatigue, fever, weight loss, malaise, tachycardia, chest pain which may be attributed to the anaemia and hypermetabolic state.

Bone marrow involvement may produce bone pain and central nervous system involvement may produce evidence of meningitis with headaches, vomiting, irritability, seizures and weakness of various cranial nerves. Enlargement of lymph nodes, spleen and liver is also found.

Diagnosis of leukaemia is by examining the peripheral blood smear in the pathology laboratory. Although the diagnosis can often be made by examining peripheral blood smear, bone marrow aspiration is usually recommended in order to assess the activity of new cell formation in the bone marrow. Prognosis for any type of leukaemia is worst in the very young and the elderly and in those patients with liver, kidney, or central nervous system involvement for a very high white blood cell count.

Treatment

Treatment for myeloid and lymphocytic leukaemia is aimed at producing total remission and restoration of normal blood counts and production of white cells in the bone marrow. Treatment will usually take the form of chemotherapy with intravenous medications such as vincristine, anthracycline or asparaginase. Other drug combinations include cyclophosphomide, methotrexate. Allogenic stem cell transplantation may also be recommended.

libido

Cause

The term libido relates to a sexual drive in men and women. The sex drive or libido is a function attended by the brain. Factors which interfere with the sex drive may include a rushed, busy life, the presence of existing children, pregnancy, illness for either male or female member of the couple (including psychiatric illness, depression, anxiety), diseases of the pituitary gland (including stroke, tumour, cancer), tumours of the adrenal glands resulting in overproduction of the steroid hormones in the body, prescriptions and over-the-counter medication including alcohol, smoking cigarettes or marijuana, sedatives, antidepressant medications, blood pressure medications, cold and flu medications, diabetes, onset of menopause, and prostate problems in men.

Rarely do people complain of excess sex drive unless it occurs in a situation where the sex drive of one member of the couple does not match the sex drive of the other. This can sometimes be a difficult problem to manage and will often require some compromise by each member of the couple.

Treatment

Patients who present complaining of problems with their libido often need the general practitioner to spend time with them to obtain a full picture of their daily life and expectations from their sex life. Investigations should be undertaken in order to rule out the possibility of any underlying medical reasons for their lack of libido. If no cause is found, explanation should be given to the individual or the couple regarding ways of improving their sex life, which may include such things as the couple spending more time together with each other, in private away from the stresses of busy life and family life. People may underestimate the importance today of relaxation time and recreation time, and need to ensure that adequate time is provided to undertake sexual activity.

lice

Cause
Head and body lice are caused by a parasite known as Pediculus humanus capitus, corporis and pubis which are transmitted from person to person by close body contact.

Symptoms
Lice are wingless bloodsucking insects which may cause local irritation, itching and a rash on the skin where the insects are located. Head lice may infect the head and eyelashes and even the beard in men.

Treatment
Treatment to eradicate head and body lice and scabies include a number of topical preparations available over the counter at chemists and include Permethrin, Lindane, Malthion, Permewthrin, Pyrethryins. For treatment of the eyelashes, either Fluorescein drops or petrolatum ointment may be applied.

liver problems

See *abdominal pain*
See *alcohol*
See *cirrhosis*
See *cystic fibrosis*
See *diabetes*
See *haemochromatosis*
See *heart failure*
See *hepatitis*

Cause
The liver is regarded as the powerhouse of the body where processing of absorbed food material occurs, and breaking down of many drugs occurs prior to being excreted from the

body either by the gut or by the kidney. The liver also produces bile salts which aid in the absorption of fats from the gut. Abnormalities may occur with production of gastric juices in the case of cystic fibrosis and cancer of the liver and pancreas, resulting in malabsorption of food material from the intestine into the body.

Diseases of the liver are many and the most commonly occurring conditions affecting the liver include tumours of the liver, cancer (either primary liver cancer or secondary cancer from tumours occurring in other parts of the body), haemochromatosis (which is an inherited condition associated with abnormality of iron storage), cirrhosis of the liver (most commonly from excess prolonged intake of alcohol), infections of the liver, e.g. hepatitis, fatty liver (which may occur in association with obesity and Type 2 diabetes), jaundice, thalassaemia (which is an inherited condition in Mediterranean countries, which results in increased fragility of the red blood cells which break down more rapidly and overload the liver's ability to process the breakdown products of the red blood cells).

Enlargement of the liver may occur in association with heart failure. Primary cancer of the liver usually occurs in patients with cirrhosis and is common when hepatitis B and C viruses are diagnosed. Cirrhosis of the liver may be caused by excess alcohol consumption, infection of the liver with hepatitis B and C, and chronic inflammatory liver conditions.

Symptoms

Symptoms of liver disease may include nausea, vomiting, jaundice, abdominal pain, abdominal distension, tiredness, lethargy, clotting disorders resulting in an increase in bruising to the skin. Symptoms of liver cancer may include abdominal pain in the right upper abdominal area, weight loss and physical deterioration in a patient known to have cirrhosis of the liver, fever, peritonitis, low blood sugar, a high calcium level, high cholesterol and high triglyceride levels.

Investigations

CT scan, ultrasound and MRI (magnetic resonance imaging) are all ways of identifying a primary liver cancer. Pathology testing for liver function tests is also essential.

Treatment

Treatment of liver disorders is aimed at treating the causative agent. If the liver cancer is less than two centimetres in diameter and is localised to a confined area of the liver, a two-year survival rate for liver cancer is still less than five per cent. Surgical resection of the cancer is possible as is injection of the tumour using special techniques; however they do not increase the life expectancy.

lung abscess

See *bronchiectasis*
See *cystic fibrosis*
See *lung cancer*
See *pneumonia*

Cause

Most lung abscesses develop from aspiration of oral secretions by patients with poor oral hygiene, alcohol intoxication, ingestion of illicit drugs, patients who have undergone anaesthetics or patients who are on sedative or opioid medication. They may also result from bronchial obstruction due to lung cancer or chronic lung infection.

Symptoms

Symptoms include persistent cough, fever, pain, sweating and weight loss, and sputum may be thick and tenacious, offensive or bloodstained.

Treatment

Diagnosis of a lung abscess is based on clinical suspicion based on the history and physical examination, chest X-ray investigation and sputum culture. Treatment for a lung abscess will require administration of intravenous antibiotics, most commonly penicillin-based antibiotic depending on the sensitivity of the organism which is isolated. On occasions, a lung abscess may require surgical intervention.

lung cancer

See *smoking*

Cancer of the lung may present as a primary lung cancer or as the site of secondary deposits from many other sites.

Cause

Smoking is the cause of most lung cancer, including some people who develop lung cancer from heavy secondary or side stream exposure to cigarette smoke. Some people may be exposed to environmental agents which increase their risk of lung cancer from asbestos, radiation, arsenic, chromates, nickel and coke oven emissions. The role of air pollution in the development of lung cancer is uncertain.

Symptoms

Symptoms of lung cancer include coughing, with or without blood, sputum production which is profuse and/or watery, bleeding from the lung with or without sputum (haemoptysis), collapse of a portion of the lung, localised wheezing.

If an obstruction occurs, infection produces fever. Chest pains, weight loss and fluid in the chest cavity may also occur. Late symptoms include weight loss and weakness. Different types of primary lung cancer exist, e.g. bronchogenic carcinoma, small cell lung cancer which spreads early in the disease and non-small cell lung cancer.

Treatment

Investigations for cancer of the lung include study of the cells in the sputum, CT of the chest, broncoscopy, biopsy of the tumour, exploratory operation of the thorax (called a thoracotomy or mediastinoscopy). Staging of the cancer is important by assessing its spread to the lymph nodes. Treatment of the tumour includes excision, followed by chemotherapy and/or radiation therapy. Cancer of the lung is particularly aggressive in elderly patients, with an average survival time of less than eight months if untreated.

lung function tests, abnormalities

See *asthma*
See *bronchiectasis*
See *bronchitis*
See *chronic obstructive airway disease (COAD)*

Cause

Lung function tests provide measures of lung volumes, gaseous exchange, function of restricting muscles, and flow rates of gases in and out of the lungs. Basic lung function tests may be carried out in the general practitioner's surgery and include spirometry and pulse oximetry (which is measured by placing a sensor usually on a finger and measures oxygen saturation of the blood. This is able to give an immediate readout of the oxygen carrying capacity in the blood).

Spirometry measures a number of important markers for lung function including a forced expiratory volume (FEV1), which is the measure of the volume of air expelled from the lungs during the first second of expiration. This test is especially useful in diagnosing and monitoring patients with obstructive pulmonary disease. The forced vital capacity (FVC) is the maximum amount of air that the patient can forcibly exhale. The peak expiratory flow (PEF) is the peak flow occurring during expiration and is used primarily for home monitoring of patients with asthma and for the detection of variations in asthma status and chronic obstructive airway disease and bronchiectasis.

Symptoms

Interpretation of these lung function tests depends on maximal effort by the patient on a consistent basis to produce reliable and reproducible assessment of lung function.

The measurement of the forced expiratory volume in the first second FEV1 and forced vital capacity (FVC) are important in distinguishing between obstructive lung conditions, e.g. asthma and restrictive lung diseases (which may be caused by loss of lung volume following partial resection of lung because of, e.g. lung cancer, bronchiectasis, lung abscess; abnormalities of structures surrounding the lung, e.g. pleural disease, kyphosis or obesity; weakness of the muscles of respiration, e.g. in neuromuscular disease; and abnormalities of the lung tissue, e.g. pulmonary fibrosis. These features are manifestations of reduced compliance or flexibility of the lung, chest wall or both.

In obstructive lung conditions as in asthma the forced expiratory volume in the first second (FEV1) and the forced expiratory volume in the first second (FEV1) divided by the forced vital capacity (FVC) are both reduced.

In restrictive lung disorders, the forced expiratory volume in the first second (FEV1) may be increased, decreased or normal, whereas the forced expiratory volume in the first second (FEV1) divided by the forced vital capacity (FVC) ratio may be increased or normal.

lymphoma

Cause

Lymphomas are a group of cancers arising in the lymphatic system of the body. The major types are called Hodgkin's lymphoma and non-Hodgkin's lymphoma. Hodgkin's lymphoma primarily involves lymph node tissue, spleen, liver and bone marrow.

Symptoms

Symptoms include painless enlargement of the lymph nodes, with fever, night sweats, unexplained weight loss, itching of the skin and hepato-spleno-megaly (enlargement of the liver and spleen). Diagnosis of lymphoma is based on chest X-ray findings followed by lymph node biopsy. There are a number of differences between Hodgkin's and non-Hodgkin's lymphoma, namely Hodgkin's lymphoma is localised to a specific group of nodes, whereas non-Hodgkin's lymphoma may be disseminated throughout the body, Hodgkin's lymphoma may be diagnosed at an early stage whereas non-Hodgkin's lymphoma may be well advanced at the time of diagnosis. Hodgkin's lymphoma tends to occur more commonly in children and have a more favourable outcome, whereas non-Hodgkin's lymphoma in children will usually be of high grade with a less favourable outcome.

Treatment

Chemotherapy and radiotherapy are used for treatment of lymphomas.

malaria

See *tropical diseases*

Cause

Malaria occurs in the tropics and is spread by an Anopheles mosquito. Infection with plasmodium is the causative agent, which comes in a number of species: falciparum, malariae, ovale and vivax.

Symptoms

The incubation period for infection varies with the type of the organism which is infected and ranges from 10 to 35 days. Symptoms include fever, headache, pains, chills and sweating. The fever will tend to come and go with a periodicity characteristic of the type of the plasmodium. The fever will last from one to eight hours and the patient will feel well until the next bout of fever. The paroxysms occur regularly over a period of 36 to 48 hours.

Treatment

Infection with malaria may be life-threatening and patients need urgent assessment with onset of the fever and a suspicion of the disease if they have been to an infected area in the preceding couple of weeks. Treatment will depend on the type of plasmodium identified, as drug resistance has emerged by the organism. Treatment of an acute attack includes quinine or tetracycline medications.

male reproductive system

See *erectile dysfunction or impotence*
See *haematospermia*
See *infertility, male*
See *penile disorders*
See *Peyronie's disease*
See *phimosis, paraphimosis*
See *priapism*
See *prostatic hyperplasia, benign*
See *scrotal mass*
See *testicular and epididymis infections*

See *testicular cancer and tumours*
See *undescended testes*

mastitis

See *breast infection*

mastoiditis

See *ear problems*
See *otitis media*

Cause

Mastoiditis is a bacterial infection of the mastoid air cells, which can follow an acute middle ear infection.

Symptoms

Symptoms include pain, tenderness, redness, swelling localised behind the ear over the mastoid bone. Pain may occur during weeks following a middle ear infection and be accompanied by fever and continuous throbbing in the area. The diagnosis is made on the clinical history and physical finding.

Investigations

Investigations may include CT scan of the mastoid air sinus, swab from the middle ear.

Treatment

Intravenous antibiotics are essential treatment of acute mastoiditis and may be followed up with oral medication for a period of time. If an abscess develops in the mastoid bone, surgical drainage may be required.

measles

Measles is a viral infection which is highly infectious and easily transferred from one patient to another who does not have immunity to the disease.

Symptoms

Measles infection is characterised by fever, cough, sore eyes, conjunctivitis, characteristic spots in the mouth and characteristic rash of the body. The diagnosis is usually a clinical one.

In children, deaths from measles is the most serious potential outcome of the disease. In some children, a long-term effect from the infection occurs in the form of a demyelinating condition of the nervous system known as sub acute sclerosing pan-encephalitis, which is progressive over a period of several years resulting in respiratory failure and death.

Treatment

Treatment for measles is supportive therapy. Prevention of measles is preferable and achieved by immunisation.

Meibomian Cyst

See *eyelid condition*

melaena *(black bowel motions)*

See *colon problems*
See *haematemesis*
See *stomach*

melanoma

See *skin problems*

Cause

Melanoma is a form of skin cancer and is potentially life-threatening if not diagnosed and treated early. Melanoma may occur anywhere in the body where pigment cells occur, including the genital area, anal area and in the pigmented areas of the eye.

Melanomas may also occur, when pigment is not a predominant factor. These are referred to as amelanotic melanomas.

Symptoms

A lesion may become a melanoma due to changes in the lesion from the effects of the ultra-violet radiation from the sun or from the exposure in solariums. Melanoma may occur at any age, but is uncommon before the second decade and the probability increases with increasing age.

Most melanoma arise in normal skin and about 40 per cent of melanoma arise in pre-existing pigmented skin lesions. Dysplastic naevi have a propensity for becoming melanoma. The features which should alert a patient to the possibility of a melanoma include change in the size, shape, contour, colour of a lesion—especially a change with red, white or blue colouration, as well as features such as a lesion which will not heal or a lesion which bleeds.

Treatment

Treatment for melanomas is surgical excision and follow-up for evidence of enlarged lymph node activity or enlargement.

The staging or thickness of the lesion is an important prognostic feature when considering the long-term survival.

Ménière's disease

Cause

Ménière's disease is a disorder of the inner ear caused by a disturbance of the vestibular system.

Symptoms

Symptoms include vertigo, sensorineural hearing loss, tinnitus, nausea and vomiting.

Treatment

Symptomatic treatment for this condition includes administration of anti-emetic medication, anti-cholinergic drugs and benzodiazepines. Diuretics and a low-salt diet may decrease the frequency and severity of episodes and for severe cases, administration of topical gentamicin or surgery may improve the condition by ablation of the vestibular system.

meningitis

Cause

Meningitis is an infection or inflammation of the meninges which are the coverings around the brain and spinal cord.

Meningitis may be classified as viral or bacterial. Agents which may cause viral meningitis include polio virus, echo virus, coxsackie virus, mumps virus, herpes simplex virus, chickenpox virus, Leptospirosis, typhus or tuberculosis.

Bacterial meningitis may be caused by neisseria meningitides, haemophylus influenza, streptococcus pneumoniae, E.coli, klebsiella, listeria. Factors such as age, head trauma and compromised immunity are important factors in determining the cause. Especially at risk are patients with alcoholism, chronic otitis media, sinusitis, mastoiditis, head injury, recurrent meningitis, pneumococcal pneumonia, sickle cell disease and asplenism (removal of the spleen).

Symptoms

Symptoms of meningitis include headache, stiff neck, fever, vomiting, drowsiness, weakness of the muscles, speech disturbance, vision defects, epileptic fits, altered conscious state to coma and death.

Treatment

Treatment for meningitis will depend on the organism which is isolated from the cerebrospinal fluid. Bacterial meningitis is treated with an appropriate antibiotic, often intravenously, with or without administration of dexamethasone (steroid). Treatment for viral meningitis is largely symptomatic management until recovery.

meningococcal disease

See *immunisation for childhood infectious diseases*

Cause

Meningococcal disease is caused by bacteria called meningococcus and it is a serious disease which causes meningitis and septicaemia and may lead to death in just a few hours if left untreated. The bacteria are spread from one person to another by close contact, by sharing water bottles in schools or sporting teams.

Symptoms

Symptoms include fever, headache, tiredness, neck stiffness, sensitivity to the light, vomiting and nausea, irritability in young children, joint pains and the onset of a characteristic red-purplish rash. Between five and 10 per cent of patients infected with meningococcus will die. Persons most at risk are close contacts of an identified case. Diagnosis of the condition is done by blood culture, examination of the spinal fluid from a lumbar puncture or by examination of the areas of skin which are affected.

Treatment

Treatment of acute symptoms is by intravenous administration of penicillin. Treatment of close contacts is by using oral rifampacin medication.

Prevention of the disease is through vaccination. A number of different strains of the disease exist and meningococcal C vaccination is advised for children in the routine vaccination schedule at 12 months. Another variant of the meningococcal vaccination protects against strains A, C, Y and W135.

menopause, problems

Cause

Menopause is a time of cessation of menstrual periods in women and hence fertility and by the age of 55 years 99 per cent of women will have reached this milestone due to decreasing function of the ovaries. Menopause does not come about overnight, but as a gradual decrease in the ovarian function commencing as early as 30 years.

Symptoms

Cessation of periods may occur with gradual changes in the periods for years preceding the menopause. Periods may become heavier or lighter. The interval between periods may become longer or shorter. Many women complain of flooding in this transition time. The most common symptom includes hot flushes during the day and at night, even in winter, as well as symptoms such as fatigue, irritability, insomnia, nervousness. These symptoms may be related to lack of oestrogen and the stress of ageing.

Lack of sleep may also be a complaint along with dizziness, pain on intercourse associated with vaginal dryness, urinary tract infections, some degree of urinary incontinence, nausea, flatulence, constipation or diarrhoea and aches and pains in the joints and muscles.

A common symptom is vaginal dryness and this is a problem for women who are sexually active. Vaginal dryness may produce painful intercourse, as well some degree of vaginal bleeding from intercourse such as contact bleeding of the penis with the cervix.

Contraception at this time is an issue as some women may still want to become pregnant, which is more unlikely to occur, whereas other women will definitely not want to become pregnant. The occasional woman will still become pregnant in the late forties (much less likely in the early fifties), but severe anxiety over becoming pregnant may occur in the peri-menopausal years.

In the longer term, osteoporosis may also develop as a result of lack of oestrogen. Before menopause women are protected from heart attacks by the presence of higher oestrogen levels, but following the menopause, risk of heart attack increases. Patients with symptomatic osteoporosis before menopause should be assessed for causes other than menopause, e.g. hyperparathyroidism, which is associated with calcium metabolism and therefore also with bone metabolism. Women who smoke are at greater risk of developing osteoporosis and in turn of developing a fracture due to osteoporosis.

Previous treatment with steroid medications is also a risk factor for developing osteoporosis, particularly following menopause. Patients with premature menopause or who have had a hysterectomy with loss of the ovaries are also at greater risk of developing osteoporosis.

Treatment

Uncomplicated menopause needs no treatment unless the woman is experiencing adverse symptoms. Not every woman needs hormone replacement therapy (HRT). HRT in the form of either tablets or skin patches will relieve symptoms such as hot flushes.

If vaginal bleeding with intercourse occurs, Pap smear screening needs to be updated. At the time of the Pap smear it may be evident that atrophic vaginitis is present, where the vaginal walls have a characteristic appearance of lack of oestrogen, look fragile and may even bleed with the contact with the brushes used to perform the Pap smear. Treatment for this condition includes topical oestrogen in the form of a vaginal tablet or vaginal cream, either one or two days per week or once per fortnight.

Sometimes women complain of breast soreness associated with the administration of vaginal oestrogen and if this happens, relief from this symptom is achieved with revision of the frequency of the vaginal medication. Topical oestrogen will also improve the frequency of urinary tract, bladder and vaginal infections and improve the tone of the vaginal muscles.

Treatment of urinary incontinence is also an issue and may require pelvic floor exercises or sometimes surgery to correct.

menorrhagia *(heavy periods)*

See *menopause problems*

Cause

Menorrhagia is said to occur when bleeding from periods is excessive in amounts or duration.

Symptoms

If excessive or prolonged bleeding occurs, iron deficiency anaemia may result. Most of the abnormal bleeding results from hormonal abnormalities. In some cases, excessive bleeding may result from an increase in the size of the uterus for women who have had one or more children, the presence of polyps or fibroids in the uterus or endocervical canal. In the case of hormonal abnormalities, ovulation may not occur and as a result the effects of oestrogen which are unopposed by progesterone stimulates excessive endometrial growth. The endometrium is being shed during the time of the period resulting in excessive, prolonged bleeding.

Treatment

Usually by the time the patient with menorrhagia attends the general practitioner, the main aim of treatment is to stop the heavy bleeding. This may be done using a hormone medication called norethisterone. The dosage of this medication may vary from one patient to another. Some patients may require up to three tablets a day in order to achieve cessation of bleeding. Once the bleeding has been controlled, a plan of action for monitoring or treating the heavy bleeding is to be developed. This may include referral to a gynaecologist for a curette procedure, even consideration of hysterectomy in the future. Sometimes performing the correct procedure will reduce the amount of heavy bleeding at least in the short term.

mesenteric artery occlusion

See *abdominal pain*
See *ischaemic colitis*

Cause

The organs inside the abdominal cavity are supplied with blood by arteries which branch from the aorta. If one of the main arteries which supply the gut becomes obstructed, severe abdominal pain may result.

Symptoms

A patient with an obstructed vessel which supplies the gut may present with anxiety, intense central abdominal pain around the navel area, profuse vomiting and bloody diarrhoea.

Treatment

It is essential that any patient with an obstruction to a vessel supplying the gut receive prompt and urgent surgical intervention. Early surgery will prevent the gut from becoming gangrenous.

migraine headache

See *flashes and floaters (in the eyes)*

Cause

Migraine is caused by a spasm in the arteries which supply the brain.

Symptoms

Not all headaches are migraine. Migraine is a specific sort of headache which is associated with nausea and vomiting, sensitivity to the light, may be preceded by an aura which means a symptom which signals the onset of a headache, e.g. flashing light in the eyes or some other visual disturbance.

Treatment

The treatment of migraine headaches takes the form of symptom relief with aspirin and/or codeine and resting quietly in a darkened room with a cold pack on the face. Medication such as naratriptan, zolmitriptan, sumatriptan, with the first signs of an attack will also relieve symptoms.

For an acute episode, treatment may include the prescription of intramuscular prochlorperazine and dihydroergotamine.

Prevention

Prevention of attacks includes avoidance of the trigger factors which a patient comes to recognise are specific for that patient, e.g. chocolate, caffeine drinks oranges, red wine, vegemite.

Long-term suppression may include prescription for beta blockers, cafergot, catapress and pizotifen daily. Oral prochlorperazine may help prevent ongoing attacks.

molluscum contagiosum

Cause

Molluscum contagiosum are wart-like structures and commonly occur in groups either on the body, legs or arms. This is a relatively common infection amongst young children.

Treatment

The structures are harmless and will resolve either spontaneously with time or by applying abrasions to the surface resulting in an inflammatory reaction followed by resolution of the lesions.

morning-after pill

See *contraception, emergency*

The morning-after pill is now available in the form of two tablets which are taken 12 hours apart and used as emergency contraception. The pills should be taken within 72 hours after the unprotected intercourse, but preferably within 24 hours.

It is recommended that the morning-after pill be taken if unprotected intercourse occurs in the middle of a menstrual cycle when the woman is not on the contraceptive pill. The middle of the cycle is the time most likely to produce a pregnancy and is termed the fertile period. The morning-after pill acts to prevent fertilisation of the ovum and implantation of any embryo which may result from the unprotected intercourse. Bleeding as a result of the taking the morning-after pill will take place within the next four to six days. The morning-after pill may sometimes produce nausea which may be treated with an anti-emetic medication .

It is recommended that if the woman is to continue with sexual activity, that ongoing contraceptive precautions are taken in order to prevent future unwanted pregnancy and to prevent the need for further emergency contraception. If condoms are the method of contraception, correct use and application of the condoms needs to reviewed also.

Practising safe sex is emphasised. Safe sex means the suppression of ovulation with one of the methods of hormonal suppression in addition to using condoms for protection from sexually transmitted diseases. Couples often feel that it is not necessary to continue with the use of condoms, once the relationship has become steady; however indiscretions do occur by either of the parties, without the other party being aware until some other emergency occurs, e.g. the male or female party contract a sexually transmitted disease, not uncommonly, genital herpes.

If genital herpes does occur as a result of unprotected sex, the person will carry the infection indefinitely and may experience outbreak of further episodes of infection, as well as pass the infection on to any future sexual partner.

There is treatment and suppression for genital herpes, but no effective cure for the disease, i.e. no means of eradicating all the signs of the infection entirely from the body once infection has taken place.

morning sickness

See *amenorrhoea (no period)*
See *pregnancy, associated problems*

Cause

Morning sickness is a symptom of early pregnancy. The name is inaccurate as the nausea may occur at any time of the day and sometimes may occur all day for a period of time in early pregnancy. The nausea is caused by increased levels of human chorionic gonadotrophin levels and oestrogen, which is produced by the developing cells of the placenta.

Treatment

If nausea and vomiting become a problem, it is recommended that the pregnant woman eat small amounts frequently of simple food (according to her taste) which is easy to digest. Fresh food is often preferable to highly processed food and fatty or spicy food is not recommended. Food such as simple carbohydrate is recommended, e.g. bread, pasta, plain rice, cracker biscuits. Eating and drinking before getting out of bed in the mornings is also helpful. Anti-nausea medication may be given if the nausea becomes excessive. Sometimes hyperemesis of pregnancy may occur where morning sickness is excessive and lasts for the duration of the pregnancy. This condition is rare and most morning sickness will subside by the beginning of the 10th to the 12th week. If hyperemesis occurs, medication will usually be needed and managed by the obstetrician in combination with the local doctor. Sometimes this may require admission to hospital for treatment of the nausea and vomiting, and fluid replacement.

Adequate nutrition is required not only for the mother, but also for the growing foetus to develop normally. Adequate rest and inactivity will also help to improve the feelings of nausea of pregnancy.

mouth ulcers

See *gingivitis*

Cause

Mouth ulcers may occur either singly or in groups and the cause is mostly unknown. There may be an association with vitamin B12 deficiencies, or iron deficiency. Stress and localised trauma may also be associated with the appearance of mouth ulcers.

Symptoms

They may present as lesions approximately one centimeter in diameter, and may last from 10 to 14 days, with larger lesions lasting for up to a month or two. Distinction should be made between aphthous mouth ulcers and oral herpes simplex mouth ulcers.

Treatment

Treatment with symptomatic agents for pain management is recommended for severe infections, otherwise there is no definitive treatment available to lessen the duration of the condition.

multiple sclerosis

Cause

Multiple sclerosis is a disease of the central nervous system which is characterised by patches of demyelisation in the brain and spinal cord, which give rise to the neurological symptoms.

Symptoms

Symptoms associated with multiple sclerosis include disturbances of vision, and coordination of eye function, disturbances of sensation, weakness, disturbances of urinary function, and sometimes mild disturbances of cognitive function.

Neurological deficits are often multiple and associated with periods of remission and exacerbation which gradually increase, resulting in an increasing degree of disability.

The most common initial symptom is abnormality of sensation either in arms or legs or on the trunk or face. Weakness in the hand or leg may also be a prominent feature in association with visual disturbance, e.g. visual field defects, pain in the eye, double vision, or paralysis of one of the muscles controlling eye movement.

Other symptoms include stiffness or unusual fatigability in the limbs, disturbances in bladder function and difficulty with bladder control, dizziness, heat intolerance, apathy, lethargy, emotional lability and depression; motor weakness is common and usually will reflect the presence of damage in the spinal cord. Deep tendon reflexes are usually increased, and progression of neurological symptoms with abnormalities in gait and balance may necessitate use of wheelchairs as the condition progresses. Painful spasms of the muscles in response to sensory stimuli may occur late in the condition.

Speech problems, tremors and nystagmus may also occur.

Involvement of the spinal cord may produce problems with bladder function causing urinary urgency or hesitancy, or acute urine retention or urinary incontinence, constipation and erectile dysfunction in men.

The history of the condition, with its periods of remission and exacerbation, are important diagnostic features. Investigations may include MRI, demonstrating lesions in the central nervous system and spinal cord.

Prognosis for the condition is variable and in some, with onset in middle age, progression of the disease is rapid. Progression of the disease is also hastened by cigarette smoking. The lifespan of patients is shortened only in patients with very severe symptoms.

Treatment

Treatment for multiple sclerosis includes administration of corticosteroids for acute exacerbations and immune modulating drugs in order to prevent ongoing exacerbations. Later in the condition additional supportive measures will be necessary in order to allow a person ongoing independence and to lead as normal a life as possible.

mumps

See *immunisation for childhood infectious diseases*

Cause

Mumps is an acute viral, contagious infection transmitted by droplet spread and direct contact with another person with the infection.

Symptoms

Mumps is characterised by enlargement of the parotid glands, and may also include inflammation of the testes, meningoencephalitis, and pancreatitis. An infection of mumps in adult males may result in swelling of the testes which may result in infertility.

Treatment

Treatment for mumps is symptomatic and supportive therapy. Prevention is achieved by vaccination with the measles, mumps and rubella vaccination. This is recommended at 12 months of age and four years of age, with boosters for adults both male and female in their second or third decade.

mycoplasma pneumoniae infection

See *pneumonia*

Cause

Mycoplasma pneumoniae infection is the most common lung infection recognised in adults and in children. Incubation period varies from about 10 to 14 days. The organism attaches to and destroys the hair cells which line the respiratory tract, and produces pneumonia, bronchitis and bronchiolitis and pneumonia.

Symptoms

Symptoms include malaise, cough, sore throat, sputum which may be bloodstained, and fatigue. Some patients may develop arthritis, rash and neurological problems.

Treatment

Treatment of choice is with tetracyclines.

myocardial infarction

See *heart attack*
See *hypertension*

nappy rash

Cause

Nappy rash occurs most commonly as a result of irritation from contact with urine and faeces. It may also arise as a result of allergic dermatitis, thrush, or psoriasis.

Symptoms

Symptoms include a red rash in the nappy area in association with redness, chafing, irritation and soreness.

Treatment

Treatment for nappy rash includes keeping the skin as clean as possible, providing moisturising cream or lotion to the area and avoiding excessive bathing as this contributes to drying of the skin. For problems with dermatitis and thrush a combination of hydrocortisone and clotrimazole will improve the problem.

neck pain

See *angina*
See *ankylosing spondylosis*
See *headache*
See *heart attack*
See *osteomyelitis*
See *polymyalgia rheumatica*
See *rheumatoid arthritis*

Cause

There are many causes of neck pain including traumatic injury, fractures and dislocations, muscle strains including repetitive injury which may arise from prolonged time spent working at a desk or over a computer (musculoskeletal headache or tension headache), cervical spondylosis, disc protrusion, rheumatoid arthritis, polymyalgia rheumatica, degenerative disease of the spine, ankylosing spondylosis, as well as angina or heart pains, meningitis, subarachnoid haemorrhage, osteomyelitis, and thyroid problems. Chewing gum or grinding teeth will cause musculoskeletal headaches, as will sleeping on a very flat pillow, or sleeping on the stomach.

Symptoms

The history of the condition will give a clue to the cause of the neck pain including a history of injury, the presence of fever, the presence of headaches, and the positioning of the headaches (e.g. headache which is present around the eye may indicate a musculoskeletal headache). The severity of the pain, as well as the amount of limitation of movement in the neck, is an indication of the nature of the pains. An elevated ESR (erythrocyte sedimentation) rate, a measure of the rate at which the red blood cells aggregate and fall to the bottom of the test tube, may indicate the presence of polymyalgia rheumatica. An X-ray or a CT scan of the cervical spine and/or skull may determine the nature of the pains.

Treatment

Treatment will depend on the cause of the pains. Patients with angina, meningitis, subarachnoid haemorrhage, osteomyelitis, fractures and dislocations may require referral to a specialist or to an emergency department for further assessment and treatment. Patients with musculoskeletal headaches will find improvement using anti-inflammatory preparations, physiotherapy to the neck, and further investigations regarding a precipitating cause for the neck problems, e.g. assessment of the work station, doing neck exercises if doing a lot of computer work, cessation of chewing gum or grinding the teeth.

needle-stick injury

See *human immunodeficiency virus (HIV)*

Accidental needle-stick injuries have come into focus since the prominence of human immunodeficiency virus (HIV) infections, hepatitis B and C. With the exception of staff treating HIV-positive patients, intravenous drug users and patients who are positive for hepatitis B and C, transmission of and acquisition of these diseases by health professionals is considered low risk.

If a needle-stick injury does occur, attempts should be made to inquire about and test the person for whom the needle was used. The person injured should be tested for HIV, and hepatitis B and C. The person should be tested again at three and six months, and again at 12 months following the injury. Each workplace will, or should have, a policy for HIV needle-stick injuries which is tailored to their particular purposes, and an incident report should be made to an occupational health and safety officer, following such an injury.

If a HIV positive person has had a needle which has accidentally injured a recipient, the recipient should be immediately referred for prophylactic antiviral agents.

nose bleed

Cause

Bleeding from the nose may occur because a small vessel has been ruptured inside the nostril. This may be related to dried secretions occurring inside the nose, and the person picking their nose.

Symptoms

It may also be related to chronic nasal congestion, an injury to the nose, may be a sign of a bleeding disorder, leukaemia, malignancies of the nasopharynx, and in adults may be related to high blood pressure. Despite what people may claim, everyone at some time picks their nose—it is part of the human condition.

Treatment

Stopping a nose bleed may be done by direct pressure to the nose using the thumb and index finger, applying ice, or diathermy to the inside of the nose under local anaesthetic. In order to achieve this treatment, referral to a specialist ear, nose and throat specialist may be required. Sometimes packing of the nose may also be required. If the bleeding does not subside with the measures that are available to the general practitioner, referral to hospital may be required.

obesity

See *diabetes*
See *hypothyroidism*
See *weight management problems*

Obesity is defined as an excess body fat. By definition obesity is measured by a body mass index greater than 30. Body mass index is measured by weight in kilograms divided by height in metres square (i.e. weight kg / height m^2).

Cause

Obesity may be caused by an excess of eating in association with inactivity and/or genetic predisposition. Genetic determinants and metabolic causes need to be excluded in cases of patients with obesity.

Overeating is more likely to cause obesity than a slow metabolic rate. Excess intake of fast food, which is high in fat and simple carbohydrates, may also lead to increased body weight and body fat content.

A sedentary lifestyle and a reduction in the amount of exercise may lead to weight gain. This is thought to be a main contributing factor for increase in weight for young people who spend prolonged periods of time either watching television, playing computer games or undertaking other computer-related activities.

Genetic factors may influence the signalling molecules and receptors in parts of the hypothalamus and gastrointestinal or digestive tracts which regulate food intake. Genetic factors may also determine the amount of energy which is expended, and have a determining effect in the distribution of body fat throughout the body, particularly associated with the distribution of abdominal fat. Prader-Willi syndrome is also associated with obesity.

Maternal obesity, paternal smoking, intrauterine growth retardation, and endocrine disorders can all produce abnormalities of weight regulation. Infant and childhood obesity are commonly associated with obesity in later life, and contribute to difficulty with weight loss in adulthood.

Cushing's syndrome produces a typical distribution of trunk and facial obesity. Corticosteroids, antidepressants, benzodiazepines, and anti-psychotic drugs may also contribute to increasing weight. Other causes of weight gain include pancreatic tumours resulting in hyperinsulinism, and hypothyroidism. Brain tumours such as craniopharyngioma or infection affecting the hypothalamus can stimulate consumption of excess calories.

Symptoms

Complications of obesity include insulin resistance, disorders of lipid metabolism, hypertension, diabetes and coronary artery disease, fatty liver which may lead to cirrhosis, obstructive sleep apnoea, degenerative arthritis particularly of the weight-bearing joints, skin disorders such as increased sweating and skin secretions, gallstones production, polycystic ovary syndrome, gout, deep venous thrombosis, pulmonary embolism, and cancer.

Diagnosis

In adults , obesity is determined by a body mass index greater than 30 kilograms per metre square. Waist circumference of greater than 101 centimetres (36.3 inches) in men, and greater than 87 centimetres (33.9 inches) in women is classified as obese. Percentage of body fat can be measured by using skin fold thickness. On average about 50 per cent of the body's fat deposits are found beneath the skin. Skin fold thickness between 0.5 centimetres to 2.5 centimetres in healthy men and 1.2 centimetres to 3.4 centimetres in women is considered to be in the normal range. In the elderly patient measurement of the skin fold thickness in the subscapular region is a more reliable estimate of body fat content.

Treatment

Weight loss of even five per cent to ten per cent improves health and decreases unwanted effects of obesity. Low-fat diets and calorie restrictions will also improve obesity and aid weight reduction. Unprocessed foods in the form of fresh fruit and vegetables should be substituted for refined carbohydrate and processed food, soft drinks and processed juices.

Physical exercise increases energy expenditure, basal metabolic rate, and diet induced thermogenesis. Exercise also regulates a moderate appetite by matching the body's needs with calorie intake. Being active improves insulin sensitivity, reduces cholesterol and serum lipids, reduces blood pressure, enhances aerobic fitness, and contributes to a feeling of psychological wellbeing. Because muscle tissue burns more calories at rest, increasing the body's muscle mass contributes to a more long-lasting increase in the body's basal metabolic rate.

obsessive-compulsive disorder

See *anxiety*

Cause

Obsessive-compulsive disorder is a form of anxiety.

Symptoms

Symptoms are characterised by thoughts or actions which become intrusive and interfere with normal daily functioning and interfere with decision making, e.g. excessive hand washing or obsession with checking that the appliances are turned off before being able to leave the house.

Treatment

Treatment consisting of anti-depressant medication will improve the condition, but often the patient will need referral for counselling or psychiatric individual or group therapy to significantly improve the symptoms.

occupational lung diseases

Cause

Occupational lung diseases such as hypersensitivity pneumonitis and extrinsic allergic alveolitis are a group of diseases of the lung which are characterised by exposure to certain allergens as part of the patient's occupation. Over 300 allergens have been identified as trigger factors for the development of hypersensitivity pneumonitis. However, only about eight of these conditions account for around 75 per cent of reported cases. The most commonly occurring examples of occupational lung diseases are associated with farming, water, birds, animals, grains, milling and construction, industry and textiles.

Farming has been associated with farmer's lung (associated with vegetable compost, mouldy grain, hay and silage), tobacco grower's lung, mushroom worker's lung (associated with mushroom compost), potato riddler's lung (associated with mouldy hay around potatoes), cheese washer's lung (associated with mouldy cheese), bagassosis (associated with mouldy sugarcane), compost lung, wine grower's lung (associated with mouldy grapes), coffee worker's lung (associated with coffee beans).

Water workers have been associated with sewer worker's lung, tap water lung, humidifier lung, hot tub lung, sauna taker's lung, due to the contamination of water associated with these occupations.

People working with animals have been associated with occupational lung diseases termed sausage worker's lung, furrier's lung, laboratory worker's hypersensitivity pneumonitis (which is associated with male rat urine and fur), fish food lung, mummy handler's lung. Bird fancier's lung is associated with contaminated bird droppings and bird feathers from pigeons, chickens, turkeys, ducks and parakeets.

People working with grains have been associated with miller's lung from infected wheat flour, malt worker's lung from mouldy barley.

Milling and construction workers are subject to wood workers' lung (from oak, cedar, pine, spruce and mahogany dust), wood trim as a disease and wood pulp worker's disease are associated with contaminated tree pulp, thatched roof worker's disease is associated with dried grass and leaves. People working in detergent, chemical and vineyard industries often have problems associated with enzymes from polyurethane foam, varnish and lacquer, and copper sulphate use. People working in textile industries are often diagnosed with byssinosis (contact with cotton, flax and hemp dust).

Symptoms

Signs and symptoms depend on whether exposure is acute, subacute, or chronic. Acute symptoms for these workers may include fever, chills, cough, tightness in the chest, shortness of breath, lack of appetite, nausea and vomiting, and tachycardia.

Treatment

Treatment of acute or subacute hypersensitivity pneumonitis is with corticosteroids for a short time. This treatment relieves the initial symptoms, but not necessarily the long-term outcome. Chronic disease has a more complicated prognosis, once fibrosis in the lung has been established. Patients may have irreversible lung changes although stabilisation of the patient's condition may occur if exposure to these agents is ceased.

oesophagitis, gastro-oesophageal reflux *(GOR)*

See *helicobacter pylori infection*

Cause

A patient with a free-flow of stomach contents back into the oesophagus due to poor control of the lower oesophageal sphincter is said to have gastro-oesophageal reflux, or GOR. This causes heartburn, indigestion, and inflammation of the oesophagus, called oesophagitis. Factors which contribute to the presence of GOR include excessive weight, fatty foods, caffeine and carbonated drinks, alcohol, tobacco smoking, and some drugs, i.e. antihistamines, tricyclic antidepressants, calcium channel blockers, progesterone, and nitrates. If persistent for a long period of time, oesophagitis may produce stricture formation and, on occasions, may result in the formation of a pre-cancer condition, referred to as Barrett's oesophagus.

Symptoms

The most common symptoms of GOR include heartburn, with or without the presence of reflux. Other symptoms include vomiting, loss of appetite, and may also result in coughing, wheezing and hoarseness of the voice.

Treatment

Treatment for GOR includes elevating the head of the bed at night, not eating within three hours of going to bed, avoiding alcohol and coffee before going to bed as well as fatty food, chocolate and smoking. Medication is recommended including proton pump inhibitors, and H2 antagonists.

Surgery is available to help reduce the effects of gastro-oesophageal reflux, most commonly offered to children, to reduce the free flow of gastric contents from the stomach back into the oesophagus. This is done by tightening the sphincter at the lower end of the oesophagus.

Barrett's oesophagus may or may not regress with medical or surgical intervention so that regular endoscopy is recommended to monitor the progress of this condition. Barrett's oesophagus may be treated by surgical removal or by laser therapy. If Barrett's oesophagus progresses to become cancer of the oesophagus, further major surgery may be indicated.

oral contraceptives

See *contraception, emergency*

The oral contraceptive pill (OC) was first used in the late 1950s and is still the most common form of contraception used. It comes in two forms: the combined pill, which contains oestrogen and progesterone (there are hundreds of products available) and the progesterone only pill, which is useful for patients with polycystic ovary, and the mini-pill, which is a progesterone only pill used during breastfeeding.

The oral contraceptive pill is around 98 per cent safe in preventing unwanted pregnancy. Some women may experience nausea with the OC, and some weight gain; however this is less likely with the progesterone only pill than for most other pills. Some pills are used specifically for the problem of acne , but also act as effective contraceptive agents. Smoking is contraindicated with the contraceptive pill as it contributed to problems of clotting disorders in women, e.g. deep venous thrombosis (DVT).

Osgood-Schlatter disease

Cause

The causes of Osgood-Schlatter disease are unknown but the condition occurs in older children and adolescents.

Symptoms

The disease causes pain and swelling below the kneecap. The symptoms are similar to arthritis, namely pain, swelling of the area, tenderness, stiffness and the area feeling hot to the touch.

Treatment

The principles of treatment are the same as for arthritis. This includes a balance between rest and exercise, heat packs to painful joints, reducing weight if overweight, gentle exercise, physiotherapy, simple analgesics, e.g. paracetamol, non-steroid or anti-inflammatory medications, e.g. ibuprofen. Sometimes surgery is required.

osteoarthritis

Cause

Osteoarthritis is the most common form of sore joints. Osteoarthritis is commonly regarded as a disease of wear and tear of joints; in fact the condition is much more complex. The cartilage surfaces lining the joints become worn away and inflamed causing pain in the joint. The most common joints involved are the weight-bearing joints of the body, including knees and hips, and are the most common joints where joint replacement is performed. Degeneration of the bones comprising the spinal column is also a common feature of osteoarthritis.

Symptoms

Whatever the cause of the arthritis, the symptoms are the same, namely pain, swelling of the joints involved, tenderness, stiffness and the joints feeling hot to the touch.

Treatment

The principles of treatment for osteoarthritis are the same irrespective of the cause. These include a balance between rest and exercise, heat packs to painful joints, reduction of weight if overweight, gentle exercise, physiotherapy, simple analgesics, e.g. paracetamol, non-steroid or anti-inflammatory medications, e.g. ibuprofen. Splinting of joints may be required in some cases of osteoarthritis, and at times referral will be necessary to specialist orthopaedic surgeons or to a rheumatologist.

osteomyelitis

Cause

Osteomyelitis is inflammation and destruction of the bone caused by bacteria or fungi.

Symptoms

Symptoms include pain, swelling of the joint or area of the bone involved, tenderness, stiffness, and the joints feeling hot to the touch.

Treatment

Treatment of osteomyelitis is first to treat the infection aggressively, and may involve surgical intervention. Treatment for some infections causing osteomyelitis may require prolonged antibiotic intervention.

osteoporosis

See *menopause, problems*

Cause

Osteoporosis is a progressive disorder of bone metabolism which decreases the bone mineral density with deterioration in the strength of the bone and the bone structure.

Symptoms

Symptoms may be absent until such time as weakness in the bone, in association with a minor accidental injury or fall, results in a fracture—most commonly to the bones in the hips (commonly called fractured neck of femur), or in the vertebral bodies of the spine. Another common place for fractures are the wrists as a person will often place their hand out to protect themselves from injury during a fall, or impending fall.

Other symptoms of progressive osteoporosis involving the spine include progressive stooping of the thoracic spine, overall decrease in height of the person, and radiographic changes in bone density. Acute or chronic back pain may also be a presenting feature of osteoporosis in the absence of any notable injury. Risk factors for developing osteoporosis include demobilisation of the body for an extended period of time, patients with low body weight, insufficient dietary intake of calcium phosphate and vitamin D, cigarette smoking and excessive intake of caffeine and alcohol. The Anglo and Asian races are more prone to this condition. A family history of osteoporosis is also an increased risk factor. Early menopause or a reduced amount of sex hormones is also a predisposing factor for the development of osteoporosis.

Causes of secondary osteoporosis include chronic renal failure, chronic obstructive airway disease, the use of corticosteroids, Dilantin or phenytoin intake for the treatment of epilepsy and the use of heparin.

These endocrine disorders associated with osteoporosis include hyperparathyroidism, hypothyroidism, hypogonadism, hyperprolactinaemia (prolactin hormone responsible for milk production), and diabetes. Liver disease, malabsorption syndromes, malignancy, rheumatoid arthritis, and sarcoidosis are also associated with an increased risk of osteoporosis.

Treatment

Treatment for osteoporosis should first begin with preventive measures such as adequate calcium and vitamin D supplementation, weight bearing exercises to improve and maximise bone and muscle strength, and to minimise the risk of accidental injury by falling episodes. Drug therapy is also available but often not until a fracture has been sustained. Medication is designed to preserve further deterioration and bony deformities and to stimulate the formation of new bone.

otitis externa

Cause

Otitis externa by definition is an infection of the external ear canal. Otitis externa may be caused by a bacterial infection, e.g. pseudomonas, or may be caused by a fungal infection.

Symptoms

Otitis externa may first present with itching, followed by the onset of pain, hearing loss, headache, pain on movement of the ear lobe, and on occasions some discharge from the ear. Swelling of the entrance to the ear canal may present in severe cases.

Treatment

Cleaning of the ear canal is most important with otitis externa. This may be done by gently syringing the ear canal, or preferably by direct suction of any debris in the ear canal, which should be done under direct vision using an operating microscope, or viewing apparatus used by a specialist ear, nose and throat surgeon. Medication may also be necessary in order to treat the infection. This may include the use of topical ear drops, and sometimes may also require oral antibiotic preparations. Sometimes an ear wick, a very small sponge, is inserted into the ear, and helps to absorb moisture and reduce inflammation and swelling in the ear canal.

otitis media

See *deafness and hearing loss*

Cause

Acute ear pain is one of the most common reasons for children presenting to a general practitioner. Otitis media or middle ear infection may be caused by viral or bacterial agents.

Symptoms

Fever, pain in the ear, headache, and body aches and pains may accompany the middle ear infection. Long-term effects of chronic otitis media may include hearing loss in children. Younger children may be seen to be pulling at the ears, or even head banging as a sign of pain in the ears. Bacterial infection causing middle ear infections is thought to occur in 60 per cent to 70 per cent of cases and if untreated, chronic hearing loss may occur. Perforation of the eardrum may follow with severe otitis media infections. Once a perforation has occurred, pain may subside as the middle ear is able to drain any fluid which may be accumulating behind the drum.

Treatment

Treatment of middle ear infection includes resting the patient, pain relief, relieving the fever, and antibiotic medication. The most common antibiotics used will be either penicillin or cephalosporins.

If chronic otitis media is allowed to develop, fluid may build up in the middle ear, or the infection may spread to the mastoid bones which lie adjacent to the ear. If either condition occurs, surgical intervention may be required either in the form of drainage of fluid from the middle ear using grommets, or a surgical procedure on the mastoid bone. Children and adults may need additional surgery, which includes tonsillectomy and removal of adenoids.

ovarian cancer

Cancer of the ovary is a very silent disease and may be well advanced before the diagnosis is made. At the time of Pap smear examination, bimanual examination of the uterus is carried out in order to determine the size of the uterus, and the presence of any enlargement of the ovaries.

Symptoms

Symptoms of ovarian cancer are often minimal, and non-specific. It may present with a lower abdominal lump or feeling of pressure, or it may present with symptoms of recurrent urinary tract infection.

Investigations

Detection of cancer of the ovary is often done using ultrasound, CT scan, or MRI scan, or estimation of tumour markers, e.g. cancer antigen 125. Diagnosis of cancer of the ovary is confirmed on histological examination.

Treatment

Surgery is the preferred treament for ovarian cancer. It requires hysterectomy, bilateral removal of the ovaries, and often chemotherapy. Treatment and long-term survival following a diagnosis of cancer of the ovary depends on staging of the disease and detection of spread of the disease.

ovarian cyst

See *ovarian cyst, acute torsion*
See *ovarian cyst, ruptured*
See *ovarian follicles*
See *polycystic ovary syndrome*

ovarian cyst, acute torsion

See *abdominal pain*

Cause

Sometimes an ovarian cyst may be attached to a stalk called a pedicle, which may twist forming what is called torsion of the ovarian cyst.

Symptoms

The symptoms of torsion of an ovarian cyst include severe cramping lower abdominal pain, and vomiting. The patient looks ill and pale. The pain may also radiate to the flank or the thigh.

Investigation

Investigation for a suspected torsion of an ovarian cyst includes an ultrasound procedure.

Treatment

Treatment for torsion of an ovarian cyst involves laparoscopic surgery, and removal of the cyst.

ovarian cyst, ruptured

See *abdominal pain*

Cause

Ovarian cysts are relatively common in all menstruating women. The ovaries are made up of numerous cysts at varying stages of development. Most ovarian cysts will resolve, even without treatment after one or two menstrual cycles, but sometimes ovarian cysts may rupture, which in turn may cause internal bleeding, shock or peritonitis. They may also become large enough to cause your ovaries to twist, which causes extreme discomfort.

Symptoms

If an ovarian cyst ruptures, sudden onset of pain may occur in the lower abdomen on either the right or left side. This may be accompanied by nausea and vomiting.

Treatment

In most instances, treatment of a ruptured ovarian cyst requires simple explanation and reassurance to the patient, and conservative management. Simple cysts less than four centimetres in diameter may require no interventional treatment; however cysts of greater than four centimetres create internal bleeding and may require laparoscopic surgery in order to remove the cyst and stop the bleeding.

ovarian follicles

See *abdominal pain*
See *periods, painful*

Ovarian cyst

Cause

An ovarian cyst is any collection of fluid, surrounded by a very thin wall within an ovary— it is a cystic tumour of the ovary, which is usually benign. Any ovarian follicle that is larger than about two centimetres is termed an ovarian cyst. Benign ovarian tumours usually grow slowly and rarely turn into malignant tumours.

Symptoms

Most ovarian cysts are asymptomatic; however some cysts may produce lower abdominal pain which at times may be severe.

Treatment

Sometimes if ovarian cysts are large, surgical intervention may be indicated; occasionally an ovarian cyst may twist and produce severe lower abdominal pain, called torsion of an ovarian cyst, and will require excision.

Ruptured (mittelschmerz)

See *abdominal pain*

Cause

Ovarian follicles rupture during the process of ovulation, hence the name mittelschmerz, which means middle of the cycle.

Symptoms

The woman may experience pain in the middle of the menstrual cycle. This may occur on either the right or left side of the lower abdomen, on average about five hours after ovulation has occurred. This may be accompanied by a heavy feeling in the pelvis, and a dull ache.

Treatment

The treatment of this condition includes explanation and reassurance of the patient, simple analgesics like aspirin or paracetamol or mild anti-inflammatory medications like ibuprofen. Other active treatment include a hot-water bottle to the lower abdomen if the pain is severe.

Paget's disease

Cause

Paget's disease is a disease of bone metabolism which causes bones to become thickened and more porous in the centre.

Symptoms

Most people with Paget's disease experience no symptoms, at least in the early part of the disease. As the condition progresses, patients may complain of aches and pains in the knees, hips and back. They may complain of problems with their hearing if the Paget's affect the bones of the skull. It may be noticeable that the patient is becoming bow-legged. Patients may notice that their head is becoming bigger; and an X-ray investigation may be able to determine the presence of Paget's disease in the skull or elsewhere. Pathology testing for an enzyme in the blood called alkaline phosphatase will also be able to help confirm or rule out the presence of Paget's disease. A bone scan will also be able to determine the presence of Paget's disease.

Treatment

Treatment for Paget's is similar to the treatment used for osteoporosis, e.g. bisphosphonate medication, but higher doses of the medication are used.

pain

Pain is a common symptom and the most common reason for patients to go to the doctor.

Cause

Pain may be acute or chronic, and may present with sensory and emotional components. Acute pain results from activation of peripheral pain receptors and occurs due to tissue damage. Chronic pain occurs due to ongoing stimulation of the receptors and is related to ongoing tissue injury.

Pain receptors are located in the skin, subcutaneous tissues, on the surface of bones and joints, and stimulation of these areas will result in sharp or dull localised pains. Pain receptors also occur in solid and in hollow organs and result in poorly localising pains, which may be described as deep aching or cramping pains.

Pain fibres enter the spinal cord from the remote regions of the body, and travel via the spinal cord to the sensory cerebral cortex. Substances released when tissue is injured can sensitise peripheral receptors.

Psychological factors are also important and may modify how pain is received. Pain modulators interact in poorly understood ways to exaggerate or reduce the perception of and response to pain.

Symptoms

Pain may be accompanied by anxiety, hyperactivity, rapid heart rate, increased respiratory rate, increase in blood pressure, and dilated pupils. Chronic pain may be accompanied by symptoms of fatigue, loss of appetite, loss of libido, depression.

Treatment

Treatment of pain is by analgesic medication such as paracetamol, aspirin, and opioids and neuromodulators, which modify the body's response to pain, including antidepressants, anti-consultants, and membrane-stabilising medication.

Treatment for pain may be administered in many ways: orally, rectally, by injection subcutaneously, intravenously, or by patches applied to the skin in a sustained release action.

palpitations and arrhythmias

See *heart attack*
See *hypertension*

Cause

Palpitations are a symptom and may be defined as a discernible irregularity of the heartbeat. Patients may describe palpitations in terms of the heart skipping a beat, an irregular beating of the heart, a fluttering sensation, a racing pulse, or rapid or slow beat of the heart.

Palpitations may be caused by excessive intake of caffeine drinks, smoking, medications, e.g. ventolin, amphetamines, cocaine. Palpitations may also be caused by irregularities of the heart, heart attack, anxiety, stressful situations, thyroid problems, fever, pregnancy, menopause, abnormalities of the electrolytes in the blood, e.g. potassium (people who take fluid tablets are prone to lose potassium in the urine).

Palpitations from an abnormal increase in heart rate may occur during exercise, or during an illness characterised by fever.

Investigations

Irregularities in the heart rate and rhythm may be detectable by performing an ECG, using a Holter monitor attached to the patient, an ECG tracing over a 12- or 24-hour period, and cardiac stress testing.

Treatment

Diagnosing a cause for the palpitations is the first step in the treatment process. The ECG and Holter monitor may be able to detect irregularities in the heart rhythm as well as show if the patient is suffering from an episode of angina or heart attack. Cessation of the caffeine products and drugs listed will also relieve the palpitations. Pathology testing will detect problems with the electrolytes in the blood and problems of the thyroid gland.

Patients who are feeling stressed may find relief with regular or intermittent administration of medication called beta blockers. This is particularly useful for those patients who find that their symptoms come on at times of having to speak to public gatherings or work gatherings. Other treatment for stress include relaxation techniques, exercise, cognitive behaviour therapy or medications prescribed by the doctor.

pancreatic cancer

See *abdominal pains*

Cause

Cancer of the pancreas may arise in a patient with no risk factors; however it has been associated with excessive alcohol intake, recurrent episodes of pancreatitis and smoking.

Symptoms

Symptoms of pancreatic cancer often appear when the tumour is well advanced and has already spread. Secondary spread is often present, even at the time of diagnosis, and may be detected in the lymph nodes, and lungs and liver. Symptoms of cancer of the pancreas may include weight loss, abdominal pain which may radiate to the back, and jaundice. An abdominal lump may be palpable. The diagnosis of the disease is best detected by a CT scan of the abdomen. A late manifestation of the disease is the presence of diabetes mellitus as the cells of the pancreas are replaced by tumour.

Treatment

Treatment for pancreatic cancer varies with the extent of the disease; however the five-year survival rate is generally less than two per cent. Surgery may be offered to patients with this condition and a Whipple's procedure (pancreatico-duodenectomy) performed.

pancreatitis

See *abdominal pain*
See *alcohol abuse*
See *pancreatic cancer*

Cause

Pancreatitis is a severe inflammation of the pancreas. The pancreas is a gland which produces pancreatic enzymes which digest food. If the pancreas becomes damaged or inflamed by infections, gallstones or cancer, the gland starts to self-destruct, resulting in very severe abdominal pain, which is termed pancreatitis.

The most common causes of pancreas problems include biliary tract disease, high and prolonged alcohol intake, drugs such as ace (angiotensin converting enzyme) inhibitors, and valproate.

The mumps virus, cystic fibrosis and pregnancy may all precipitate an episode of pancreatitis. Patients with gallstones and abnormalities of the biliary duct system may present with symptoms of pancreatitis or it may follow an endoscopic retrograde cystopancreatogram or ERCP investigation.

Repeat episodes of pancreatitis may result in pancreatic cancer.

Symptoms

The symptoms of acute pancreatitis include severe abdominal pain, nausea and vomiting. Shock with a fall in blood pressure and multi-system organ failure may follow. Severe abdominal pain might also be accompanied by a haemorrhagic rash on the abdomen in the area around the navel.

Treatment

Diagnosis of acute pancreatitis is based on an elevated level of serum amylase, which is an enzyme released from the pancreas during an episode of pancreatitis. Treatment of acute pancreatitis involves provision of intravenous fluid, pain relief, and a nasogastric tube to keep the stomach free of any contents until the pancreas recovers. Any underlying cause will need to be addressed, e.g. removal of gallstones or cessation of alcohol intake.

When the cause of pancreatitis involves cancer, the progress of the disease is often rapid and fatal. Patients will require significant pain relief in the form of pethidine, morphine, and anti-nausea medication. Progress of the patient's condition may be done by monitoring the white cell count, serum amylase, plain X-ray of the abdomen, and CT scan of the abdomen.

panic disorder

See *anxiety*
See *depression*

Panic disorder or a feeling of some impending disaster for no apparent reason is treated with medication called Selective Serotonin Re-absorption Inhibitors (SSRIs) and will often require referral for cognitive behaviour therapy treatment. Hypnotherapy is a useful tool to help improve the disorder.

papillomavirus *(HPV)*

See *human papillomavirus*

Parkinson's disease

Cause

Parkinson's disease is caused by a deficiency of a particular neurotransmitter called dopamine in the brain.

Symptoms

The deficiency of the neurotransmitter causes symptoms of stiffness in the muscles, tremor in the hands, head, neck and legs, and reduction in the quality of movement. People who have Parkinson's disease often have a shuffling gait, and shaking of the hands, head or legs. People with Parkinson's disease may find it difficult to write as the disease progresses, which occurs because of the rigidity in the muscles in the hands. Not uncommonly, they may appear to have a 'wooden' appearance of the face due to rigidity of the muscles of the face, and have difficulty with speech, and a tremor of the lower jaw.

Treatment

Treatment is in the form of medication to replace the reduced amounts of dopamine in the brain. Medication, e.g. levodopa, will help, but not cure the disease. In the future, treatment with embryonic cells may minimise the effects of Parkinson's disease or perhaps result in a cure.

paronychia

Cause

Paronychia is defined as an infection in the tissue around the margins of the fingernails or toenails. This may be caused by any of the bacteria which cause skin infections, staphylococcus or streptococcus.

Symptoms

Symptoms include pain, redness, localised swelling, and a collection of pus.

Treatment

Treatment of the condition is to incise the localisation of the pus and release it. This may or may not require anaesthetising the finger or toe with local anesthetic in the form of a ring block. The incision of the area may then be followed with oral antibiotics and pain relief. As soon as the pus is released, the pain will improve. A further diagnosis of diabetes needs to be excluded in some patients.

Care and hygiene of the hands and nail beds is important, and biting of the fingernails should be avoided.

pelvic adhesions

See *abdominal pain'*

Cause

Pelvic adhesions are mainly due to infection, previous surgery, or endometriosis.

Symptoms

Symptoms for pelvic adhesions include pelvic pain, infertility, and painful periods.

Treatment

Pelvic adhesions may be treated by laparoscopic removal of the adhesions.

pelvic inflammatory disease

See *abdominal pain*
See *sexually transmitted diseases*

Cause

Pelvic inflammatory disease (PID) refers to a chronic infection in the fallopian tubes and is most commonly caused by ongoing infections of chlamydia or gonorrhea, or following termination of pregnancy or a curette procedure.

Symptoms

Symptoms include lower abdominal pain, fever, backache. As a result of pelvic inflammatory disease, patients may experience pain with intercourse, infertility, and/or ectopic pregnancy, heavy or painful periods, vaginal discharge, and pain on urinating. Following termination of pregnancy or curette, antibiotics will be recommended in order to prevent the onset of PID.

Treatment

Treatment for PID includes prescription of one or more antibiotics depending on the bacteria which is isolated from the vaginal swab.

penile disorders

See *erectile dysfunction*
See *Peyronie's disease*
See *phimosis, paraphimosis*
See *priapism*
See *prostate cancer*

peptic, perforated or gastric ulcer

See *abdominal pain*

Cause

A peptic ulcer is an ulcer anywhere in the gastrointestinal tract. A gastric ulcer refers to an ulcer in the stomach. A patient with a perforated peptic ulcer is indeed a sick patient. Perforation may occur either in the stomach or in the duodenum, in an existing ulcer or inflammatory condition of the gut.

Symptoms

The patient will present with abdominal pain or abdominal distention. The patient will describe sudden severe pain, will appear anxious, will want to remain as still as possible, and will appear grey, sweaty, with nausea and vomiting. A chest X-ray will show that there is gas under the diaphragm. In order to demonstrate the gas, the patient needs to be in an upright position for 15 minutes prior to the X-ray.

Treatment

Treatment for a perforated peptic ulcer requires immediate referral to hospital and surgical closure of the perforation. Often the patient will need to be resuscitated as part of the initial treatment with intravenous fluids, pain relief, and antibiotics, and may require a period in treatment and observation in the intensive care unit.

perichondrititis

Cause

Perichondrititis is an infection of the cartilage, gristle part of the ear lobe. It may become infected with the insertion of earrings which pierce the cartilage portion of the ear.

Symptoms

Symptoms may include pain and localised swelling, redness and tenderness in the ear. On occasions an abscess may also form, which may require drainage.

Treatment

Treatment of perichondrititis involves the use of oral antibiotics, such as penicillin. An abscess will need to be drained, and earrings may need to be removed.

periods, painful

See *endometriosis*

Cause

Dysmenorrhoea or period pain is caused by spasms in the vessels within the uterus before menstruation. Other causes include onset of menopause, the presence of an intrauterine contraceptive device, infection in the fallopian tubes, endometriosis, uterine fibroids, or uterine polyps in the endocervical canal. In addition, dysmenorrhoea may be produced by uterine prolapse, or a tight endocervical canal where a build-up of pressure from menstrual blood at the time of menstruation occurs inside the uterus causing pain. Dysmenorrhoea will often improve after the delivery of the first child.

Symptoms

Symptoms of lower abdominal pain may be accompanied by headache, malaise, and a general feeling of being unwell. Not uncommonly, women may need to take time off school and work because of the severity of period pain.

Treatment

Identification of a treatable cause is important to help reduce the incidence of dysmenorrhoea. Pain relief such as an anti-inflammatory, e.g. ibuprofen or a combination of aspirin and codeine or, mefenamic acid will relieve the pain. Other measures include a hot-water bottle to the lower abdominal area, sitting in a warm bath, and regular physical exercise.

The oral contraceptive pill may also improve the severity of dysmenorrhoea. The provision of the oral contraceptive pill allows for some periods to be skipped, particularly if there are special events where the woman wishes to remain period and pain free. Apart from the provision of the oral contraceptive pill, injectable forms of female hormone may also provide an option for minimising period frequency, i.e. injectable progesterone will often result in no periods for the duration of the implant which can last up to three years.

There are new devices which may be inserted into the uterus which will also help to improve the symptoms of dysmenorrhoea.

The patient may require antibiotics for an infection in the fallopian tubes, repair of the uterine prolapse, or removal of the uterine/cervical polyp. Education of the patient is also important since the presence of periods is likely to continue in a woman's life into her fourth or fifth decade.

period problems

See *amenorrhoea*
See *periods, painful*
See *menorrhagia*
See *polycystic ovary syndrome*
See *pregancy, associated problems*

Perthe's disease

See *hip pain*

Peyronie's disease

Cause

Peyronie's disease is caused by increasing amounts of fibrous tissue in the muscle of the penis, called the cavernous sheath. The cause of this condition is unknown.

Symptoms

The fibrous tissue leads to a contracture of the penis resulting in a deviation of the penis to one side, painful erections, and problems with sexual intercourse.

Treatment

Treatment for this condition is unpredictable. Treatment with high potency corticosteroids into the lesions has been effective in some patients. Supplementation with vitamin E and vitamin K para-aminobenzoate has had some success; however surgical correction will usually result in the development of further scar tissue.

phaeochromocytoma

See *adrenal gland, problems*

Cause

Phaeochromocytoma is a tumour in the adrenal gland of cells which produce adrenalin and noradrenalin.

Symptoms

Symptoms include the presence of persistent or alternatively paroxysmal episodes of significantly elevated blood pressure, with or without the presence of other symptoms such as severe headache.

Treatment

Treatment involves removal of an identifiable tumour producing the excess amounts of adrenalin and noradrenalin from the adrenal gland.

phimosis, paraphimosis

Cause

Phimosis is the inability to retract the foreskin, while paraphymosis refers to a tight band of tissue around the foreskin in the retracted position.

Symptoms

In children the foreskin is fairly adhered to the head of the penis until the age of about four years when spontaneous separation occurs, allowing retraction of the foreskin. Gradual separation of the foreskin and head of the penis in children is sometimes accompanied by burning and stinging on urination and may be mistaken for symptoms of urinary tract infection.

Treatment

Treatment of the foreskin with topical steroid cream three times a day will often resolve the phimosis. Circumcision is another option for a chronic condition. If a paraphimosis occurs, this should be regarded as a medical emergency as constriction of the penis may lead to impairment of the blood supply. Referral to a specialist or an emergency department should be made.

pigeon toes

See *knock knees*

Cause

Pigeon toes is a term applied to children who walk or run with their toes pointing towards the centre. This is often the cause of frequent falls as they are seen to stumble or fall over their feet. The reason for the deformity in the alignment of the legs is based on the fact that children with pigeon toes are often found sitting on the floor 'between their knees', which results in torsion or mal-alignment of the bones of the lower limb originating from the hips and knee.

Treatment

Treatment for this condition simply involves encouraging a child not to sit with this particular posture but to sit on the floor cross-legged. Given time this condition will resolve itself spontaneously without significant other intervention.

piles

See *haemorrhoids*

pill, the

See *contraception, emergency—morning after pill*
See *oral contaceptives*

pituitary gland abnormalities

See *hyperpituitarism*
See *hypopituitarism*

The pituitary gland is a small gland which sits in the middle of the skull and, along with interacting with the hypothalamus which is part of the brain, it regulates the function of the endocrine glands of the body. The endocrine system is an integrated system of small organs that involve the release of extracellular signalling molecules known as hormones. The endocrine system is instrumental in regulating metabolism, growth, development and puberty, tissue function, and also plays a part in determining mood.

The pituitary gland is divided into anterior pituitary and posterior, and may present as a problem with overactivity or underactivity.

platelet dysfunction abnormalities

Cause

Platelets are small cell fragments which act as anticoagulant (or anti-clotting) agents. The number of platelets circulating at any one time may be influenced by the production of platelets, or by the phases of the menstrual cycle. Numbers of platelets will be reduced in the end stages of pregnancy, and increase in response to inflammatory processes in the body. Platelets are eventually destroyed by the spleen.

Platelet abnormalities include thrombocytosis, which is a reactive phenomenon, a decrease in platelets (thrombocytopenia), and platelet dysfunction.

Causes of thrombocytopenia include failed platelet production, increased destruction of platelets in the spleen, the dilution of platelets. The risk of bleeding is inversely proportional to the number of platelets present in the circulating blood. In patients with thrombocytopenia, a peripheral blood smear may suggest a cause.

Symptoms

Platelet dysfunction results in characteristic skin manifestations, e.g. multiple petechiae or pinpoint areas of haemorrhage on the skin—usually most evident in the lower limbs, scattered ecchymoses at sites of minor trauma, mucosal bleeding, e.g. nose bleeding, vaginal bleeding or bleeding from the digestive gastrointestinal tract.

Treatment

Patients with thrombocytopenia or platelet dysfunction may require a platelet blood transfusion, and any drugs which may be thought to be contributing to the condition should be withdrawn, especially aspirin and nonsteroidal anti-inflammatory preparations.

pleurisy

See *bronchitis*
See *lung abscess*
See *pneumonia*

Cause

Pleurisy is an infection or inflammation of the outer covering or the pleural lining of the chest wall. Pleurisy may result from an infection in the underlying lung, or from problems caused by tuberculosis, uraemia (renal failure), malignancies (including mesothelioma), rheumatoid arthritis, or a fracture of the rib.

Symptoms

Symptoms start with sharp stabbing pain which is made worse by breathing, associated with coughing, and sometimes rapid, shallow breathing.

Treatment and Investigations

Treatment of pleurisy is directed towards the underlying medical condition. Pleurisy may be diagnosed clinically by the practitioner hearing the sound of friction when the patient breathes in and out, and signs of inflammation, infection or a malignancy may be evident on chest X-rays.

Pain relief is indicated. The pain may be improved by supportive bandaging of the entire chest. Antibiotics and inhaled bronchodilators are indicated for infection processes, and deep breathing is indicated to help clear the infection in the lung.

pneumococcus

Pneumococcal infections are caused by bacterial infection with a bacterium called streptococcus pneumoniae.

Symptoms

Pneumococcal infections are primarily infections of the lungs, but may also involve middle ear infections, sinus infections, meningitis, endocarditis, septic arthritis, and rarely peritonitis.

Treatment

Treatment of pneumococcal infections involves administration of an appropriate antibiotic, most commonly in the penicillin group. The choice of antibiotic will depend on the sensitivity of the bacteria. Prevention of the disease is achieved by vaccination, e.g. Prevenar which is recommended at two-, four- and six-months of age. People over the age of 65 also qualify for pneumococcal vaccination, which should be repeated every five years.

pneumonia

See *bronchiectasis*
See *pleurisy*
See *respirstory system diseases*

Cause

Pneumonia is an acute inflammation in the lung caused by an infection. The infection can be bacterial, viral, fungal or parasitic. Pneumonia may be acquired in the community or in hospital. Community-acquired pneumonia is most likely due to streptococcus, haemophilus, chlamydia, mycoplasma, and legionella. Hospital-acquired pneumonia is more commonly due to staphylococcus aureus (or golden staph).

Symptoms

Symptoms of pneumonia include coughing, shortness of breath, chest pain, malaise, fever, or upper abdominal pain if the lower lobes of the lung are involved. Symptoms in young children may include non-specific irritability and restlessness and elderly patients' symptoms may present as confusion states.

In hospital-based patients with hospital-acquired pneumonia, symptoms may be suspected on the basis of worsening oxygenation levels, and increased respiratory secretions. Non-infectious causes of pulmonary deterioration such as acute respiratory distress syndrome (ARDS), pneumothorax and pulmonary oedema (or fluid on the lung) must be excluded.

Treatment

Investigations and treatment for pneumonia will vary according to whether the patient is community- or hospital-based and the nature of the infecting organism. The mortality in hospital-based patients has a less favourable prognosis due to the existence of other co-morbidities. Treatment for bacterial pneumonia is in the form of antibiotic medication administered either orally or intravenously depending on the sensitivity of the organism to the antibiotics. The diagnosis may be made and monitored using chest X-ray, sputum cultures, and pathology testing.

pneumothorax

Cause

Pneumothorax results from a break in the outer covering of the lung and may occur spontaneously or in response to trauma to the chest, fracture of the rib, following surgery, lung cysts or bleb, and in asthma and emphysema. Tension pneumothorax may occur where air enters the pleural space and is trapped, pushing the lung and heart to one side causing increasing difficulty in breathing, and is usually in response to an injury and requires urgent medical intervention.

Symptoms

Symptoms include chest pains and shortness of breath. Diagnosis is made on the patient's past history, clinical examination and chest X-ray.

Treatment

Treatment for pneumothorax includes re-inflation of the lung with a chest drain. Sometimes surgical intervention will be required to prevent recurrence.

polio

See *immunisation*

Cause

There are three different types of virus which cause polio (also called infantile paralysis, or by its full name poliomyelitis). They belong to a group of viruses called picornaviridae. Poliovirus is acquired by direct exposure to an infected individual.

Symptoms

Symptoms of polio vary from a minor illness and include fever, malaise, headache, sore throat, vomiting, to a life-threatening illness with fever, malaise, neck stiffness, deep muscle pains, weakness and paralysis of groups of muscles, and problems with swallowing.

Treatment

Treatment includes antibiotics and symptomatic relief of pain and headache. Prevention is achieved by vaccination commencing at two, four and six months of age and at four years of age. A polio booster is recommended in adult years.

polycystic ovary syndrome

See *amenorrhoea*
See *obesity*
See *infertility, female*

Cause

Polycystic ovary syndrome is caused by an enlargement of the ovaries with small, thickened capsules. The cause is unknown.

Symptoms

Ovaries commonly contain many follicles and sometimes large cysts. Oestrogen levels are found to be elevated in polycystic ovary syndrome, and the patient has an increased risk of developing an endometrial hyperplasia, and endometrial cancer. Polycystic ovary is a syndrome which is characterised by obesity of varying degrees, irregular periods or even amenorrhoea (no periods) which is otherwise unexplained. Androgen levels may also be increased, signs of which include acne, and facial hair, which increase the risk of developing metabolic syndrome. The diagnosis of the condition is confirmed by demonstration of large follicles in the ovaries by ultrasound technique. Blood testing is also done.

Treatment

Treatment for polycystic ovary syndrome is directed at diagnosing the presence of anovulatory cycles. For women who are contemplating pregnancy, the provision of fertility treatments may be required in order to produce ovulatory cycles and hence pregnancy. For women who are not contemplating pregnancy, treatment with progesterone medications, either by injection or by the oral contraceptive pill, should be administered in order to reduce the possibility of endometrial hyperplasia or endometrial cancer, and to reduce the amount of circulating androgens. Weight management to prevent obesity is an important part of treating this condition.

polymyalgia rheumatica

See *temporal arteritis*

Cause

Polymyalgia rheumatica is an autoimmune disease.

Symptoms

The symptoms of polymyalgia rheumatica include pain and stiffness in the neck, shoulders, and pelvic muscles. It commonly affects patients in their 50s and 70s and is more common in women than men. Early morning stiffness is a problem, associated with loss of appetite, weight loss, and malaise. Headache is associated with temporal arteritis and a loss of pulsation in the temporal arteries.

Treatment

Treatment is with corticosteroids, which improve the condition, but relapses are not uncommon.

pregnancy, associated problems

Cause

Pregnancy occurs with the fertilisation of the ovum with a sperm. The fertile period of the female cycle occurs 14 days prior to the commencement of the next period, so that in a normal 28 day cycle, the fertile period will occur at around day 14, which coincides with the middle of the cycle. If the woman has a 21-day cycle, the fertile time of the cycle will occur again 14 days prior to the anticipated next cycle, i.e. at around day seven of the cycle. Dating of a pregnancy by convention occurs from the date of the last normal menstrual period (LNMP), and pregnancy will be expected to conclude 40 weeks from the time of the last normal period.

Symptoms

Diagnosis of the pregnancy will usually be possible when the period is late by a week. The best time to perform a pregnancy test is with the first urine of the morning, because this is the time of day when the pregnancy hormones are likely to be most concentrated in the urine. In some women, a positive pregnancy test may not occur until the period has been missed by more than a week. In this case, blood testing for the presence of human chorionic gonadotrophin is possible in order to confirm or exclude case of pregnancy. Home pregnancy kits are available for testing for pregnancy and are as good as those available at the local doctor.

Symptoms which are common in pregnancy include nausea (or morning sickness which may occur at any time throughout the day), vomiting, lower abdominal pain, spotting or vaginal bleeding in the early part of the pregnancy (which sometimes is an indication of a threatened miscarriage), anorexia, indigestion, fussy eating, tiredness, lethargy, disruption to sleep, breast enlargement and tenderness, weight gain, elevation in blood pressure, gestational diabetes and swelling of the feet.

Incidental maternal medical problems may occur in pregnancy including problems with constipation (often from taking iron tablets, but also from the feeling of pressure as the foetal head increases in size), nausea (should have resolved by week 12), heartburn, indigestion, urinary tract infections, vaginal discharge, varicose veins and haemorrhoids (both of which may become worse with each successive pregnancy), heat intolerance, problems finding a comfortable sleeping position at night, fatigue, some food intolerance or alternatively, unusual food cravings, urinary incontinence, intolerance for some household smells particularly smells from cooking foods, swelling of the feet and hands, lack of libido (which may be more of a problem for the male partner), forgetfulness, emotional irritability and obsessiveness (care should be taken if these symptoms occur prenatally for the development of postnatal depression).

Tender breasts are one of the earliest signs of pregnancy with engorgement of the breasts, along with urinary symptoms of urinary urge and urinary tract infections.

In the presence of a positive pregnancy test, an abnormality of pregnancy still may occur in the form of a blighted ovum or ectopic pregnancy, which will not result in a normal outcome of pregnancy. At around six weeks following the last normal menstrual period, an ultrasound will be able to confirm that there is a live intra-uterine pregnancy.

A combination of excess weight gain, elevation in blood pressure, and swelling of the feet in pregnancy is a condition known as pre-eclamptic toxaemia, and requires urgent medical intervention and supervision as it may lead to maternal epileptic fitting and compromise to the safety of the foetus. Patients with pre-eclamptic toxaemia are required to rest in bed either at home or in hospital to prevent or minimise the risk to the baby, until delivery has occurred. Sometimes medical risk to the mother may continue for another seven to 10 days following the delivery of the baby, and the mother should be monitored during this time if she is considered at risk.

Diet in pregnancy is important, and women need supplementary folic acid and iron. Dieting for weight reduction however is not recommended in pregnancy, irrespective of the woman's body mass index (BMI) or body weight. Alcohol consumption and smoking are not recommended from the earliest time of the pregnancy, and women contemplating a pregnancy should also abstain from alcohol in anticipation of a pregnancy. Foetal alcohol syndrome may result from a pregnancy where alcohol consumption has occurred.

Consumption of some cheeses and exotic cold meats is not recommended.

Regular antenatal visits are important throughout the duration of the pregnancy, in order to monitor the health of the mother and growth of the foetus. The size of the uterus may be calculated. By 20 weeks the uterus will have reached the level of the umbilicus, and by 30 weeks the uterus will have reached half-way between the umbilicus and the xiphisternum. Foetal movements will be felt by the mother from anywhere around 20 weeks onwards, firstly as flutters in the abdomen. Then with each passing week, stronger kicks will be felt, along with general movement of the foetus.

Intercourse during pregnancy is not contraindicated except in the presence of bleeding, vaginal pain, or leakage of amniotic fluid. Sometimes bleeding, particularly early in the pregnancy, may indicate a threatened miscarriage. If bleeding occurs late in the pregnancy, medical attention should be sought immediately as abruption of the placenta may impair blood flow in the placenta, and therefore endanger the oxygen flow to the foetus. Bleeding and early uterine contractions may be signs that a premature delivery is imminent, and medical supervision is required.

Exercise is not contraindicated, although vigorous exercise should be moderated through the course of the pregnancy. Fitness levels should be maintained with gentle exercise and nutrition levels kept at an optimum. Excess weight gain due to either overeating or excess fluid build-up, is also not desirable, and should be managed by the treating practitioner. Weight gain in the pregnancy should not exceed a total of more than 13 to 15 kilograms depending on the build of the woman, and most of the weight gain will occur in the third trimester. It is also not recommended that pregnant women be exposed to the increased temperatures of saunas and hot tubs.

Although neonatal care these days is excellent, unplanned early delivery still carries with it risk to the baby. If the pregnancy is less than 34 to 36 weeks, some induced maturation of the baby's lungs may be necessary for an early delivery. It is generally regarded that a pregnancy less that 25 weeks of the anticipated 40 week duration of the pregnancy is not compatible with life because of the immaturity of the baby's lungs and other organs to sustain it independently outside of the uterus.

Maturation of the foetal lungs will normally be done by administration to the mother of some injectable steroids over one or more days at the discretion of the treating obstetrician prior to the delivery.

Early warning signs of potential problems in pregnancy include headaches, persistent nausea and vomiting, dizziness, visual disturbance, lower abdominal aches and pains, strong contractions, vaginal bleeding, rupture of the membranes, swelling of the hands and feet, reduced urinary output, and any infections. Any of these problems should be reported to the treating practitioner, and a course of action planned.

The signs of imminent delivery include low back pains or lower abdominal pains with contractions occurring at regular intervals, and rupture of the membranes.

Treatment

Early assessment of foetal maturity enables an accurate prediction for the date of delivery; however it is not uncommon for delivery to occur up to a couple of weeks early. If however the duration of the pregnancy extends beyond 42 weeks estimated gestation, delivery is recommended because the placenta after that time begins to become nonfunctional.

Prenatal diagnosis is available for central nervous system abnormalities, using nuchal translucency (an ultrasound investigation), and ultrasound examinations to detect the presence of gross abnormalities in the foetus. Amniocentesis is also available during pregnancy for high-risk pregnancies to determine the presence of other chromosomal abnormalities, e.g. Down syndrome.

Nuchal translucency investigation is also available for mothers at risk of foetal abnormality. This investigation is undertaken at around 13 weeks.

In the vast majority of cases, pregnancy will run a normal course of 40 weeks from the time of the last normal menstrual period. Early intervention in a delivery of a baby is indicated in the case of a diabetic mother (where the complication rate in the newborn is much higher), women with pelvic disproportion, a history of a previous caesarian for any reason, and for foetal distress, where emergency caesarian may be indicated.

premature ejaculation

Cause

Premature ejaculation refers to circumstances where ejaculation frequently occurs too soon to produce sexual gratification. Ejaculation may occur during foreplay or even prior to or just before vaginal penetration.

Premature ejaculation or loss of an erection may occur at times for a variety of reasons including inappropriate interruptions, but if ejaculation occurs on a regular basis prior to either or both of the sexual partners feeling sexual gratification, then premature ejaculation is said to be a sexual arousal or performance problem.

Symptoms

The male and female sexual arousal response curve is very different in nature. Men are able to become sexually aroused more quickly and are able to reach an orgasm more quickly than females. In a mutually satisfying sexual relationship, reaching orgasm is desirable enabling both partners in the relationship to achieve a satisfactory response. Where the response of one of the partners is not concordant with the other, sexual disparity may occur. It is more often the case that the male partner will need to learn how to delay orgasm in order for the female partner to become sufficiently aroused to also achieve sexual orgasm, and sexual satisfaction. Delaying ejaculation so that intercourse may take place is then the aim of treating premature ejaculation.

Treatment

Treatment for premature ejaculation involves a progressive educational process of the couple, as they become more relaxed sexually with each other. Medication is also of assistance, such as beta blockers, usually in low doses.

pressure in the eye

See *glaucoma*

priapism

Cause

Priapism is a term used to describe persistent, painful, abnormal erections, and may result from the use of injectable or oral medication for erectile dysfunction.

Treatment

Treatment for priapism includes the use of injected vasoconstrictor agents, or pseudo ephedrine in tablet form or alternatively, intramuscular injection with pethidine or morphine will allow the erection to subside.

prostate cancer

See *breast cancer*
See *erectile dysfunction or impotence*
See *incontinence*

Cause

The cause of prostate cancer is uncertain. Some famlies carry BRCA gene 1 or 2, which is associated with prostate cancer in men as well as breast cancer in women.

Symptoms

Symptoms of benign prostatic hyperplasia and prostate cancer are similar; however in the case of prostate cancer symptoms may also include pain resulting from spread of the disease to the bones, most commonly those of the vertebral column.

Investigations

Prostate cancer is more likely to feel hard to the touch on digital examination, and is irregular in outline; however this alone is not sufficient for a diagnosis of prostate cancer.

Treatment

For patients with prostate cancer, staging and grading of the malignancy is necessary in order to define the extent of disease. Elevation of an enzyme called acid phosphotase indicates the presence of secondary cancer deposits either in the lymph nodes or in the bones. A bone scan may be more sensitive in determining the presence of bony secondaries.

A diagnosis of prostate cancer need not mean a death sentence and many elderly men die with prostate cancer rather than die from the effects of prostate cancer. Grading of prostate cancer is also a means of predicting prognosis for an individual patient; this is done by histological assessment of the tumour tissue.

Following treatment for prostate cancer, both the acid phosphotase and prostate-specific antigen levels decrease. These parameters are used to monitor progression of the disease and the possibility of spread to other parts of the body. For many patients, control of the disease is certainly possible. Treatment for the disease depends on the tumour's stage and grade.

Surgical intervention for prostate cancer is a likely possibility for most patients. Watchful waiting though is an option, particularly if patients are asymptomatic and older than 70 years of age. This approach yields the same overall survival rate as prostatectomy in elderly men. Complete prostatectomy is the treatment of choice for men less than 70 years of age. Complications from the procedure, however, includes the possibility of urinary incontinence, stricture formation in the bladder neck and urethra, erectile dysfunction (which has been estimated from 30 per cent to 100 per cent of men following prostate surgery), and faecal incontinence.

Treatment may also include cryotherapy (or destruction of the prostate cancer by freezing), and radiotherapy. Some problems are experienced by patients following prostatic radiotherapy and include proctitis, cystitis, diarrhoea, fatigue, and rectal bleeding.

Radiotherapy is also used as palliative treatment for pain relief in patients with symptomatic deposits of prostate cancer in the bones, most commonly in the vertebral column. Some patients are also treated with androgen deprivation by surgical castration. Treatment may also include the provision of luteinising hormones.

Androgen deprivation may lead to low energy levels, osteoporosis, anaemia, and loss of muscle mass with long-term treatment. For high-grade tumours, chemotherapy with or without hormonal therapy is used before surgery in some protocols along with radiation in others. The choice of regime will largely depend on the recommendation of the specialist managing the patient.

prostate infection or prostatitis and prostate abscess

Cause

Prostatitis refers to a group of disorders that present with symptoms of urinary obstruction and perineal or pelvic pain. Prostatitis may be caused by acute or chronic bacterial infections. The means by which prostatitis occurs is really unknown but a prostate abscess may form following an acute episode of prostatitis.

Symptoms

Some of the symptoms may result from the presence of infection of the prostate gland as well as spasms of the muscles of the floor of the pelvis. Symptoms may include urinary irritation, urinary frequency and urgency, a feeling of incomplete bladder emptying and pain either in the tip of penis, lower back, or in the testicles. Pain may also be experienced with ejaculation. If the prostatitis is caused by an acute bacterial infection, symptoms such as fever, malaise, muscular aches and pains, tachycardia, rapid respiratory rate, and even hypotension may occur.

Abscess formation may be suspected in patients with ongoing or recurrent urinary tract infections with persistent lower pelvic pain, despite antibiotic therapy. Patients experiencing these symptoms should be further investigated with either ultrasound or cystoscopy examinations.

Treatment

Prostatitis is treated with antibiotics, anti-inflammatory medications, and pain relief.

Treatment for prostate abscess involves appropriate antibiotic therapy as well as drainage by trans-urethral evacuation, or by aspiration and drainage of the abscess.

prostatic hyperplasia, benign

See *prostate cancer*
See *prostate infection or prostatitis and prostate abscess*

Cause

Benign prostatic hyperplasia is the enlargement of the prostate in men. The risk of prostate enlargement increases with age, and most men over the age of 50 years will have some degree of prostate enlargement. Some drugs may add to the symptoms of prostate enlargement. These include antidepressants, alcohol consumption, drugs used for Parkinsonism, and some adrenaline-like medications used for coughs and colds.

The cause of benign prostatic hyperplasia is uncertain but it is probably associated with hormonal changes in association with the process of ageing. The prostate gland surrounds the urethra and produces fluid which contributes to ejaculatory fluid. As the prostate increases in size, it exerts pressure on the urethra until it reaches the size where outflow obstruction to the bladder occurs during urination. This may precipitate an episode of acute urinary retention or may come about gradually with symptoms of chronic urinary retention over a period of time.

Symptoms

The symptoms of prostate enlargement include difficulty initiating urination, poor urine stream, urinary hesitancy, the urge to pass urine more frequently, particularly during the night, and urgency of urination. This condition may become painful in the presence of a large distended bladder. The risk of acute urine retention is increased with consumption of alcohol. Infections of the bladder and of the prostate may occur.

Symptoms of benign prostatic hyperplasia include urinary frequency, urgency, hesitancy, incomplete emptying of the bladder, overflow incontinence, poor stream of urine, dribbling of urine, and urinary retention—either chronic or acute. Straining during urination may cause congestion of the superficial vein of the prostatic urethra and cause rupture of a vessel resulting in blood in the urine, production of haemorrhoids, and inguinal hernia. Straining during urination may also produce feelings of fainting and even collapse. Acute urinary retention may be precipitated by periods of decreased mobility, climatic conditions such as cold weather, post-anaesthesia, alcohol ingestion, and some drugs, e.g. antidepressants.

The presence of benign prostatic hyperplasia may coexist with prostate cancer, producing similar signs and symptoms. Patients with significant symptoms, particularly in the presence of blood in the urine, should be referred to a urologist for further assessment in order to eliminate the possibility of prostate cancer.

Investigations

Diagnosis of benign prostatic hyperplasia and prostate cancer is based initially on physical examination, e.g. rectal examination at which time the texture, size and feel of the prostate is noted. Other investigations include prostate specific antigen levels (PSA), cystoscopy, transrectal ultrasound, and prostate biopsy.

Treatment

Treatment for benign prostatic hyperplasia or hyperplasia includes the use of surgery where complete obstruction occurs, review of any medications which may promote urinary retention such as anti-cholinergics, sympathomimetics, and opiates. Any coexisting infection should be treated with antibiotics. For patients with mild to moderate obstructive symptoms some preparations may improve the obstructive symptoms.

Drugs are available to improve the urine flow, e.g. transulosin hydrochloride, and restruction of evening fluids will improve sleep disturbance. If it is determined that prostate cancer is present, prostate operation may follow.

pseudomembranous colitis

Cause

This condition may be caused by the use of some antibiotics, and is due to an overgrowth in the bowel of an organism called clostridium difficile, which produces toxins causing inflammation of the bowel.

Symptoms

Symptoms include profuse, watery diarrhoea, abdominal cramping, fever, which may commence up to six weeks following the administration of the antibiotics.

Treatment

Firstly the antibiotic treatment should be discontinued and replaced with metronidazole or alternatively, vancomyacin for up to 10 days.

psoriasis

Cause

Psoriasis is a skin condition where the cells in the skin are being produced at a faster rate than normal, and the skin on the surface becomes flaky and is exfoliated more rapidly than normal. Psoriasis is more commonly thought of as a skin condition but can produce pain and swelling in joints as well. The cause of psoriasis is unknown.

Symptoms

The skin often looks rough and flaky on the outside, and red and raised underneath. It is usually not painful. Some people with psoriasis may develop arthritis in association with the skin condition, called psoriatic arthritis. Psoriasis may develop at puberty or menopause. Whatever the cause of the arthritis, the symptoms are commonly pain, swelling of the joints involved, tenderness, stiffness and the joints feeling hot to the touch.

Treatment

The condition usually improves in the summer and deteriorates in the winter so treatment includes exposure to ultraviolet light. Topical steroid creams will improve the condition as will tar-based soap preparations. Treatment of psoriatic arthritis is treatment of the psoriasis with dithranol, and cytotoxic drugs such as methotrexate.

psychiatric conditions

See *anxiety*
See *depression*
See *disturbed patients*
See *obsessive-compulsive disorder*
See *panic disorder*

puberty, problems

See *adolescent health, problems*

Cause

During puberty, a portion of the brain called the hypothalamus sends signals to the pituitary gland to start producing male and female hormones from the testes and ovaries respectively which will trigger the development of secondary sexual characteristics such as penis size, testicle size and beard growth in males, and breast development and the onset of periods in females, and pubic and underarm hair growth.

Delayed

Changes of puberty may be delayed as a result of chromosomal abnormalities, e.g. Turner's syndrome, Noonan's syndrome, and Klinefelter's syndrome, or it may result from primary pituitary failure.

Precocious

Changes of puberty may also commence early, and this is known as precocious puberty. Precocious puberty is characterised by the development of secondary sexual characteristics before the age of eight years in girls and nine years in boys. Tumours of the ovary, testes, brain, or pituitary gland may result in the onset of precocious puberty.

Symptoms

Female secondary sexual characteristics include the development of the vulva, pubic hair development, breast development, commencement of periods, and increased fat deposition on the hips. Secondary sexual characteristics in boys include growth of the testicles and penis, voice changes and facial hair growth. Both sexes develop auxiliary and pubic hair and the potential for increased body odour.

Investigations

Confirmation of the diagnosis of precocious or delayed puberty is made by X-ray examination of the left hand and wrist to assess the degree of sexual maturation and the acceleration of bone growth. In adolescent males, bone age may be delayed. In this case, there is often a family history of similar delay in the onset of puberty. Assessment by a paediatric or adolescent trained endocrinologist may be necessary in order to determine the best course of action. Measurement of levels of sex hormones and adrenal hormones will also confirm a diagnosis of precocious or delayed puberty. Females who have not commenced periods by the age of 16 or 17 years of age should be investigated for a cause of delayed puberty. Chromosomal abnormalities in both males and females will result in infertility, and the need for replacement of deficient hormones.

Treatment

If the development of the signs of puberty is within one year of the population standards, treatment is not required . If this is not the case, female sex hormone can be suppressed until the time of normal puberty. Response to treatment must be monitored. If precocious puberty is due to testicular tumour in boys, the tumour should be excised.

pyloric stenosis

Pyloric stenosis is a condition which occurs in infants at around eight to 10 weeks of age. It is accompanied by characteristic projectile vomiting increasing with every feed. This condition may come on acutely, or a baby may have a prior history of vomiting prior to the diagnosis of pyloric stenosis.

Cause

This condition is caused by an increased development of the muscle which allows the material to leave the stomach. The diagnosis can be made by the medical practitioner who will feel a small lump in the upper abdomen.

Treatment

The most common form of treatment with this condition is surgical release of the muscular sphincter. This will usually require a minor operation.

Q fever

Cause

Q fever is caused by a bacterium called Coxiella burnetii and associated with contact with infected urine and faeces of sheep, cattle, goats. Transmission is by inhalation of infected aerosols. The condition may also be perpetuated by tick bite with an incubation up to 28 days.

Symptoms

Symptoms include fever, headache, chills, malaise, chest pains, non-productive cough, pneumonia, hepatitis with an increase in the size of the liver, abdominal pains and jaundice. Endocarditis sometimes occurs.

Treatment

Treatment is with tetracyclines and chloramphenicol.

rabies

Cause

Rabies may be acquired by a bite from an infected domestic or wild animal. Luckliy Australia is free of animals that carry the virus but if you are considering travelling overseas to countries where rabies is endemic in domestic and wild animals, vaccination against rabies should be considered prior to travel.

Symptoms

Rabies is characterised by involvement of the nervous system, where the virus travels from the site of inoculation to the spinal tract and brain where it multiplies. It may lie dormant for up to two months before manifesting as depression, restlessness, malaise, fever and profound thirst. Restlessness increases to excitement and excessive salivation as the virus may selectively infect the salivary glands. Painful muscle spasms of the larynx and pharynx follow, and death may occur due to exhaustion and general paralysis in three to ten days.

Treatment

If rabies develops, treatment involves symptomatic measures to the cardiovascular and respiratory systems.

rectal bleeding

Cause

Causes of rectal bleeding include anal fissures, angiodysplasia or new vessel formation in the wall of the gut causing intermittent bleeding, colitis, carcinoma of the colon, colonic polyps, diverticular disease, inflammatory bowel disease, haemorrhoids.

Symptoms

Rectal bleeding may or may not be accompanied by other symptoms of abdominal pain, and abdominal cramps. Other symptoms may include pain on passing bowel motions, or bleeding associated with bowel motions.

Investigations

Rectal examination represents the first line of investigation; however this alone has limitations and colonoscopy should be considered to exclude serious causes for rectal bleeding.

Treatment

The treatment for rectal bleeding will depend on establishing a diagnosis.

red eyes

See *eyes, red, bilateral*
See *eyes, red, unilateral*

refractive error

Cause

Refractive error is said to occur when the patient requires glasses in order to read. A person may be long-sighted or short-sighted, have astigmatism or presbyopia.

Refractive errors occur because the eyeball is either too long for the light rays to accurately converge on the retina at the back of the eye—this is called being short-sighted; or when the eyeball is too short and the rays of light entering the eye focus behind the retina—this is called being long-sighted.

Astigmatism results when the eye is asymmetrical in its measurements from front to back and from side to side. Presbyopia occurs as a person ages and the lens inside the eye is unable to flatten itself sufficiently in order for the person to be able to see close objects without the assistance of reading glasses.

A refractive error is common after cataract surgery and requires the use of reading glasses, even in the presence of an intraocular lens. A special form of refractive error which presents as a conical shape of the cornea is called keratoconus.

Symptoms

Symptoms include an inability to clearly see objects either up close or at a distance. Sometimes patients may not be aware that their field of vision is at all abnormal, and may need formal eye testing before the problem is identified.

Treatment

Refractive errors may be corrected with appropriate glasses or contact lenses. Short-sightedness may also be treated by an ophthalmologist using special surgical technique to correct the condition.

Treatment for keratoconus involves the use of specialist contact lenses which flatten the cornea and also correct for refractive error. In some cases, patients with keratoconus may require corneal grafting.

renal colic

See *abdominal pain*
See *renal stones*
See *urinary tract infection*

Cause

The ureter is the tube which leads from the kidney to the bladder. If a stone or blood clot occurs in the ureter, severe colicky pain will occur on that side.

Symptoms

Renal colic pain arises as a severe constant pain in either the right or left side. The pain of renal or ureteric colic is very intense and may be accompanied by small or large amounts of blood in the urine.

Investigations

The diagnosis of renal or ureteric colic may be made by detecting the presence of small or even large amounts of blood in the urine. Plain X-ray of the abdomen may demonstrate the presence of stones in the kidney. Over about 75 per cent of stones will be detectable in this way. A special X-ray of the kidney called an intravenous pyelogram where dye is injected into the bloodstream and then concentrated in the kidney may demonstrate a stone in the kidney and also indicate kidney function. An ultrasound may be utilised to locate a stone and then to exclude the possibility of obstruction of urine flow.

Treatment

The treatment of renal and ureteric colic almost always requires pain management. This is usually done by administration of a strong analgesic such as morphine, and the administration of an anti-nausea medication such as prochlorperazine or metoclopromide, usually by intramuscular injection.

renal dialysis

Renal dialysis is a treatment for patients with renal failure. Techniques include intermittent haemodialysis, continuous chemofiltration and haemodialysis, and peritoneal dialysis to remove elements from the blood that are normally excreted in the urine. All techniques involve pumping the patient's blood through a dialyser, exposing it to a semipermeable membrane and returning the cleansed blood via the circuit back to the body.

renal failure, chronic

See *kidney failure*

Cause

Chronic renal failure is a long-standing progressive deterioration of renal function. Causes of chronic renal failure include haemorrhage or severe fluid loss due to excessive use of diuretic medications, low cardiac output due to cardiomyopathy, heart attack, and pulmonary embolism. Other causes include septicaemia, liver failure, some antihypertensive agents, and renal artery obstruction.

Acute infections including glomerulonephritis and interstitial nephritis might also lead to renal failure. Destruction to the outflow of urine from the kidney, obstruction located in the bladder, and obstructions to the outflow from the bladder due to an enlarged prostate or cancer of the bladder or prostate, may also lead to renal failure.

Symptoms

Symptoms of chronic renal failure usually develop slowly over time and include loss of appetite, nausea, vomiting, lack of energy, fatigue, generalised itching, decreased mental alertness, muscle twitches, muscle cramps, water retention, and malnutrition. Some patients may experience peptic ulceration and bleeding, abnormalities of sensation in the extremities called peripheral neuropathy, and sometimes fitting or seizures.

The diagnosis is based on the patient's history, laboratory findings from pathology tests for renal function and not uncommonly, renal biopsy.

Treatment

Treatment for chronic renal failure is directed towards treating the underlying condition, and attention must be paid to fluid and electrolyte balance, often with the provisions of dialysis and sometimes with consideration of renal transplantation.

renal stones

Cause

Renal or kidney stones are relatively common and may or may not be symptomatic. Stones are caused by super-saturation of the urine with stone-forming salts or reduced urine excretion. Calcium oxalate crystals are the most common point of origin for the formation of kidney stones.

Symptoms

Severe back, loin or lower abdominal pains are the most commonly occurring symptoms, along with blood in the urine. Pain may be associated with nausea, vomiting, abdominal distension, fever, chills and urinary frequency. Renal colic is experienced when the stones move from the kidney down the ureter to the bladder. Rarely is a stone isolated from the urine, although occasionally this does happen. When the stone is passed, the pain subsides. Most renal stones may be demonstrated on X-ray.

Treatment

Kidney stones pass spontaneously or may be fixed in the pelvis of the kidney (staghorn kidney stone). The presence of a fixed stone may cause kidney infection to occur and if possible it is desirable for the stone to be removed. Removal of stones may occur with the aid of high frequency sound waves (lithotripsy) which destroys the stone. If the stone is causing obstruction of the ureter and the kidney, it may be necessary to place a stent in the ureter or kidney (to prevent the kidney from failing due to back pressure of the obstruction from the stone) until such time as destruction of the stone may occur. Long-term antibiotics may also be necessary to prevent infection. Treatment of an acute episode of renal colic includes pain management, increased fluid intake and relief of vomiting and infection. Occasionally open surgery to remove the stone may be necessary.

renal vascular disorders

See *kidney/renal failure*

respiratory system diseases

Diseases of the respiratory system, including the sinuses, nose and throat are referred to below:

See *asthma*
See *bronchiectasis*
See *bronchiolitis*
See *bronchitis*
See *lung abscess*
See *lung cancer*
See *occupational lung diseases*
See *pleurisy*
See *pneumonia*
See *respiratory system cancer*

respiratory system cancer *(nasopharynx, larynx, tonsils and tongue)*

See *lung cancer*
See *smoking*

Cause

Smoking of cigarettes, pipes or cigars is a very potent predisposing factor leading to cancer of the respiratory system, tongue, nasopharynx, and tonsils. Chewing tobacco is also a cause of oral cancer. Cancers of the nasal mucosa and the throat are common in Asian countries. Malignant melanoma lesions may occur in the mouth. Sometimes Epstein Barr virus may result in predisposition to cancer of the head and neck.

Symptoms

Nasopharyngeal cancer may first present with nasal or eustachian tube blockage, and later with bloody discharge from the nose, with nose bleeds and cranial nerve palsies and lymph node swelling of the cervical nodes. Symptoms of persistent lumps in the mouth require biopsy to exclude the possibility of a cancer. Sore throat is the most common presenting symptom of cancer of the tonsil, the second most commonly occurring cancer of the respiratory tract after cancer of the larynx.

Treatment

Treatment of nasopharyngeal cancer is radiation therapy. Treatment of cancer of the tonsil includes surgery and irradiation. Cancer of the tongue is treated with a combination of surgery and radiation. Cancer of the larynx is treated with laryngectomy and radiation.

retention of urine, acute

See *prostatic hyperplasia, benign*
See *prostate cancer*
See *prostate infection or prostatitis and prostate abscess*
See *ovarian follicles*

Cause

The most common cause of acute urinary retention is prostate gland problems in men. The prostate gland is located at the base of the penis and produces seminal fluid which is ejaculated. When the prostate gland enlarges, obstruction to the flow of urine may occur. If the obstruction becomes total, or if the obstruction becomes chronic, retention of urine will occur in the bladder.

Other causes include cancer of the prostate, prostatitis, blockage from a stone, an injury of the urethra (tube in the penis), and damage to the nerve supply to the bladder. This condition is much more common in males than females.

Some medication may cause urinary retention, e.g. some antidepressants.

Symptoms

Symptoms of acute retention of urine will present with varying degrees of inability to pass urine, and may present more chronically with an increasingly poor stream of urine. When the obstruction becomes complete and the bladder starts to enlarge, increasing discomfort and pain will occur. Before total obstruction occurs, some dribbling from the bladder may occur at times when the patient has no control of his or her bladder.

Treatment

Treatment of acute retention of urine necessitates catheterisation to drain the bladder of its contents. Anyone who has had an acute episode of retention of urine will require a referral to a specialist urologist for an opinion regarding the ongoing treatment. Ongoing treatment may involve an operation on the prostate. If the episode of urinary retention has been caused by a drug, the drug should be immediately withdrawn and the catheter should remain in place for 48 hours to ensure that a repeat episode does not occur.

retracted nipples

Cause

Retracted nipples are simply an anatomical variation in some women, where the erectile tissue in the nipples is tethered in some way, preventing the nipples from standing out from the chest.

Treatment

Surgical intervention to correct retracted nipples is unsuccessful. Women with retracted nipples who wish to breastfeed their babies may need to use a breast pump.

rheumatic fever

Cause

Rheumatic fever is caused by a complication of a streptococcus A infection. It occurs most commonly following streptococcal sore throat in young children.

Symptoms

Arthritis is the most common symptom, and chorea (rapid, jerky, involuntary movements) may occur as part of the acute illness.

Longer-term symptoms include damage to the heart valves resulting in heart murmurs and sometimes requiring valve repair or even replacement of damaged heart valves.

Treatment

Treatment of streptococcal throat infections with antibiotic preparations will prevent the onset of rheumatic fever.

rheumatoid arthritis

Cause

Rheumatoid arthritis is an autoimmune disease, where the body produces antibodies to the linings of joints.

Symptoms

Rheumatoid arthritis is a common cause of sore joints and stiffness. This disease commonly involves symmetrical pain and deformity of joints, i.e. pain involving joints in the hands and the feet equally. This disease can affect any joints in the body. The disease results in swelling and deformity of joints, along with pain and loss of function. In the past this has been most common in joints in the hand;

however with better treatment options today these deformities are less commonly seen. It might occur at any age, and in children it is known as juvenile rheumatoid arthritis.

Whatever the cause of the arthritis, the symptoms are commonly pain, swelling of the joints involved, tenderness, stiffness and joints feeling hot to the touch.

Treatment

The principles of treatment for arthritis are the same irrespective of the cause. These include a balance between rest and exercise, heat packs to painful joints, reducing weight if overweight, gentle exercise, physiotherapy, simple analgesics, e.g. paracetamol, non-steroid or anti-inflammatory medications, e.g. ibuprofen. Splinting of joints may be required in some cases of rheumatoid arthritis, and at times referral will be necessary to specialist orthopaedic surgeons or a rheumatologist who may also recommend disease-modifying anti-rheumatoid drugs (DMARDs), e.g. hydroxychloroquine, minocycline and methotrexate.

Ross River virus

Cause

Ross River fever is caused by a virus, and transmitted from person to person by mosquitoes.

Symptoms

Symptoms in the initial phase are flu-like with fever, lethargy, muscle and joint aches and pains, and sometimes a skin rash. The illness can continue for a prolonged time with the lethargy and aches and pains. Having once been infected, lifelong immunity is conveyed from that time onwards.

Treatment

There is no specific treatment for this viral condition, and symptomatic treatment for the fever and aches and pains in the form of paracetamol or ibuprofen is recommended. Prevention is possible by using mosquito repellent, long-sleeved clothing when outdoors, staying indoors at dawn and dusk, and avoidance of mosquito breeding grounds.

rubella

See *immunisation*

Cause

Rubella or German measles is an infectious viral disease caused by the ribonucleic acid or RNA rubella virus.

Symptoms

Symptoms of rubella include a characteristic rash, lymph node enlargement, mild fever and feeling unwell. Infection during pregnancy may lead to miscarriage, or may lead to congenital rubella syndrome in the infant, characterised by problems of vision, hearing, heart abnormalities, and varying degrees of intellectual retardation.

Effective protection is conveyed by immunisation in the measles, mumps, rubella vaccination, which is recommended at 12 months and four years of age, with a booster in the second or third decade. German measles may potentially be fatal to young children. It may also lead to a condition called subacute sclerosing pan-encephalitis some years following infection with the wild strain of German measles. This progressively leads to weakening of the muscles of the body and ultimately death from respiratory failure as a result of weakness of the respiratory muscles.

Treatment

Treatment for German measles is symptomatic and prevention is preferable. There is no cure or treatment for subacute sclerosing pan-encephalitis.

salivary gland, stone

Cause

Stones may obstruct the secretions of the salivary gland resulting in an infection. Why these stones form is not known.

Symptoms

Patients may present with a history of localised pain or more widespread pain if there is significant infection and abscess formation, localised swelling, inability to chew on the affected side. Localised sensitivity to hot or cold food in the mouth also results in pain in the salivary gland.

Investigations

Investigations for stones in the salivary glands are made by CT scan of the gland, ultrasound, or by canulating the duct of the gland and injecting dye. This investigation is called a sialogram, which is not only diagnostic but also therapeutic in that it may clear the gland of the stone.

Treatment for a stone in the salivary gland is with oral antibiotics, usually amoxilicillin, and pain relief. Relief of the obstruction is essential and elimination of other causes for an obstruction, e.g. tumour, is essential. If a tumour exists, surgical removal by a surgeon of the tumour and gland is necessary.

scabies

Cause

Scabies is caused by a parasitic mite which burrows under the skin.

Symptoms

The mite causes irritation, redness of the skin, and often tracks appear where the burrowing in the skin may be visible. People who are infected complain of itching and irritation. It is highly infectious and may spread throughout whole households. It most commonly occurs on the hands, between the fingers, around the waistline, but may occur all over the body. Not uncommonly scabies infections may spread rapidly in places such as nursing homes and hostels.

Treatment

Treatment includes application of a body wash and various preparations that are available, e.g. medication containing permethrin. This is applied to dry skin, left overnight and washed off the next morning. The whole family should be treated at the same time. A repeat treatment may be necessary one week from the first application.

scarlet fever

Cause

Scarlet fever is caused by a beta haemolytic streptococcus, usually from a sore throat, but it is relatively uncommon today.

Symptoms

Symptoms include sore throat, and a rash which is a diffuse red–pink in colour and covers the body.

Treatment

Treatment is with antibiotics, preferably penicillin.

schizophrenia

Cause

Schizophrenia is a psychiatric condition termed a psychosis or loss of contact with reality. The cause of schizophrenia is unknown but is thought to be genetic. The use of hallucinogenic drugs, including marijuana, may also induce a state of altered mental capacity similar to an acute episode of schizophrenia.

Symptoms

Schizophrenia is characterised by hallucinations, delusions, abnormalities of behaviour, a limited range of emotions, impaired reasoning and problem solving, and social dysfunction.

Treatment

Treatment of schizophrenia in the short and long term includes medical management with drug therapy, psychotherapy, rehabilitation and, where appropriate, cessation of precipitating hallucinogenic drugs such as marijuana.

scrotal mass

See *testicular cancers and tumours*

Cause

Scrotal masses may be due to inflammation, trauma, tumours of the testis or epididymis, scrotal abscess, urethral strictures, hydrocoele (which is an accumulation of fluid in the scrotum), haematocoele (which is an accumulation of blood in the scrotum), spermatocoele (a spermatic cyst), inguinal hernia, varicocoele (a collection of large veins in the scrotum), or lymphoedema.

Symptoms

Symptoms of the lump may be accompanied by anxiety, fever, aches and pains.

Treatment

Scrotal masses should always be investigated. Trauma to the scrotum should assess for damage to the testicles, whilst tumours should be treated aggressively.

Scrotal abscesses may arise from infections of the testicle and epididymis and should be treated vigorously. Drainage of the abscess will hasten recovery.

Urethral strictures may be accompanied by swelling of the scrotum, pain, redness, and accumulation of urine, and may be treated by dilatation and endoscopic investigations.

Treatment for a hydrocoele or accumulation of fluid in the scrotum is both therapeutic and diagnostic in that fluid which is drained from the scrotum may be sent to pathology for examination. Accumulation of fluid in the scrotum is not uncommon and drainage of the fluid may need to be repeated at regular intervals. Surgery may prevent fluid from reforming.

Haematocoele is usually the result of trauma and may be treated by draining the fluid and provision of antibiotics in order to prevent secondary infection.

Spermatocoele may be difficult to diagnose and distinguish from a hydrocoele; however if concern arises regarding the nature of the lump, excision and subsequent histological examination will provide the diagnosis. Aspiration of fluid from the scrotal lump may be sent to pathology to assist with diagnosis.

Inguinal hernia is common in men and a lump from the inguinal canal would usually extend into the scrotum. The lump will often reduce when pressed either by the patient, practitioner or spontaneously when the patient is lying down. Inguinal hernia commonly results from strain injuries during lifting and often require surgical repair. Varicocoele or large blood vessels will normally disappear when the patient is lying down; however surgery may be indicated for symptomatic treatment or if the vessel is impinging significantly on the testicle in children.

scrotal pain

See *scrotal mass*
See *testicular cancer and tumours*
See *testis, torsion*

Cause

Causes of scrotal pain include torsion of the testis (twisted testes), infections in the testis or local trauma to the testis. A diagnosis of torsion of the testis is the most commonly occurring cause for scrotal pain in children.

Symptoms

Symptoms include sudden onset of pain in the case of torsion of the testis, accompanied by nausea and vomiting, or fever in the case of infection in the testis. It is important to seek medical advice as sometimes it may be difficult to distinguish the conditions.

Treatment

Torsion of the testis is a medical emergency requiring urgent surgical correction in order to prevent loss of the testis. Treatment for infection of the testis is with appropriate antibiotics

seborrhoeic keratoses

See *skin problems*

Cause

Seborrhoeic keratoses are pigmented skin lesions which are waxy in texture and appear as wart-like structures anywhere on the body. The cause is unknown, but some people are more prone to these lesions than others and they commonly occur in older people.

Treatment

Treatment is often only for cosmetic purposes as the lesions are not dangerous and do not proceed to a malignant state. Treatment may be diathermy, liquid nitrogen, and some success may be gained by using fluorouracil cream, used for other forms of sun-damaged skin.

septic arthritis

See *hip pain*

Septic arthritis is caused by bacterial infection in a joint.

Symptoms

Whatever the cause of the arthritis, the symptoms are commonly pain, swelling of the joint involved, tenderness, redness, stiffness and the joints feeling hot to the touch.

Treatment

Treatment of septic arthritis is first to identify the sourse of the infection. If possible, a culture should be sent to the pathologist. Treating the infection with appropriate antibiotics and surgical intervention may be required. Sometimes surgical intervention with irrigation of the joint, and surgical cleaning of the joint, may be required. If it is found that in addition to septic arthritis, osteomyelitis of the bone is also present, ongoing antibiotic treatment, either intravenously or orally, may be required for a prolonged period of time.

septic shock

Cause

Most cases of septic shock occur while the patient is in hospital, commonly in newborn babies and pregnant women, and is due to an overwhelming infection in the blood. Shock is a clinical state characterised by hypotension resulting in reduced blood flow to the organs, cellular dysfunction and ultimately death, but the mechanism of action of septic shock is not entirely understood.

Common organisms which cause septic shock include staphylococci and meningococci. Common sites where infection may lead to bacterial or septic shock include the urinary system, the gall bladder and biliary ducts, and digestive or gastrointestinal systems.

Patients with heart attacks may sometimes present with signs of hypovolaemic or low cardiac output shock which is distinctive from septic shock. Causes may include decreased circulating volume of blood, and diminished cardiac output.

Symptoms

Symptoms include fever, tachycardia (abnormally rapid heart rate), and rapid breathing. If the patient is also starting to show signs of confusion and altered conscious state, hypotension and reduced urine output, septic shock should be considered. In bacterial or septic shock symptoms often begin with chills and fevers, with shaking and an inability to feel warm.

Other predisposing factors to septic shock include patients with diabetes, cirrhosis, low white cell count, if the patient is suffering from cancer or undergoing treatment for cancer with cytotoxic drugs or is being treated with an endotracheal tube, indwelling catheter draining the bladder, drainage tubes following abdominal or chest surgery, and patients who are receiving corticosteroid treatment.

If untreated, toxic shock results in the decrease in oxygen delivery and carbon dioxide removal, causing organ dysfunction. Eventually capillaries are bypassed resulting in decreased oxygen delivery particularly to vital organs, which in turn impairs the removal of carbon dioxide and waste products of metabolism and eventually leads to organ failure.

Provided the signs and symptoms of septic shock are recognised early, the overall mortality rate remains favourable. Poor outcomes often result from delayed recognition and treatment.

Symptoms of hypovolaemic shock include clamminess, pallor, cyanosis, rapid respiratory rate, lethargy and confusion.

Treatment

Treatment of septic shock includes aggressive resuscitation with intravenous fluids, intravenous antibiotics, and frequently intensive care unit support and correction of the underlying cause.

A rare form of septic shock includes sepsis due to staphylococcal infection and is termed toxic shock. This condition has been linked to the use of tampons.

sexually transmitted diseases

See *anal itch*
See *chlamydia*
See *gonorrhoea*
See *hepatitis*
See *herpes simplex virus (lips and genital area)*
See *human immunodeficiency virus (HIV)*
See *scabies*
See *syphilis*
See *testicular and epididymis infections*
See *vaginal discharge*

shingles (herpes zoster)

See *eyes*
See *herpes zoster*

Cause

Shingles is caused by the same organism which causes chickenpox, namely varicella zoster. It most commonly occurs in adults, and results from reactivation of the chickenpox virus.

Symptoms

Shingles produces a rash which may affect any portion of the body, is commonly confined to one side of the body front and back, in a pattern which follows the embryological dermatomes of the body, i.e. the segments of the body which develop in the foetus. If shingles infection presents on the face, it commonly involves the upper half of the face and scalp in a distribution which follows that of the branches of the trigeminal nerve. Sometimes this infection is so severe in older patients that admission to hospital is warranted.

Treatment

Early diagnosis of shingles is the key to successful treatment, which takes the form of antiviral agents called acyclovir. In order to achieve best effectiveness, the medication should be administered within 72 hours from the appearance of the rash of shingles. Pain relief may also be required in the acute phase, and sometimes medium to long term to relieve the post-herpetic pain from shingles infection.

sinusitis

See *headache*
See *halitosis*

Cause

Sinusitis is an inflammation of the sinuses due to viral, bacterial or fungal infections, or due to allergic reactions. Bacterial infection causes sinusitis, and culture of the nasal passages may reveal haemophylus, staphylococcus or streptococcus. In children it is important to suspect a foreign body up the nose. Patients with sinusitis usually present with an upper respiratory tract infection which is followed by a secondary bacterial infection as part of the disease.

Symptoms

The symptoms of sinusitis include nasal obstruction and congestion with profuse nasal discharge, cough, facial pain and headache, fever and malaise, and possibly muscular aches and pains and lethargy.

Symptoms also include localised pain and tenderness over the affected sinuses, referred dental pain to the affected side, nasal discharge, which may be yellow, green or bloodstained, some degree of nasal congestion and obstruction. However, sometimes sinusitis may occur with minimal symptoms of obstruction to the nasal passages, cough, fever and bad breath.

Treatment

Sinusitis is treated with antibiotics, most commonly with penicillin-based antibiotics as a first choice, decongestant preparations, steam inhalation, nose blowing, and symptom relief from the aches and pains and headache. Exclusion of nasal polyps is sometimes necessary. Referral to an ear, nose and throat surgeon may be necessary if the infection does not clear, for surgical washout of the sinuses. Not uncommonly, a specialist may recommend the addition of corticosteroids (either as a nasal inhalation or as oral tablets) for a period of time.

skin problems

See *acne*
See *dermatitis/eczema*
See *impetigo*
See *keratoacanthoma*
See *melanoma*

Most people do not think of skin as an organ of the body, but it is a very active organ and is producing new cells every single day of a person's life. Every day we discard cells from the outer layers of the skin, and these are replaced by new cells which are generated from the deepest layers of skin on a continuous basis.

Skin covers the body from head to toe, containing receptors for touch, detection of temperature and pressure and conveys information to the brain about the world around us. It contains the blood vessels, sweat glands, and oil producing glands which help to keep the skin nourished and moisturised.

The skin also contains fine hairs which assist in sensory detection and discrimination. The skin is subject to a vast array of chemicals at home and at work, and environmental elements of sun, wind and hot and cold conditions. The skin provides a method of cooling the body by sweating and, providing the skin is intact, provides a barrier between these elements and the body.

The skin is not a homogeneous covering of the body, but varies in thickness, pigmentation and distribution of sensory organs. The variation in pigmentation produces lesions in the skin, commonly referred to as moles, of varying shape, size and the potential to be harmful. When skin is subject to the effects of ultraviolet radiation from the sun either during normal everyday activities, sporting activities or by lying in the sun, changes occur in the skin which may not be fully appreciated for several decades. Ultraviolet radiation produces skin cancers, called basal cell carcinomas and squamous cell carcinomas. Other forms of skin cancer include malignant melanomas and keratoacanthomas. Malignant melanomas may occur anywhere in the body which contains pigment cells (called melanocytes). They may even occur in the eye, genital area, and around the anus.

Some families have more pigmented skin lesions than others, and their skin lesions should be assessed from an early age. It is best to look for a good general practitioner to assess skin lesions on a regular basis.

The skin is also affected by smoking, alcohol consumption, and ingestion of prescribed and recreational drugs and medications. A combination of these internal and external environmental factors may contribute to significant ageing of the skin's appearance, and the quality of the skin and its effectiveness in maintaining a barrier to infection as the body ages.

slipped femoral epiphysis

See *hip pain*

smoking

See *emphysema*
See *heart attack*
See *lung cancer*
See *osteoporosis*
See *pancreatic cancer*
See *sudden infant death syndrome*

Cigarettes
Cigarette smoking has an effect on almost every organ system in the body, e.g. heart, lungs, brain, kidneys, peripheral arteries, skin, and leads to considerable morbidity and mortality. It adds to the risks of developing complications from atherosclerosis, hypertension, elevation in cholesterol, obesity and diabetes, There has been significant evidence that smoking leads to emphysema and lung cancer, and causes excessive ageing of the skin, which is particularly

noticeable on the skin of the face. Patients who smoke also have a greater risk of suffering from heart attack or stroke.

Passive smoking may contribute to respiratory problems in members of the same household as a smoker. Children in a household where there are smokers can experience a range of health problems, mostly relating to respiratory and ear, nose and throat problems. Sudden infant death syndrome is also more common in a household where one or more people smoke on a regular basis. Smoking in the workplace is now prohibited by government legislation.

Marijuana

Users of marijuana may also experience lung damage. Marijuana produces a dreamy state, distortion in time, colour, space, and the feelings of exhilaration may be overtaken by feelings of panic. Coordination is impaired with the use of marijuana in much the same way as a person may experience if intoxicated with alcohol. Short- and long-term use may induce schizophreno-like symptoms which require urgent treatment and which usually resolve with withdrawal of the marijuana. The metabolites of marijuana may remain present in the urine for up to some months, and are detectable on testing.

Some pre-employment medical examinations require that the patient be tested for not only recreational drug consumption, but also for the use of marijuana.

snoring and sleep apnoea

See *obesity*
See *weight management problems*

Cause

Snoring is a noise caused by the vibrations of the muscles of the soft palate and other soft tissues in the upper airways as air passes over the tissues during respiration. The soft tissues of the palate fall back into the air space at the back of the throat causing an obstruction to the passage of air, in much the same way as air would be let out of a partially obstructed neck of an inflated balloon causing noise and vibration.

Snoring occurs most commonly when the person is lying on their back and the noise causes disruption for the person sharing the bed with the snorer.

The mechanics involved with snoring may also cause obstruction to the passage of air in and out of the lungs thus impairing oxygenation of the blood during sleep, and also causing episodes of apnoea (or cessation of breathing). This is called sleep apnoea. Obesity is a common cause of sleep apnoea.

Symptoms

Symptoms of snoring may not be reported by the patient but the sleeping partner may complain and many a partner has retreated to the second bedroom because of the snoring. Snoring may contribute to daytime sleepiness, fatigue, and the snorer often wakes in the morning not feeling refreshed.

The patient may complain of tiredness during the day, nodding off in front of the television, while sitting at the dining room table or sometimes nodding off while driving. Such patients should be advised to seek assessment as a matter of priority, and should be advised not to drive until a treatment plan has been devised for them.

Investigations

Investigations for sleep apnoea may be undertaken to assess the degree and frequency of obstructed episodes the patient may be experiencing each night. These tests may be undertaken either at the patient's home or in a sleep laboratory.

Treatment

Various regimes are available for the treatment of snoring including weight reduction, attention to the support of the head and neck with pillows, and sleeping positions in the bed, and avoidance of certain substances prior to going to bed, e.g. smoking, alcohol, muscle relaxants and sleeping tablets.

A C-pap (or nocturnal positive pressure device) machine may significantly improve sleep apnoea and sleeping positions in the bed.

solar keratoses

See *skin problems*

Cause

Solar keratoses result from the skin receiving an excessive amount of exposure to ultraviolet light.

Treatment

Treatment for solar keratoses includes diathermy, liquid nitrogen, and topical preparations such as fluorouracil. Other forms of treatment include those available through dermatologists for cosmetic surgery involving intense pulsed light (IPL) for extensive areas to be treated, particularly on the face.

spleen disorders

The spleen is an abdominal organ which is involved in immune protection of the body.

Cause

Increased activity in the spleen may result from myeloproliferative diseases, lymphoproliferative diseases (lymphomas such as Hodgkin's lymphoma), leukaemia (especially chronic lymphocytic leukaemia and chronic myeloid leukaemia), storage diseases (Gaucher's disease, amyloidosis, Niemann-pick disease), haemolytic anaemia (sickle cell anaemia, spherocytosis, thalassaemia) and connective tissue diseases.

In tropical climates infectious diseases such as malaria may also be responsible for increased activity in the spleen resulting in splenomegaly. Other causes of splenomegaly include cirrhosis of the liver, and thrombosis of the portal or spleen veins. Trauma to the spleen may also result in an increase in size as a result of a haematoma surrounding the spleen itself, and may require surgical intervention. Rupture of a haematoma of the spleen before surgery may produce a rapid fall in blood pressure.

Treatment

Treatment of problems in the spleen is directed at the underlying disease. An intact spleen protects against serious infections by filtering the bacteria. Following splenectomy, patients are more at risk of developing sepsis and precautions should be observed to avoid patients developing a fever at any time. It is sometimes recommended, that patients who have had their spleen removed receive vaccinations—such as meningococcal, pneumococca—prior to the operation or immediately following the operation for rupture of the spleen. Patients should then ensure that all vaccinations are maintained from that point.

sprains

Cause

The most commonly occurring sprain (or ligamentous injury) is a sprained ankle, from a fall or twisting injury from sporting activities.

Symptoms

Symptoms include swelling of the area, bruising, pain, and difficulty with weight bearing.

Treatment

Treatment is to first exclude a fracture, then apply ice, rest, elevation and pain relief. A compression bandage will help control the swelling, and strapping will support the injury. An ultrasound from the physiotherapist will assist with healing and mobility, reduce swelling and help disperse the bruising.

staphylococcus aureus

See *endocarditis*
See *gastroenteritis*
See *impetigo*
See *osteomyelitis*
See *pneumonia*
See *toxic shock syndrome*

Symptoms

Staphylococcus aureus or golden staph, is responsible for skin infections including infections in wounds, and impetigo in children. The reservoir for infection is located in the nasal passages, and resistance to various antibiotics is not uncommon. MRSA (multi-resistant staph aureus) is common following operations in hospitals and is becoming more and more problematic. Staphylococcus aureus is also a cause of pneumonia, endocarditis, osteomyelitis, gastroenteritis and toxic shock syndrome.

Treatment

Treatment for staphylococcal infections is with penicillin, and where resistance to penicillin has been proven, vancomycin is the antibiotic of choice.

stomach

See *haematemesis (vomiting blood)*
See *melaena (black bowel motions)*

stomach cancer

See *helicobacter pylori infection*
See *peptic, perforated or gastric ulcer*

Cause

The causes of stomach cancer are many but smoking and helicobacter pylori play a significant role in its onset.

Symptoms

Symptoms of stomach cancer include bleeding anywhere along the digestive tract from the mouth to the anus.

The symptoms of haematemesis, bleeding which originates from the stomach, depends on the amount and the rate of blood loss. If bleeding is sudden, the patient may become hypotensive and require resuscitation. If the bleeding is slow and over a period of time, the patient may present with symptoms of anaemia. The patient may also present with black bowel motions (melaena) as the first sign of bleeding from the bowel.

Investigations

Investigations of bleeding from the bowel require an endoscopy and/or a colonoscopy to determine if the cause is stomach cancer.

Treatment

Treatment for bleeding from the bowel firstly requires attention to resuscitation measures, with fluid replacement and blood transfusion, depending upon the amount of bleeding which has taken place.

Specific therapy will depend on the bleeding site. If endoscopic measures fail to stop the bleeding, surgical intervention may be required.

Treatment for stomach cancer consists of surgery and chemotherapy, but long-term survival is poor except for the presence of local limited disease.

stroke

See *transient ischaemic attack*

Cause

A stroke is defined as a neurological problem causing loss of either motor or sensory function of the body or a combination of both, e.g. loss of function of one side of the body, loss of speech, or vision.

Stroke may include haemorrhagic stroke, where the cardiovascular event presents as a bleed into the brain tissue, or may take the form of occlusive stroke, where the blood vessels supplying parts of the brain are occluded thus depriving the brain of blood flow, oxygen and function.

Symptoms

Symptoms of a stroke may include headache, problems with coordination of parts of the body or total loss of function of parts of the body, loss of consciousness. High blood pressure is a risk factor for the development of stroke, as is the deposition of cholesterol in the cerebral arteries.

Treatment

Treatment for stroke patients include determining the cause of the stroke, controlling hypertension, maintaining fluid hydration to the patient, prevention of the stroke from extending to become a more major event, anticoagulant therapy (with heparin or warfarin, in the case of occlusive stroke), quitting smoking, physiotherapy, speech therapy and rehabilitation.

Urgent diagnosis, assessment and referral help to improve the outcome in stroke patients.

sty

Cause

A sty is caused by an infection at the base of the eyelashes.

Symptoms

Symptoms include redness of the eyelid, swelling and mild pain.

Treatment

Treatment is based on removing the infected eyelash. Heat applied to the area will help, and topical antibiotics will assist if the infection is severe.

sudden infant death syndrome

See *smoking*

Sudden infant death syndrome (SIDS) is a distressing event for all. To assist in the prevention of SIDS, babies should be placed on their back or sides for sleeping, and not on their stomach.

Cause

The cause of SIDS is not really known, but it is felt that there is an association with babies who are exposed to cigarette smoke.

Treatment

Treatment for the family following a sudden infant death involves comfort and support and often counselling. SIDS support groups are available and provide positive support to families where a sudden infant death has occurred.

sunburn

See *skin problems*

Cause

Sunburn is caused by damage to the skin from the effects of ultraviolet light. Solariums are no different to lying out in the sun, and may be considered even more damaging to the skin.

Symptoms

Sunburn causes redness, pain and blistering of the skin, followed by peeling of the top layer of skin. It is felt that burning to the skin in early childhood is sufficient to cause sun cancer later in life, and that all sun exposure is cumulative lifelong. Sun exposure, even small daily exposure, will result in increased ageing of the skin compared to those people who minimise their exposure to the sun and who regularly use sunblock.

Treatment

Treatment of severe sunburn includes pain relief. At times symptoms may be improved with the application of a one per cent hydrocortisone cream to the affected areas of skin.

Prevention is desirable, by avoiding lying in the sun, particularly in the day between 10 am and 3 pm, wearing a wide brim hat, frequent application of 30+ sunblock when outdoors and particularly during swimming and outdoor water sports. Cover-up clothing is also desirable.

sweating

Cause

Sweating is a mechanism of the body to enhance cooling. Some people sweat more than others, and in some people sweating is induced by nervousness or anxiety. Increased production of sweat is called hyperhydrosis.

Symptoms

Symptoms include excessive production of sweat in the armpits, on the hands and feet, on the face, or on the whole body. People sweat more when they are under psychological or physiological stress or in response to an infective illness, acute blood loss or heart attack, acute perforated peptic ulcer and other forms of serious acute illness.

Treatment

Excessive sweating most commonly of the hands and/or feet and of the armpits may be effectively treated surgically by an operation called sympathectomy of the nerve supply to the glands. Excess sweating may also be treated with administration of Botox injections. Botox however needs to be repeated at regular intervals, and is expensive.

Treatment of underlying infection or of the symptoms of physiological stress in response to blood loss or heart attack will minimise the effects of sweating.

syphilis

See *sexually transmitted diseases*

Cause

Syphilis is a sexually transmitted disease caused by an organism from the group of agents called a spirochete, called treponema pallidum.

Symptoms

Symptoms include genital ulcers, meningitis, skin rash, aortic disease and neurological abnormalities.

The disease has three distinct phases if left untreated. The first stage or acute primary phase occurs with sexual contact. After an incubation period of between three to four weeks, an ulcer, called a chancre, will develop at the site of the inoculation such as the penis, anus, rectum, perineum, vulva, cervix, or on the mouth.

In the secondary phase of the infection, symptoms occur such as fever, malaise, anorexia, nausea, fatigue accompanied by headache and aches and pains. Almost any organ of the body can be affected in the secondary phase.

The tertiary or third phase of the condition develops some years later when cardiovascular and nervous system degeneration occurs. This stage of the disease may occur up to 10 years following the primary infection.

Treatment

The treatment of choice at any stage of the disease involves prescriptions of sustained-release penicillin.

systemic lupus erythematosus

Cause

Systemic lupus erythematosus (also called lupus or SLE) falls into a group of diseases known as autoimmune diseases or connective tissue disorders. The cause is unknown, but it may have a genetic basis. The disease may be induced by some drugs.

SLE attacks and injures the body's own organs and tissues and almost every system of the body can be affected. SLE may be the cause of arthritis.

Symptoms

Systemic lupus erythematosus may involve a number of organs of the body. The most commonly affected organs are the joints, heart, lungs, kidneys, liver, and nervous system. Whatever the cause of the arthritis, the most common symptom is pain in the joints. Other symptoms include swelling of the joints, tenderness, stiffness and the joints feeling hot to the touch.

Treatment

Treatment for systemic lupus erythematosus includes prescription with steroids and sometimes the use of immunosuppressive drugs.

The principles of treatment for systemic lupus erythematosus is the same as for arthritis. These include a balance between rest and exercise, heat packs to painful joints, reducing weight if overweight, gentle exercise, physiotherapy, simple analgesics, e.g. paracetamol, non-steroid or anti-inflammatory medications, e.g. ibuprofen. Splinting of joints may be required in some cases of SLE, and at times referral will be necessary to a specialist such as a rheumatologist.

tantrums

Cause

Tantrums are a manifestation of behaviour problems in children, often involving public displays of oppositional behaviour.

Symptoms

Tantrums do not occur when the child is alone, and are induced by the child as a means of attention seeking and achieving their own demands.

Treatment

Consistent, sensible parenting is the secret behind prevention or elimination of temper tantrums in children.

tarsal tunnel syndrome

See carpal tunnel syndrome

Cause

Tarsal tunnel syndrome is caused by the entrapment of the nerves to the foot caused by pressure from the surrounding fibrous tissue bands.

Symptoms

Symptoms of this condition include pain in the foot or toes, numbness, and weakness in the muscles of the foot.

Treatment

Treatment for this condition is successfully achieved by a simple operation releasing the nerves.

tearduct blockage

Cause

Tearduct blockage occurs in babies, and represents a developmental phase where the tear duct has not yet canalised. Given time, most blockages will resolve spontaneously and not require any intervention, except supportive measures.

Symptoms

Most commonly, the child will present with discharge from the eyes. Frequent washing with warm water is required.

Treatment

If there is significant discharge, topical antibiotic drops may be prescribed, in addition to regular washing of the eyes with warm water and drying with clean cotton balls for each eye.

If problems continue, referral to an ophthalmologist for probing of the tear duct may be necessary.

teething

Teething is defined as a developmental milestone of infancy consisting of the eruption of primary teeth, usually from the age of six months onwards, until 20 primary teeth have erupted. The same degree of discomfort is not necessarily associated with eruptions of the secondary teeth, starting from the age of six when front teeth top and bottom begin to be replaced by the secondary teeth. X-ray of the jaws during late childhood and adolescence will demonstrate the presence of erupted teeth inside the jaws, and the presence of wisdom teeth.

Symptoms

Teething does not cause ear infections, fevers, diarrhoea or vomiting, but may be associated with irritability, discomfort and pain.

Treatment

Simple analgesic pain relief may be necessary during this time of teething.

temporal arteritis

See *polymyalgia rheumatica*

Cause

Temporal arteritis is thought to be an autoimmune-type condition where the vessels in the area of the temporal bone become inflamed and thickened with resulting reduction in blood flow. It can cause visual defects or blindness if untreated.

Symptoms

Temporal arteritis is a unilateral headache associated with local tenderness in the area of the forehead. Inflammation in the blood vessels may be accompanied by pain and tenderness of the arteries involved.

Treatment

Treatment for this condition is the administration of oral corticosteroids and it is monitored by serial pathology testing of the ESR (erythrocyte sedimentation rate) which measures the amount of inflammation in the body.

temporomandibular joint

See *arthritis*
See *dental problems*
See *facial pain*
See *headache*
See *tension headache*

Cause

Temporomandibular joint (TMJ) problems often have many factors, but most are related to abnormal movements of the jaw in socket.

The TMJ is the joint which opens and closes the mouth. Pain in the area may be due to mechanical problems with the joint, e.g. arthritis, abnormalities of the dental bite, frequent chewing of gum, or grinding or clenching of the teeth.

Symptoms

Pain in the temporomandibular joint or side of the face is a common symptom and may be accompanied by ringing of the ears, pain in the ear caused by irritation or inflammation of the temporomandibular joint, and some tinnitus or ringing of the ear may occur on the affected side.

Other symptoms include pain when pressure is applied to the joint when the mouth is open, and sensitivity of one or more of the teeth on the same side. The temporomandibular joint may also exhibit noises on opening and closing the mouth.

Investigations

Direct viewing of the ear drum is essential and examination of the temporomandibular joint will often reveal the diagnosis. In order to exclude a more sinister cause, auditory brain stem responses, as well as pure tone or audiometry should be performed.

Treatment

Treatment of pain in the area of the temporomandibular joint needs to exclude dental cavities as a cause for the pain. Treatment may also include provision of a mouth splint for night use to correct the abnormal bite action of the jaws (from a dentist or orofacial specialist), and cessation of the use of chewing gum.

Treatment of temporomandibular joint dysfunction includes addressing any precipitating cause, e.g. dental problems, mal-occlusion, teeth grinding. Pain relief may be required, in the form of either simple paracetamol, or anti-inflammatory preparations.

tension headache

See *migraine*

Cause

Tension headache or musculoskeletal headache is often referred to by patients as migraine headache, but it is not a migraine. Tension headaches are common among people who spend prolonged periods sitting in front of the computer, at a desk either as part of work or as a student. Tension headache can be precipitated by people who chew gum or who chew for prolonged periods of time, and people who grind their teeth. Tension headache may be brought on by spasm in the muscles of the region of the cervical spine, by poor posture (either in a sitting, standing or lying position), trauma to the cervical muscles (whiplash), or by inappropriate bedding, e.g. a sagging mattress or a poor quality pillow.

Symptoms

Headache, nausea, vomiting, feeling unwell, tiredness and lethargy may accompany a tension headache. Tender areas in the muscles around the head and cervical spine are also characteristic of a tension headache.

Treatment

The diagnosis is made during the course of the physical examination when the patient is found to have multiple tender areas around the head and neck region. People often think they must have a brain tumour because of the severity of the pain and need to be reassured.

Learning how to prevent the symptoms, and learning how to stop the symptoms from progressing to become very severe are also important. Physical treatment including massage and physiotherapy to the cervical region are helpful. It is also important to try to identify the triggering factors producing the headache, as the symptoms are likely to return. Identification of trigger points and application of pressure to these points will often help to relieve the pain.

Physical exercise is an important preventative measure, as well as stretching the muscles of the neck, back, thighs and lower legs. Strengthening the muscles in this region is also important. One of the precipitating factors may be the pillow on which the patient sleeps every night, and attention should be paid to this. The pillow needs to be supportive of the cervical spine (neck areas) during the period of sleep, as the head is heavy and the cervical spine needs support against the weight of the head during the night.

testicular and epididymis infections

See *testicular cancer and tumours*

Cause

Testicular and epididymis infections (epididymo-orchitis) may be caused by a range of bacterial infections including gonorrhoea and chlamydia. This may result in abscess formation or even compromise the blood supply to the testicle. A common cause is related to the presence of indwelling catheters, in particular following prostate surgery. An infection primarily in the testis of viral origin is most commonly due to the mumps virus.

Symptoms

Symptoms of scrotal pain or lower abdominal pain may present with this condition. The patient may be feverish. The presence of urethritis suggests the possibility of a sexually transmitted disease for either gonorrhoea or chlamydia. In cases involving pain in the testis, the possibility of testicular torsion (or twisting of the testicle) should always be considered. Testicular torsion should be regarded as a medical emergency because unless treated early, loss of one or both of the testicles may result from lack of blood supply.

Treatment

Investigation of testicular tumours may include a Doppler ultrasound. Once testicular torsion as a diagnosis has been excluded, treatment for epididymo-orchitis includes bed rest, scrotal ice packs, anti-inflammatory analgesics, antibiotic therapy and, if necessary, intravenous antibiotics should be administered. Testing for sexually transmitted diseases should be performed and treatment prescribed as necessary. A urological follow-up is recommended.

testicular cancer and tumours

See *scrotal mass*

Cause

The cause of testicular cancer is unknown, but the risk of testicular cancer is increased in cases of undescended or partially undescended testicles. Other tumours of the testicles include tumours of the epidermis and spermatic cord, which are usually fibromas or lipomas.

Symptoms

Most testicular tumours will present with a lump in the scrotum, which may or may not be painful and most testicular masses will result in a diagnosis of cancer. If a testicular mass is found, staging of the cancer may be done using abdominal and pelvic CT scan.

Prognosis for testicular cancer depends on the stage of the disease and the presence of secondary spread.

Treatment

Treatment for testicular cancer involves surgical excision. Some cancers may be suitable for radiation therapy or chemotherapy. In some cases radiotherapy to the chest is recommended to minimise the effects of secondary spread of the tumour.

testis, torsion

See *scrotal pain*
See *testicular and epididymis infections*

Cause

Torsion of the testis occurs when the testicle twists around and cuts off the blood supply.

Symptoms

Pain may occur in both testicles and in the lower abdomen.

Treatment

Torsion of the testis constitutes a medical emergency. In order to preserve a functioning testicle, the patient will need urgent referral to hospital for treatment to be carried out.

testosterone, low *(hypogonadism)*

Cause

Hypogonadism in males is defined as a testosterone deficiency with decreased or no sperm production. It may result from a disorder of the testes, called primary hypogonadism, or it may result from secondary hypogonadism involving the hypothalamus and pituitary gland.

Both primary and secondary hypogonadism may be congenital or acquired as a result of the ageing process, due to disease, drugs, or other factors. Congenital causes of hypogonadism include Klinefelter's syndrome, the absence of testicles, myotonic dystrophy, enzymatic defects in testosterone synthesis, Noonan's syndrome, and secondary or hypothalamic/pituitary causes including Kallmann syndrome, Prader-Willi syndrome.

Primary acquired causes include chemotherapy or radiation therapy, following virus infections including mumps, echovirus and group B arbovirus. Secondary acquired causes include any systemic illness, hypopituitarism, haemochromatosis, drugs containing oestrogen, metoclopramide, opioids, Cushings syndrome, cirrhosis, severe obesity, alcoholism and liver failure.

Symptoms

Primary hypogonadism may range from a child being born with male chromosomes yet with female external genitalia, or ambiguous genitalia, or microphallus and undescended testes. In some cases, hypogonadism is not detected until a delay in the onset of puberty is recognised. If left untreated at this stage, secondary sexual characteristics will fail to develop. As a result, affected males will present with poor muscle tone, high-pitched voice, small scrotum, small or infantile size of the penis and testicles, and sparse body hair including facial and pubic hair. If testosterone deficiency develops in adult life, the symptoms will depend on the duration of the deficiency, e.g. decreased libido, erectile dysfunction, sleep disturbance, mood changes, increased visceral fat and osteoporosis may occur.

Treatment

Treatment of hypogonadism is directed towards testosterone replacement, either in the form of testosterone patches, or by injection on a regular basis. Injections may need to be given every two to four weeks intramuscularly. One of the side effects of administration of testosterone in men over the age of 50 include acne, increase in breast size, prostate enlargement, and on occasions may promote growth of prostate cancer (without actually causing prostate cancer).

Oral forms of testosterone are available; however these medications carry risk of liver dysfunction and hepatic adenoma. Infertility due to primary hypogonadism may use intratesticular sperm which may be harvested for fertilisation of an egg with the assistance of in-vitro fertilisation (IVF).

tetanus

Cause

Tetanus is an acute condition caused by toxins released from a bacterium called clostridium tetani.

Symptoms

Symptoms include muscle spasms, which commence around the face and lower jaw and give the condition the name lock jaw. Tetanus is a ubiquitous organism and infection may result from a seemingly trivial injury, e.g. a rose thorn from the garden. Vaccination for tetanus occurs in accordance with the immunisation schedule for children starting at two months of age and, regular boosters are recommended up until the age of 50. If this regime has been followed, the National Health and Medical Research Council advises that subsequent vaccinations after the age of 50 is regarded as unnecessary. The effects of tetanus, if untreated, are life-threatening. The incubation period for acute tetanus ranges from two to 50 days (with an average of five to 10 days).

Treatment

Treatment for the disease, once established, includes administration of tetanus immuno-globulin and intensive care support to relieve the muscle spasms.

thalassaemia

Cause

Thalassaemia is a genetically inherited abnormality of haemoglobin. People from countries surrounding the Mediterranean are more likely to inherit this condition. It may be inherited as thalassaemia minor or thalassaemia major.

Symptoms

Most often symptoms of thalassaemia are negligible. The diagnosis may be made on routine pathology screening with a full blood count. Sufferers of thalassaemia major may experience severe anaemia, breathlessness, jaundice, enlargement of the spleen and sometimes physical and mental retardation.

Treatment

For thalassaemia minor, no treatment is required. For thalassaemia major, treatment may be required in the form of blood transfusion and bone marrow transplantation.

thoracic outlet syndrome

Cause

Thoracic outlet syndrome represents a group of conditions affecting the nerves which supply the arm and the arteries which supply the arm.

Symptoms

Symptoms include pain, tingling, and numbness in the arm, hands and fingers.

Treatment

Surgical treatment to relieve the pressure on the nerves may be required in order to relieve the symptoms.

thrombophlebitis

See *leg pains*

Cause

Thrombophlebitis is an inflammation of a vein resulting in clot formation.

Symptoms

Symptoms include pain and swelling overlying the area of inflammation, associated with tenderness and sometimes fever.

Treatment

Treatment for the condition includes antibiotics, pain relief, heat packs, and sometimes anticoagulant medication.

thrush

See *vaginal discharge*

Cause

Thrush may present as an oral or vaginal infection with yeast called Candida albicans. Vaginal thrush is common in adult females who are sexually active. A reservoir of the organism may live in the adult gut, which acts as a source of self-recurrent inoculation.

Symptoms

Symptoms may occur following sexual intercourse, or following antibiotic administration with vaginal discharge, itchiness, and soreness and redness. Oral thrush may accompany the use of inhaled corticosteroid for asthma.

Treatment

Treatment for oral thrush includes oral nystatin drops for babies. For adults, amphoteracin lozenges may be taken for seven days.

For vaginal thrush, clotrimazole pessaries or creams may be used. For persistent infections, oral metronidazole tablets three times a day may be necessary.

thyroid cancer

See *hyperthyroidism*

Cause

The cause of thyroid cancer is unknown.

Symptoms

The most common presentation resulting in a diagnosis of thyroid cancer is that of a painless lump in the neck in the region of the thyroid gland. Thyroid cancers are not highly malignant, and following treatment patients usually make a good recovery for a normal life expectancy. Thyroid cancers are more common in young females.

Treatment

Treatment for thyroid cancer includes removal of the tumour. The patient is then given thyroid hormone replacement to suppress the production of the patient's own thyroid hormone. Large tumours require total removal of the thyroid gland with post-operative radiotherapy to remove any remaining thyroid tissue. Secondary deposits of the cancer of the thyroid may appear in bones.

thyroid problems

See *goitre*
See *hyperthyroidism*
See *hypothyroidism*
See *thyroid cancer*

The thyroid gland is an endocrine gland that sits in the front of the neck and is important in determining the metabolic rate of the body. Problems with the thyroid may be classified into overactivity (hyperthyroidism), or underactivity (hypothyroidism). The thyroid gland is also a common site for cancer.

thyrotoxicosis

See *hyperthyroidism*

tinea

Cause

Tinea is a fungal infection of the skin caused by tiny organisms called mycosporum, trichophyton, and epidermophyton. The fungus lives in the outer layers of the skin, hair and nails and commonly occurs on the feet, groin, body and nails. Ringworm is a form of tinea contracted from infected cats. Tinea of the feet is commonly transmitted from one person to another in areas of common bathing such as showers in gyms, and public swimming pools.

Symptoms

The infection causes symptoms of itching, irritation of the skin, a raised scaly inflammatory rash which spreads.

Treatment

Treatment of tinea is by topical anti-fungal preparations, e.g. imidazole or by oral preparation for severe infections with griseofulvin. If patients are taking griseofulvin, care should be taken not to fall pregnant during the treatment.

tiredness

See *anaemia*
See *arrhythmia*
See *depression*
See *hypothyroidism*
See *infections*
See *jet lag*

Cause

Tiredness is one of the most common complaints as a presenting symptom in general practice. It is a very non-specific symptom and the causes range from lack of sleep to serious medical problems.

Symptoms

Tiredness in itself is a very general symptom with causes ranging from lack of sleep to anxiety and depression, stress-related symptoms, pre-event nerves, sleep apnoea, the effects of shift work, pre- or post-acute illness including infections, and chronic fatigue syndrome. Following infection with some viruses, e.g. Epstein Barr virus and Ross River virus, tiredness may persist for some months. Tiredness may be accompanied by anaemia, and heavy periods.

Treatment

Identifying a cause for the tiredness will sometimes help with the anxiety which exists over the condition. Treatment is specific for anxiety and depression, and sleep studies may identify sleep apnoea for which appropriate treatment may be recommended. A treatment plan for anaemia and heavy periods will also improve the symptoms of tiredness.

tonsillitis

Cause

Tonsillitis is caused by a variety of bacteria including streptococcus and haemophilus. Sometimes Epstein Barr virus may cause severe tonsillitis.

Symptoms

Symptoms of tonsillitis include sore throat, soreness when swallowing, fever, headache, muscular aches and pains. Severe tonsillitis may sometimes require admission to hospital for intravenous antibiotics. Tonsilar abscess may occur at times (called quinsy) and may require surgical drainage in hospital.

Treatment

Antibiotics are required for the treatment of tonsillitis, unless the patient is allergic to penicillin. Symptomatic relief of pain and fever may be given with paracetamol or ibuprofen.

toxic diffuse goitre

See *hyperthyroidism*

toxic nodular goitre

See *hyperthyroidism*

toxic shock

Cause

Toxic shock is a clinical condition caused by the effects of a staphylococcus infection, most commonly with tampon usage, and may be associated with a forgotten tampon.

Symptoms

Symptoms include fever, vomiting, diarrhoea, muscle aches and pains, skin rash, low blood pressure as the condition progresses, followed by altered state of arousal if not treated.

Treatment

Treatment includes removal of all vaginal foreign bodies, and antibiotic therapy, intravenously in hospital if the patient develops the effects of shock.

transient ischaemic attack *(TIA)*

See *stroke*
See *hypertension*

Cause

Transient ischaemic attack (TIA) and stroke are closely related, and a TIA may progress to a stroke if treatment is not sought.

Symptoms

Symptoms may include transient motor weakness or sensory disturbance. Transient ischaemic attacks are sometimes accompanied by atrial fibrillation (irregular twitchings of the heart).

Investigations

Investigations for a transient ischaemic attack (TIA) include a full pathology assessment including cholesterol, blood sugar level, liver and kidney function, ECG, carotid Doppler (to determine patency of the arteries in the neck), thyroid function, and a CT of the head and neck.

Treatment

TIA symptoms must be treated as a medical emergency, with referral to an emergency department or specialist as soon as possible for assessment.

Treatment for TIA is aimed at preventing a more serious cardiovascular event such as a paralysing stoke. Treatment of TIA attacks include attention to existing hypertension, diabetes, electrolytes disturbances, and thyroid problems.

Anti-coagulant therapy is considered appropriate for some, and in most cases anti-platelet (with aspirin) therapy is recommended. Quitting smoking is essential, if reducing risk factors for further attacks is a concern.

transplantation

Symptoms

Symptoms or organ failure, e.g. kidney, lung, heart, liver, or problems with corneal opacity may warrant consideration for organ transplantation.

Treatment

Transplantation is a procedure or treatment of last resort for medical problems where organ failure has occurred. Not every patient or medical condition is suitable for transplantation. Transplantation may occur in one of a number of ways, e.g. using the patient's own tissues, as in bone or skin grafts, using genetically identical material from, for example, an identical twin, or using genetically dissimilar material from other tissue organ donors. Transplanted tissue may consist of either cell or stem bone marrow donations organ donation as in kidney, heart or lung.

All recipients of organ donation from genetically dissimilar tissue are at risk of rejection of the tissue or organ, because the recipient's immune system recognises the presence of foreign tissue. This is called a host versus graft disease.

Human leucocyte antigen (HLA) typing matches as many human HLA antigens as possible, reducing the rejection rate and therefore improving the survival of the graft in the recipient.

Prior to selecting a donor and recipient, exposure to common infections is screened to minimise the risk of infection in the recipient. Evidence of past infection with cytomegalovirus, Epstein Barr virus, herpes simplex virus, varicella zoster virus, and hepatitis B and hepatitis C viruses, and HIV virus as well as tuberculosis are screened prior to transplantation. Prior history of a malignant condition, e.g. malignant melanoma, or skin cancer or any other cancer will automatically disqualify a person from donating tissue or organs.

All recipients of donor organs need assistance to minimise rejection using immunosuppressive therapy. Immunosuppressive therapy is able to reduce the rate of organ rejection and is largely responsible for the success of organ transplantation. Immune suppression, however, is not specific and the entire immune response is depressed which may potentially result in problems of overwhelming infection, and sometimes lead to the death of the patient. Corticosteroids, cyclophosphomide, cyclosporine and tacrolimus are commonly used drugs for heart and lung, and kidney, liver and pancreas transplantation.

travel illness

See *tropical diseases*
See *immunisation*
See *infectious diseases of adults*
See *diarrhoea*
See *influenza*
See *travel sickness*
See *jet lag*

A review of individual immunity and all appropriate vaccinations should occur well in advance of travel to foreign destinations. Prevention of exposure to potential infections is essential once arriving at the destination. This includes, not drinking the local water, not eating food washed in local water, not consuming ice cubes made from local water. Eat only cooked food or food which is packaged or water which is packaged in bottles, even for cleaning teeth, do not open your mouth under the shower.

travel medicine

See *jet lag*

Travel can be a demanding and exhausting time. Not only does it involve doing unfamiliar activity, but often involves doing unfamiliar activities in unfamiliar places, with unfamiliar protocols and procedures which can be stressful.

Crossing time zones also adds to the physical stress on the body, and requires time for recovery for the body to catch up, and regain a normal diurnal rhythm of day and night. Artificially inducing sleep on planes can be a hazard for the passenger, cabin crew and other travellers potentially creating an additional risk should an emergency occur.

People thinking of travelling to exotic places should consult with their doctor well in advance of the anticipated time of departure in order to allow time for vaccinations, which may require as much as six months' lead time prior to departure. After a trip, an early visit to a doctor is recommended if the patient is unwell.

travel sickness

Cause

Travel or motion sickness is caused by constant motion or vibration from any means of transport.

Symptoms

Symptoms include nausea and vomiting; a sick, knotted feeling in the abdomen; salivation; pallor; and loss of appetite. The thought of the journey may heighten the degree of the motion sickness symptoms.

Treatment

Treatment for travel sickness is with atropine-like preparations, avomine and kwells. Patients prone to travel sickness should take the medication an hour before embarking on a journey, and then at regular intervals during the journey.

tremor

See *anxiety*
See *Parkinson's disease*

Cause

Tremor may be defined as a rhythmic movement of parts of the body, including the hands, arms, legs, head, and muscles of the face. A tremor may be caused by conditions such as anxiety, cerebral palsy and cerebellar ataxia, familial tremor, liver failure, mercury poisoning, multiple sclerosis, Parkinson's disease, thyrotoxicosis (or hyperthyroidism), and Wilson's disease (a disorder of copper storage).

Treatment

The diagnosis is a clinical one and the treatment varies depending on the cause of the tremor. Specific applications are available for the treatment of Parkinson's disease. Betablockers are sometimes used to reduce the effects of tremor associated with anxiety and also essential familial tremor.

tropical diseases

See *immunisation*
See *infectious diseases*

Cause

Tropical disease medicine is a speciality in it's own right, and it may be difficult in temperate climates to establish a definite diagnosis for such diseases. Not uncommonly, travellers to tropical areas may return home with an infection which they have contracted during their holiday or travels, and may require the expertise of a tropical disease physician in order to determine the nature of their symptoms. Some diseases are destination specific, others are less destination specific but more common in some parts of the world e.g. HIV, and other sexually transmitted diseases.

Some tropical diseases do not have vaccinations

These conditions may be difficult to diagnose for those unfamiliar with diagnosing tropical diseases. Some travel diseases acquired in tropical areas do not have vaccinations as a means of prevention prior to travel. These diseases include dengue fever, lymphatic filiariasis, leishmaniasis, leptospirosis, plague, schistosomiasis, trypanosomiasis. Repeated exposure to dengue fever not infrequently proves to be fatal.

Some tropical diseases have vaccinations which reduce risk of infection prior to travel.

See entries on immunisation, and infectious diseases.

Some tropical diseases have prevention methods other than vaccination

Malaria infection has a high mortality rate for those infected. For those who live in malaria areas, some degree of tolerance to the disease is achieved. However they may experience recurring bouts of the disease. Malaria prevention is achieved by using appropriate antibiotics during exposure time in tropical regions, as well as continuing the medications for a month after leaving the malaria area. Research is currently being done to develop a malaria vaccination, but is not available at present. Additional precautions are recommended for physical risk reduction and exposure minimisation to mosquitoes infected with malaria parasites by the use of protective clothing, insect repellent, and avoiding being out at dawn or dusk.

Other travel diseases are commonly causes by unfamiliar surroundings from biting animals and insects. Bites and stings from native and domestic animals, snakes, scorpions, spiders, mosquitoes and other stinging insects.

Symptoms

Infections may be accompanied by high fevers, skin rashes or irritation, of coughing, of weight loss, of respiratory distress, diarrheoa and vomiting symptoms, and of general malaise.

Treatments

Treating tropical diseases starts with prevention and avoidance of the diseases in the first place. Making the correct diagnosis is often the most challenging part of the treatment process.

tropical ear

See *otitis externa*
See *swimmer's ear*

Tropical ear is an infection of the external ear canal and it does not just occur in the tropics. It is more correctly called otitis externa. Most commonly it is a fungal infection or a combination of a fungal infection and a bacterial infection. It is important with this condition that the ear canal be cleaned out, best done by suction. Sometimes it is necessary to place a wick into the external canal to assist with keeping the canal dry and allowing administration of eardrops to be kept in contact with the ear canal.

tuberculosis

Cause

Tuberculosis is a chronic progressive infection caused by mycobacterium tuberculosis.

Symptoms

Tuberculosis is primarily a disease of the lungs, and is associated with cough and sputum production, chest pain, and shortness of breath which may be related to progression of the disease into the lung tissue.

Other symptoms include spontaneous pneumothorax (or rupture of the outer lining of the lung) which may cause total or partial collapse of the lung. Bloodstained sputum may result as the disease progresses and erodes the substance of the lung. If erosion of the lung continues and disrupts a major blood vessel, heavy bleeding and potentially fatal bleeding may occur.

The diagnosis of tuberculosis is made from sputum culture and examination and isolation of the bacterium on a smear test. In an active case of tuberculosis of the lungs, the patient may experience little or no symptoms or discomfort or feeling of being unwell. The sputum may be yellow or green in colour and most productive after rising in the morning. Patients may also complain of night sweats.

Tuberculosis presents a public health emergency in that on identification of a case of tuberculosis, contacts for that patient need to be traced and tested for evidence of the disease in order to prevent further spread.

Treatment

Treatment protocols for patients with tuberculosis are often complex and require the involvement of a tuberculosis specialist in order to devise the most appropriate antibiotic regime to contain the infection, as well as eradicate the infection from the lungs and elsewhere in the body. These drugs include isoniazid, rifampin, ethambutol, pyrazinamide.

typhoid

See *tropical diseases*

Cause

Typhoid fever is a systemic disease caused by salmonella typhi with an incubation period of between eight and 14 days following an acute infection. Notification of the local health department is required.

Symptoms

Symptoms such as high fever, aches and pains, meningitis, constipation, anorexia, arthralgia, abdominal pain, and a rose-coloured rash are all part of typhoid fever. Increase in the size of the spleen and liver occurs along with elevated liver function tests and an abnormality in the pathology tests. The bowel motions become loose and watery and may contain blood. Pneumonia may occur secondary to an infection with pneumococcus.

Treatment

Without antibiotics, rapid progression of the disease follows with a high mortality rate. Antibiotics are recommended, either intramuscularly or intravenously with, e.g. ciprofloxin or chloramphenicol, amoxicillin, trimethoprim. Steroids may be added to antibiotic treatment in the presence of severe toxicity.

undescended testes

See *testicular cancer and tumours*

Cause

Developmentally, the testicles develop inside the abdominal cavity and migrate during the process of development from the abdominal cavity through the groin and into the scrotum. Undescended testes occur when the testicles are located in a position other than in the scrotum.

Undescended testes occurs in about three per cent of full-term male infants, and in about 30 per cent of pre-term infants. In most cases the testes will descend spontaneously within the first four months of life.

Symptoms

An undescended testicle may be detected by a paediatrician or by a parent during routine care for the child and developmental checks during monitoring of child development. If the testicles cannot be palpated into a position in the scrotum, this is said to constitute an undescended testicle.

Treatment

Undescended testicles pose a threat to the integrity of the testicle either from the point of view of exposure to trauma in the groin, or the risk of malignant change at some time later in life. Treatment for an undescended testicle is surgical. Ideally, correction of undescended testicles should occur before the age of 18 months or as soon as possible after it is detected.

Undescended testes are a cause for concern for the development of cancer, infertility, and torsion of the testis. Gentle examination of the patient is necessary in order to confirm the presence of a normal testis. If it is found that no testicle can be palpated in the scrotum at the inguinal ring, it may be an atrophic undescended testis.

If neither testicle can be palpated, a test called human chorionic gonadotrophin stimulation (HCG) test may be performed. Patients with testicles will respond by producing testosterone, whereas those without testes (including females) produce none. In patients where neither testicle can be palpated, abdominal laparoscopy may be indicated in order to determine if the testicles are still located within the abdominal cavity.

urinary incontinence

See *diabetes*
See *menopause, problems*
See *pregnancy, associated problems*
See *prostate cancer*
See *prostate infection or prostatitis and prostate abscess*
See *prostatic hyperplasia, benign*
See *retention of urine, acute*
See *urinary tract infections*
See *vaginitis, atrophic*

Cause

Urinary incontinence may be due to either increase in the urge to urinate before uncontrolled leakage occurs, called urge incontinence, or stress incontinence, due to an abrupt increase in intra-abdominal pressure due to coughing, sneezing, laughing, bending, or lifting. Stress incontinence is the second most common cause of incontinence in women, most commonly after the effects of childbirth. It is more severe in women who are overweight

Overflow incontinence is the dribbling of urine from the bladder, functional incontinence refers to a loss of urine due to cognitive or physical impairments as with the elderly or following a stroke, and mixed incontinence is any combination of the above. Some medication may increase the likelihood of incontinence, e.g. diuretics.

Symptoms

Incontinence may present in one of four different ways. Urge incontinence (or an urgent irrepressible need to urinate); stress incontinence, which is a leakage of urine due to a sudden increase in intra-abdominal pressure, e.g. from coughing, sneezing, laughing or lifting; overflow incontinence with the dribbling of urine from the bladder; and functional incontinence which is associated with physical impairments, e.g. dementia or following stroke.

Treatment

Assessment for urinary incontinence may be done using urodynamics, where the bladder is filled with fluid and the pressure measured while the patient's ability to maintain continence is observed. General measures to improve bladder functioning include pelvic floor exercises, modifying fluid intake at certain times of the day, avoiding fluids which irritate the bladder, e.g. caffeine-containing drinks. Some drugs are useful in treating incontinence, such as drugs which improve sphincter tone, and oestrogen which is used to treat atrophic urethritis in women.

urinary tract infections

See *diabetes*
See *dysuria, incontinence*
See *prostatitis*
See *sexually transmitted diseases*
See *urinary retention*
See *vaginitis, atrophic*
See *vaginal discharge*

Cause

The most common causes of urinary tract infection are E. coli, chlamydia and gonorrhoea. However a wide range of organisms may be isolated from the urine of patients complaining of urinary tract infections. Urinary tract infection in women is one of the most common presentations in general practice. Predisposing factors in women include reproductive age, sexual activity, and the oral contraceptive pill. Urinary tract infections include bladder infections as well as infections of the kidney.

Symptoms

Symptoms include urinary frequency, a feeling of discomfort, burning or stinging on urination, and at times urgency incontinence, stress incontinence and nocturia or waking at night with the need to pass urine, and passing blood in the urine. Symptoms may be aggravated by vaginal intercourse. At times, recurrent urinary tract infections may be the presenting complaint of a bladder cancer or cancer of the ovary, and may be detected with appropriate ultrasound investigation.

Urinary tract infections may occur in men, and may be related to co-existing prostate problems. Urinary tract infections are more common in both men and women with diabetes. Urinary tract infections are more common for people who present with kidney or renal stones. Patients presenting with kidney infections are more likely to present with loin pain, while patients with bladder infections are more likely to present with lower abdominal pain.

Patients who may present with a urinary catheter infection in association with kidney or renal stones may present with a combination of these symptoms, as well as severe abdominal pain or colic associated with the passing of the stone from the kidney to the bladder. Patients with severe infections may present with symptoms of passing varying amounts of blood in the urine.

Children who present with recurrent urinary tract infections should be investigated for abnormalities including reflux of urine into the ureter, which may progress to cause renal failure if unrecongnised and not treated adequately.

Treatment

Treatment of a urinary tract infection includes antibiotic medication as well as an alkalinisation agent (such as cranberry or sodium citrate), which is effective in flushing out the bladder and reducing the population of bacteria in the bladder, increasing the fluid intake and sometimes pain relief.

The choice of antibiotics depends on the organism which is isolated from the urine and on the sensitivity of that organism to available antibiotics. Most commonly used antibiotics include trimethoprim, keflex, amoxicillin, norfloxacin and nitrofurantoin.

Prophylaxis for prevention of recurrent urinary tract infections, particularly in the presence of kidney or renal stones, includes a daily dose of medium- to long-term medication such as nitrofurantoin.

uterus cancer

See *bleeding*
See *menopause problems*

Cause

Endometrial cancer is more common in women with oestrogen-producing ovarian tumours, delayed menopause or patients with abnormal menstrual history or infertility. Obesity, hypertension, diabetes mellitus, breast cancer and a family history of breast or ovarian cancer can possibly predispose a person to the condition.

Symptoms

The most important symptom is that of post-menopausal bleeding or prolonged heavy periods in the pre-menopausal patient.

Treatment

The treatment of choice is that of total hysterectomy, with a possibility of ongoing progesterone therapy. Chemotherapy using cyclophosphamide, doxorubicin, cisplatin intravenously, with megestrol acetate orally can improve the overall response rate.

vaginal bleeding

See *cervical cancer*
See *child abuse*
See *domestic violence*
See *ectopic pregnancy*
See *polycystic ovary*

Cause

Vaginal bleeding may be caused by intercourse (due to mechanical friction or pressure on the cervix), irregular bleeding in between periods called intermenstrual bleeding and may be caused by a loss of hormonal control (particularly if the oral contraceptive pill has not been taken at the same time each day or missed altogether on the occasional day), irregular periods which may be due to anovulatory cycles (i.e. not ovulating in a cycle).

Both intermenstrual bleeding and irregular periods may be due to variation in the natural hormones in the body. Irregular bleeding will occur for women on the pill who do not take the pill at the same time even within a cycle, or who have been taking an antibiotic for an infection, or who have had diarrhoea during a cycle. The pill is processed more quickly in the liver in the case of taking antibiotic medication or is not absorbed as well in the case of diarrhoea and vomiting during a cycle.

PCO (or polycystic ovary), cancer of the cervix or uterus or ectopic pregnancy may also result in abnormal vaginal bleeding. Ectopic pregnancy may result in some vaginal bleeding and should be suspected if it occurs in a woman four to eight weeks into the pregnancy, and can be diagnosed on pelvic ultrasound. With polycystic ovary syndrome, irregular bleeding may occur, and further investigation should occur particularly if the patient is overweight, or experiencing problems of infertility.

Some patients may experience bleeding during a Pap smear, which in itself is not of concern, but sometimes if contact bleeding occurs on a regular basis, e.g. during intercourse, further investigation is warranted.

Sexual abuse in children may also be a cause of vaginal bleeding. Vaginal bleeding will occur at the time of first intercourse as a result of breaking the hymen at the entrance to the vagina and is called 'losing one's virginity'.

Symptoms

Symptoms which may accompany vaginal bleeding include lower abdominal pain, particularly with ectopic pregnancy, intermenstrual and irregular bleeding. Irritation or the onset of thrush may follow intercourse. Behavioral problems may be found in children for whom sexual abuse is the cause.

Treatment

Adequate lubrication during intercourse is essential to reduce discomfort and bleeding associated with intercourse. Regulation of the periods may be achieved with the oral contraceptive pill. Investigation for polycystic ovary (PCO) may confirm the diagnosis, and for women with this condition who do not wish to become pregnant, intermittent administration of progesterone only contraceptives is recommended. For women who are having anovulatory cycles who have excess hair and who do not wish to become pregnant, treatment consists of administration of dehydroepiandrosterone (DHEAS) (and are precursors of oestrogens and progesterones) in order to reduce the body hair. The benefits of DHEAS are said to be improvement in mood, energy, sense of wellbeing, the ability to function well under stress, improved physical performance, sleep quality, lower body fat, lower cholesterol, reverse aging, improved brain functioning.

For women who desire pregnancy, infertility treatments are used such as clomiphene.

vaginal discharge

See *bacterial infections*
See *menopause problems*
See *pelvic inflammatory disease*
See *pregnancy problems*
See *sexually transmitted diseases*
See *thrush*

Cause

Vaginal discharge may be categorised as either physiological, i.e. normal production of vaginal secretions in a mature female, or abnormal. Physiological discharge is normal and may change in character throughout the menstrual cycle, particularly if the patient is not on the oral contraceptive pill. The discharge may be clear to white and thick in the first half of the cycle and then watery in the second half of the cycle.

Abnormal vaginal discharge may be caused by a number of different factors including bacterial vaginitis (from a retained or forgotten tampon or pelvic inflammatory disease), pelvic inflammatory disease, trichomas. Other infections are from sexually transmitted diseases such as gonorrhoea, chlamydia, genital herpes. Thrush causes a very characteristic discharge.

Other causes include malignancy in the vaginal canal, and fistula formation between the vaginal canal and the rectum may occur which leads to faecal contamination of the vaginal discharge. It may also be associated with an intra-uterine contraceptive device, endometriosis, ectopic pregnancy, a threat of miscarriage, loss of hormonal control using either the contraceptive pill or depo-progesterone preparations. Vaginal discharge may be due to poor genital hygiene, atrophic vaginitis, contact bleeding following intercourse, post-menopausal bleeding.

Symptoms

The character of vaginal secretions may be used as a guide to the fertile time of the month in women who want to become pregnant.

Symptoms associated with the vaginal discharge along with the history of the symptoms give ample clues to be nature of the condition. Infections such as candida or thrush, trichomonas, sexually transmitted diseases such as gonorrhoea, chlamydia, genital herpes, pelvic inflammatory disease may be accompanied by a discharge which is either white, yellow, green or grey in colour.

Some patients may complain of offensive odour with infection, and patients with ectopic pregnancy or threatened miscarriage may complain of lower abdominal pain and even feeling faint. If abdominal pain and feeling faint are part of the symptoms, urgent investigation is warranted and may even require urgent referral to an emergency department or gynaecologist.

The discharge caused from thrush is watery with clumps of white cottage cheese-like material. Women complain of variable amount of pain associated with thrush, and pain on intercourse or on attempts to perform Pap smears. The symptoms from bacterial infection, forgotten tampon, and pelvic inflammatory disease may be watery in consistency, profuse, bubbly or frothy with offensive smell. Symptoms from chlamydia, human papilloma virus (HPV) or genital herpes may be minimal. Genital herpes infection will present as sores or blisters on the genital area associated with pain, and potentially may recur at any time from the initial infection.

Treatment

There is no treatment required for normal physiological vaginal discharge as it is normal.

For thrush, a number of products are available, including a once only tablet, vaginal pessaries, creams and, for more severe infections, oral medications, e.g. metronidazole, three times a day for a week.

Bacterial vaginitis from a retained or forgotten tampon, pelvic inflammatory disease, or trichomonas is treated with metronidazole pessaries once daily for a week.

Gonorrhoea is treated with intramuscular administration of penicillin.

Genital herpes infection is treated with antiviral agents, e.g. acyclovir for an acute attack, as well as ongoing suppression of further episodes.

HPV causing genital warts is treated with electrocautery or burning to the area involved or by the application of topical agents, e.g. imiquimod. HPV causing abnormalities in the cervical Pap smear is treated with diathermy, which is most commonly treated by the gynaecologist. Cone biopsy or excision of areas of the cervix may be done if abnormal cells have progressed to cause cancer of the cervix. The patient will need more extensive treatment involving a procedure called Lletz which removes a portion of the cervical canal affected. Sometimes hysterectomy may be required for more advanced form of disease. Before this is undertaken, the patient will require testing for pregnancy.

For infections such as gonorrhoea and trichomonas, treatment of the sexual partner is also essential. Treatment for trichomonas includes metronidazole for seven days. Treatment of gonorrhoea may be achieved using a simple antibiotic regime, either orally or by injection.

vaginitis, atrophic

See *incontinence*
See *menopause, problems*
See *urinary tract infections*

Cause
Atrophic vaginitis is caused by a lack of female hormones on the vaginal mucosa in the post-menopausal years, and in women who have had a hysterectomy, including removal of the ovaries.

Symptoms
Patients with atrophic vaginitis may experience vaginal pain or discomfort, particularly with intercourse, and at times pink discharge after intercourse, vaginal dryness and discharge, and recurrent vaginal and urinary infections. Atrophic vaginitis may be accompanied by bloodstained discharge at times other than after intercourse. Bacterial vaginitis (infection of the vagina) may follow.

Treatment

Atrophic vaginitis is treated with topical vaginal oestrogen, either in tablet or cream form, which may be applied twice daily in the first two weeks followed by a weekly application thereafter. If bacterial infection is found to co-exist, treatment with clotrimazole may be required.

valvular disorders of the heart

Cause

The valves of the heart include the aortic, mitral, pulmonary and tricuspid. The aortic and mitral valves are located on the left side of the heart and the pulmonary, and tricuspid valves are located on the right side of the heart.

In general terms, each of these valves may demonstrate either partial blockage in the outflow of blood, called stenosis, or a leakage of the valve, called regurgitation. Stenosis and regurgitation of any of the valves of the heart, if severe enough, will lead to symptoms of inefficient pumping action of the heart which may become symptomatic for the patient in the form of reduced exercise tolerance, shortness of breath, fatigue, or sleep disturbance because of shortness of breath.

Symptoms

Major cardiac symptoms include chest pain or discomfort, shortness of breath, weakness, fatigue, palpitations or discernible irregularities of the heart, a feeling of lightheadedness and, a feeling of being faint. These symptoms may occur in cardiovascular as well as non-cardiac disorders.

Investigations

Investigations of the heart valves may be undertaken by using echocardiography, exercise stress echocardiography studies, and cardiac catheterisation.

Treatment

Treatment for abnormal valves of the heart may involve surgical repair or replacement of the valves, most frequently a mitral valve or aortic valve. Patients with a disorder of the heart valves should receive antibiotics prior to any dental procedures.

viral infections

Cause

Viruses are small particles of nucleic acids with outer coverings of protein and lipid combinations. There are several hundred viruses which infect people and are capable of penetrating human cells and creating an infection. It is often difficult to know which of the many viruses are present at any one time.

Symptoms

Some viruses have a pattern of physical signs with prodromal symptoms such as fever, headache, lethargy. Many of these symptoms are non-specific and common to many infections.

The appearance of a rash may assist in diagnosing an illness. Infections such as measles, German measles and chickenpox all have characteristic rashes, but diagnosis is difficult in the early stages of the disease.

Influenza virus A, B, C and Para influenza viruses cause acute bronchitis, pneumonia and croup. Adenoviruses cause adult respiratory disease, conjunctivitis and diarrhoea. Epstein Barr virus causes infectious mononucleosis. Rhinovirus causes the common cold. Enteroviruses cause meningoencephalitis, neonatal sepsis, myocarditis, adult respiratory disease. Epidemic gastroenteritis viruses cause vomiting and diarrhoea. Rubeolar virus causes measles, rubella virus causes German measles. Varicella virus causes chickenpox and herpes zoster. Herpes virus causes herpes infections on the lips and genital area and keratoconjunctivitis in the eyes. Hepatitis viruses cause hepatitis A, B, C, D. Papilloma virus causes common warts, genital wart and genital cancer. Flaviviruses cause yellow fever, dengue fever, Japanese encephalitis, Murray valley encephalitis. Rabies virus causes rabies.

Slow viruses are associated with the onset of diseases years after infection, e.g. measles is associated with subacute sclerosing pan-encephalitis leading to respiratory failure and death up to 10 years after infection. Jakob-Creutzfeldt disease, with symptoms like mad cow disease, is associated with central nervous system degeneration years after the initial infection.

Treatment

Treatment of most viruses consists only of symptomatic measures, e.g. pain relief, treatment for fever, runny nose, sore throat, and aches and pains. Some anti-viral agents exist and have proven successful in the treatment of conditions such as genital herpes and its suppression and in the treatment of HIV.

vision, sudden loss of

See *migraine headache*
See *stroke*
See *temporal arteritis*
See *transient ischaemic attack*

Cause

Sudden loss of vision may be total or partial in an eye. Partial loss of vision may indicate the presence of pressure on the optic nerve, due to reduced blood supply to the optic nerve, a tumour, particularly of the pituitary gland, cancer, or an abscess or infection of the optic nerve or brain, or migraine. Total loss of vision in an eye may indicate a stroke or blockage of the retinal artery or vein.

Treatment

Immediate referral to an ophthalmologist or emergency department is recommended with any sudden loss of vision.

visual acuity, problems

See *blindness or loss of vision*
See *cataract*
See *multiple sclerosis*

Cause

Visual acuity is the term given to the accuracy with which a patient can read the standardised Snellen eye chart. Visual acuity may be influenced by a refractive error, or eye disease, i.e. cataracts, retinal detachment, macular degeneration, inherited eye conditions, e.g retinitis pigmentosa. Optic neuritis, glaucoma, and bleeding into the vitreous humour part of the eye, which may occur in patients with severe diabetes, may cause loss of vision.

Optic neuritis may come and go, requiring treatment intermittently in order to preserve sight. Bleeding into the eye as a result of either trauma or from diabetes may require the intervention of an eye specialist, to remove the bloodstained material from the eye, and in the case of diabetes, laser treatment to the retina may be required.

Colour blindness is most common in men. It is an inherited condition and is carried on the x-chromosome of mothers of affected men. It is possible to have colour blindness in a female where the father is colour blind, and the mother is a carrier for the gene. This, however, is an uncommon occurrence.

Amblyopia or lazy eye occurs in children, and it is important to identify as early as possible in the child's life. It may present as a turned eye, and treatment may include patching the good eye in order to make the weak eye stronger. Alternatively, an eye specialist may recommend the application of dilating drops in the good eye for the same reason. In the case of amblyopia, the brain switches off the sensory information which it receives from the weaker eye, as the images from the two eyes do not fall on corresponding parts of the retina, thus producing a blurred image. The brain finds this blurred image difficult to interpret and it is confusing for the patient. As a result the brain suppresses the image from the weaker eye causing it to lose its power to process incoming sensory information, and the visual acuity decreases. If this is not reversed by the time the child is two years (some people say younger), the reduced vision in the affected eye is permanent. The purpose of this treatment is to achieve equal vision in both eyes resulting in binocular vision.

The pinhole test is a quick and easy and useful test in determining a cause for reduced visual acuity. A hole is made in a piece of paper one to two millimetres in diameter, and given to the patient to hold up to the affected eye. The patient is then asked to read the eye chart and the best recorded vision is noted. If the patient's vision improves with the pinhole test, most likely the reduction in visual acuity is the result of a refractive error. Alternatively, if the vision does not improve, some other factor for the reduction in vision is acting.

Treatment
When a vision problem is identified, immediate medical consultation should be sought.

vomiting blood (haematemesis)

See *haematemesis*
See *stomach*

warts or human papilloma virus *(HPV)*

There are numerous strains of papilloma virus which cause common warts on the hands or feet. Other strains cause genital warts, and still other strains cause abnormailities in cervical cells in women and are thought to be responsible for around 70 per cent of abnormal pap smears.

Treatment

Treatment for common warts is achieved by topical preparations, diathermy, liquid nitrogen, or excision.

Treatment for genital warts includes topical preparations, e.g. imiquimod cream, diathermy, liquid nitrogen, or excision.

Vaccination is now available in various strains of human papilloma viruses or HPV which will give protection from the development of abnormal Pap smears in women, and also convey protection in men for carcinoma of the penis which is also thought to arise from infection of human papilloma viruses or HPV.

weight management problems

See *anorexia nervosa*
See *diabetes*
See *hypothyroidism*
See *obesity*

Cause

Weight management is a balance of energy intake and energy expenditure. Losing weight can occur by increasing energy expenditure. Modern lifestyles have placed most of us in the fast lane for everything—transport, communication, information, labour-saving devices in the home and pre-packaged food. By utilising many of these labour-saving devices and shortcuts, we also have bypassed a lot of energy utilisation in order to spend more time either at work, in front of the computer, or watching various forms of entertainment.

People have forgotten how to prepare a home-cooked meal (or have never learnt how to cook a meal from fresh produce). The fresh produce lane at the supermarket is grossly overshadowed by a huge selection of pre-packaged, pre-prepared food with labelling which is difficult to fully comprehend. Fast food which used to be consumed as 'treat food' has been normalised and is now accepted as everyday food. However it comes at a hidden cost of less control over methods of preparation and knowledge of its preparation, and more calories.

Symptoms

People have for years now been focusing on their cholesterol levels, and most patients want to know this and write it down for posterity, but many have little appreciation of the fact that it is not just cholesterol which is a potential problem here. As we have more time to eat fast food, we also eat more. We eat more high energy food with more calories than if we took time to prepare the food ourselves. In addition, low fat has been replaced by high carbohydrate and high sugar content of food, with the net result that overall we are still overeating, and under exercising.

Every magazine has the latest miracle diet with celebrities endorsing the benefits of the program, and telling how they lost vast amounts of weight in the shortest possible time. Everyday people are also expecting to achieve the same results overnight as their favourite celebrity and are disappointed when this does not happen. If food intake to the body is grossly restricted, however, the metabolic rate of the body (or the rate at which the body processes food material) slows down and at the same time switches to storing available food as fat. When a normal diet is resumed, storage of food material as fat goes into full swing and the body rebounds with restoring the weight previously lost. This is called yo-yo dieting and is quite counter-productive to achieving long-term normal body weight.

It has also been demonstrated that the position of the body fat is an important factor in healthy body metabolism. More and more research has been done regarding metabolic syndrome where emphasis has been placed on truncal obesity. It has been shown that this is a greater risk indicator for the development of diabetes, and the development of insulin resistance and impaired glucose tolerance which are precursors of diabetes mellitus.

Not only has fast food become the norm, but fast drink has also become commonplace and a daily intake of some sort of carbonated drink is not uncommon. Children at a very young age have become juice-aholics where they should be drinking full cream milk and laying down calcium in the bones as an insurance policy against osteoporosis for the future.

Adults and children alike have also become coke-aholics and juice-aholics where soft drink and excess packaged fruit juice consumption on a daily basis have become accepted as the norm. Exercise is important for children and adults for prevention or reversing of insulin resistance, developing and maintaining strong bones and healthy weight, and is recommended as a safeguard for prevention of osteoporosis.

Potato crisps and other high energy foods are stocked even in pharmacies, and labeled as 'all natural ingredients' and are enticing for the young, and used as shorts cuts for parents to assist with compliance of children with good behaviour when out in public or, e.g. when visiting the doctor. Not uncommonly, the general practitioner has to look over or beyond the debris of potato crisps in the mouth of the child in order to assess upper respiratory complaints.

This is not only sending the wrong messages to the parents regarding 'treat food' but is seen as chemists endorsing these products. It is also seen as an alternative to positive parenting where the child must receive a treat for doing as the parent wants, often before the desired behaviour has occurred.

Treatment

If a healthy weight is to be achieved, exercise and a calorie-controlled diet are essential. If the weight loss target is substantial, this process may be assisted with the help of meal replacement formulae, in the form of shakes which provide predictable amounts of calorie intake and provision of added vitamins and minerals which ensures that the body's metabolism does not go into 'starvation mode'. It is essential however for the patient to be aiming for changes in lifestyle habits in eating and exercising. Rather than thinking of dieting, a change of mindset should be directed to thinking of changes in lifestyle and eating and exercising habits. In that way the weight which is lost is less likely to be regained in the future.

whooping cough

See *immunisation for childhood infectious diseases*

Whooping cough or pertussis is regarded as one of the childhood infectious diseases. It is a highly infectious disease in children and teenagers, and is caused by an organism called bordetella pertussis.

Symptoms

Symptoms of whooping cough are initially those of a non-specific upper respiratory tract infection which is then followed by a characteristic cough. The cough consists of paroxysms of prolonged coughing followed by a large inspiratory high-pitched whoop, which lends its name to the condition. Whooping cough in young children may be life-threatening; however protection may be conveyed to children in the form of vaccination in accordance with the vaccination schedule recommended by The National Health and Medical Research Council. Diagnosis of the condition is made using a nasopharyngeal culture.

Treatment

Treatment of whooping cough is achieved using appropriate antibiotics.

X-linked conditions

Cause

X and Y chromosomes constitute the chromosomes which denote the sex of the individual. XX denotes female gender, and XY denotes male gender. Some genetic disorders are carried on the female X-chromosome. X-linked recessive chromosome if transmitted to a male child will result in a condition being expressed in the individual.

Symptoms

Conditions such as colour blindness, diabetes insipidus, haemophilia, hydrocephalus, duchene muscular dystrophy, retinitis pigmentosa, testicular feminisation syndrome and albinism are examples of x-linked recessive conditions which are transferred from mother to son. In these conditions as well, sons have a one in two chance of acquiring the x-chromosome condition, and daughters may also have a one in two chance of being a carrier of the condition.

Treatment

There is no treatment for these conditions.

X-rays

X-rays are a form of electromagnetic radiation which is used both diagnostically and therapeutically. X-rays are used primarily to detect abnormalities of radio opaque substances in the body, e.g. fracture of bones, as well as soft tissue abnormalities. X-rays are also used therapeutically in the treatment of various forms of cancer.

X-rays as a diagnostic medium are being supplemented or replaced by other forms of diagnostic modalities, including ultrasound, CT scans (or computer tomography), and magnetic resonance imaging (MRI).

xanthelasma

Cause

Xanthelasma are fatty deposits of cholesterol which occur around the eyelids near the top of the bridge of the nose.

Symptoms

These lesions cause no symptoms apart from appearing as yellowish raised deposits which patients dislike. They produced no harmful effects; however where they occur in patients, a cholesterol check should be undertaken.

Treatment

Treatment for these lesions is achieved by excision of the plaques; however they do tend to recur and do tend to be bilateral.

yellow fever

See *tropical diseases*

Cause

Yellow fever is caused by a virus called flavivirus, and is transmitted by mosquito bites. The mosquito types Aedes aegypti and haemagogus are the vectors which carry the virus.

Symptoms

Patients who contract yellow fever have a high mortality rate of up to 50 per cent with haemorrhagic fever. Symptoms include fever, chills, headache, dizziness, muscular aches and pains, nausea, vomiting, constipation, restlessness, irritability, jaundice, abdominal pain and tenderness, vomiting blood, skin rash, confusion. The disease may last a week and in severe cases, delirium seizure, coma and multiple organ failure result in death.

Treatment

Treatment is mainly symptomatic and supportive with prophylaxis against gastrointestinal bleeding with proton pump inhibitors to help prevent the degree of bleeding from the gut. Prevention is by way of immunisation and programs to reduce mosquito populations, the use of mosquito nets and protective clothing. Infected patients should also be isolated in rooms that are well screened and sprayed with insecticides.

QUICK REFERENCE LIST OF CONDITIONS

Is the condition you are looking for in this book? This quick reference guide will help you.

A

Abdominal aortic aneurysm 14

Abdominal lumps 14

Abdominal pain 15

Abscess 16

Acne 17

Addisonís disease 18

Adenitis, mesenteric 19

Adolescent health, problems 19

Adrenal crisis 20

Adrenal gland, problems 20

Adrenal virilism (adrenogenital syndrome) 21

Alcohol abuse 22

Aldosteronism (Connís syndrome) 23

Allergic reactions and hypersensitivity disorders 23

Alopecia (hair loss) 25

Amenorrhoea (no period) 26

Anaemia 27

Anal itch 28

Anal pain 28

Anaphylaxis (acute allergic reaction) 29

Aneurysm 30

Angina 30

Ankylosing spondylitis 31

Anorexia 32

Anorexia nervosa 32

Anxiety 33

Appendicitis 34

Arm and hand pain 35

Arrhythmia 35

Arthritis 36

Aspergerís syndrome 37

Asthma 37

Atherosclerosis 39

Atrophic vaginitis 39

Autism 39

B

Baby, problems 40

Back pain 40

Bacterial infections 41

Bad breath (halitosis) 42

Balanitis 43

Bed sores 43

Bed-wetting (enuresis) 44

Belching, bloating 45

Bellís palsy or facial weakness 46

Benign prostatic hyperplasia (BHP) 46

Biliary colic 46

Bipolar disorder 47

Bites and stings 47

Bladder cancer 48

Bladder problems 49

Bleeding 50

Blepharitis 52

Blindness or loss of vision 52

Blisters 53

Blood disorders 55

Blood in the urine 55

Blood pressure 55

Body odour 56

Boils 56

Bowel motions, black 56

Bowel obstruction, large 57

Bowel obstruction, small 57

Brain tumours 58

Breast cancer 59

Breast cysts and lumps 60

Breast discharge 60

Breastfeeding 61

Breast infection and abscess (mastitis) 62

Breast pain and tenderness 63

Breath holding 63

Bronchiectasis 64

Bronchiolitis 65

Bronchitis 65

Brucellosis 66

Bruising 66

Burns 67

C

Calluses, corns 68

Cancer 68

Cardiomyopathies 71

Cardiopulmonary resuscitation 72

Cardiovascular system problems 73

Carpal tunnel syndrome 74

Cataracts 74

Cellulite 75

Cerebral palsy 75

Cervical cancer 76

Chest pain 77

Chickenpox 80

Child abuse 80

Childhood infectious diseases 81

Children, common problems 84

Chlamydia 85

Cholera 85

Cholesterol 86

Chronic obstructive airway disease 87

Cirrhosis of the liver 88

Clotting disorders 89

Coagulation disorders 89

Coeliac disease 89

Cold sores 90

Colds and flu, or viral upper respiratory tract
    infection 91

Colic, baby 92

Colonic cancer 92

Colon polyps 93

Colon problems 94

Coma 94

Confusion 95

Congenital dislocation of the hip 95

Conjunctivitis 95

Constipation 96

Contraception 98

Contraception, emergency—morning-after pill 100

Convulsions 101

Coordination 102

Corneal ulcer 103

Coronary artery disease and atherosclerosis 104

Coronary syndrome 104

Cough 105

Coughing blood (haemoptysis) 106

Cramps 107

Crohnís disease 107

Croup 108

Crying baby 109

Cryptosporidium 109

Cushingís syndrome 110

Cystic fibrosis 110

Cytomegalovirus 112

D

Dandruff 112

Deafness and hearing loss 113

Dementia 116

Dengue fever 117

Dental problems 117

Depression 118

Dermatitis/eczema 119

Diabetes 120

Dialysis 122

Diarrhoea 122

Diphtheria 123

Disturbed patients 123

Diverticular disease 124

Diverticulitis 125

Dizziness 126

Domestic violence 127

Dry Hair 128

Dry skin 128

Dysmenorrhoea (painful periods) 129

Dysuria (pain on passing urine 129

E

Ear diseases 130

Ear infections 130

Ear lobes, infected (perichondrititis) 130

Ear pain 131

Ear wax 131

Ears, pressures problems 131

Eating disorders (anorexia, bulimia) 131

Ectopic pregnancy 132

Ectropion 132

Eczema 133

Emphysema 133

Endocarditis 134

Endometriosis 135

Entropion 136

Enuresis 136

Epilepsy 136

Epistaxis (bleeding nose) 137

Erectile dysfunction or impotence 138

Ewingís tumour 139

Eye inflammation 139

Eye or eyelid infection 140

Eye trauma 140

Eyes 141

Eyes, pressure in 141

Eyes, red, bilateral (both eyes) 141

Eyes, red, unilateral (one eye) 142

F

Facial pain 143

Factor V Leiden 143

Female reproductive system 144

Fever 144

Fevers in children 145

Flashes and floaters (in the eyes) 146

Flatulence (passing wind) 146

Floppy baby 147

Flu 147

Folliculitis 148

Foot odour 148

Foot pain 148

Foot strain 150

G

Gall bladder problems 151

Ganglion, wrist, forearm 152

Gastro-oesophageal reflux 152

Gastroenteritis 153

Gastroenteritis, viral 153

Genital herpes, herpes simplex infection 154

Genital warts 155

Giardia 155

Gingivitis 156

Glandular fever 156

Glaucoma 157

Glomerulonephritis 158

Goitre 159

Gonorrhoea 160

Gout 160

Gravesí disease 161

Groin pain 161

H

Haematemesis (vomiting blood) 162

Haematemesis and melana 162

Haematospermia 162

Haematuria (blood in the urine) 162

Haemochromatosis 163

Haemophylus influenza B 164

Haemorrhoids 164

Hand, foot and mouth disease 165

Hangover 165

Hay fever (rhinitis) 166

Head lice 166

Headache 167

Hearing loss 168

Heart attack 168

Heart failure 172

Heartburn 174

Heel pain 174

Helicobacter pylori infection 174

Hepatitis 175

Hernia 176

Herpes simplex virus (lips or genital area) 176

Herpes zoster (shingles) 177

Hip pain 178

HIV 179

Hodgkinís disease 179

HPV 180

Human immunodeficiency virus 180

Human papillomavirus 181

Hyperpituitarism 182

Hypertension 183

Hyperthyroidism 184

Hypopituitarism 184

Hypotension 185

Hypothyroidism 186

I

Immune response 187

Immunisation 188

Immunisation for childhood infectious diseases 189

Impetigo 191

Impotence 192

Incontinence 192

Infections 193

Infectious diseases of childhood 195

Infectious diseases of adults 195

Infertility, female 197

Infertility, male 198

Inflammatory bowel disease 199

Influenza (flu) 200

Ingrown toenails 200

Injuries to the ligaments 201

Insect bites 201

Insomnia 202

Intercourse, problems 202

Intussusception 203

In-vitro fertilisation 204

Iron deficiency 204

Irritable colon/bowel 205

Ischaemic colitis 205

J

Jaundice 207

Jet lag 208

Jock itch/rash 208

K

Keloid scar 209

Keratoacanthoma 209

Keratoses (skin condition) 209

Kidney cancer 210

Kidney disorders 210

Kidney/renal failure 210

Kidney stones 212

Knee pain 212

Patello-femoral syndrome 212

Knock knees 213

L

Laryngitis 214

Leg pains 214

Leptospirosis 217

Leukaemia 217

Libido 218

Lice 219

Liver problems 219

Lung abscess 221

Lung cancer 221

Lung function tests, abnormalities 222

Lymphoma 223

M

Malaria 224

Male reproductive system 224

Mastitis 225

Mastoiditis 225

Measles 225

Meibomian cyst 226

Melaena (black bowel motions) 226

Melanoma 226

Ménièreís disease 227

Meningitis 227

Meningococcal disease 228

Menopause, problems 229

Menorrhagia (heavy periods) 230

Mesenteric artery occlusion 231

Migraine headache 231

Molluscum contagiosum 232

Morning-after pill 232

Morning sickness 233

Mouth ulcers 234

Multiple sclerosis 234

Mumps 235

Mycoplasma pneumoniae infection 236

Myocardial infarction 236

N

Nappy rash 237

Neck pain 237

Needle-stick injury 238

Nose bleed 239

O

Obesity 240

Obsessive-compulsive disorder 241

Occupational lung diseases 242

Oesophagitis, gastro-oesophageal reflux 243

Oral contraceptives 244

Osgood-Schlatter disease 244

Osteoarthritis 245

Osteomyelitis 246

Osteoporosis 246

Otitis externa 247

Otitis media 248

Ovarian cancer 248

Ovarian cyst 249

Ovarian cyst, acute torsion 249

Ovarian cyst, ruptured 250

Ovarian follicles 250

P

Pagetís disease 252

Pain 252

Palpitations and arrhythmias 253

Pancreatic cancer 254

Pancreatitis 255

Panic disorder 256

Papillomavirus 256

Parkinsonís disease 256

Paronychia 257

Pelvic adhesions 257

Pelvic inflammatory disease 257

Penile disorders 258

Peptic, perforated or gastric ulcer 258

Perichondrititis 259

Periods, painful 259

Period problems 260

Pertheís disease 260

Peyronieís disease 260

Phaeochromocytoma 261

Phimosis, paraphimosis 261

Pigeon toes 262

Piles 262

Pill, the 262

Pituitary gland abnormalities 262

Platelet dysfunction abnormalities 263

Pleurisy 264

Pneumococcus 264

Pneumonia 265

Pneumothorax 266

Polio 266

Polycystic ovary syndrome 267

Polymyalgia rheumatica 267

Pregnancy, associated problems 268

Premature ejaculation 271

Pressure in the eye 272

Priapism 272

Prostate cancer 272

Prostate infection or prostatitis and prostate
    abscess 274

Prostatic hyperplasia, benign 274

Pseudomembranous colitis 276

Psoriasis 276

Psychiatric conditions 277

Puberty, problems 277

Pyloric stenosis 278

Q

Q fever 279

R

Rabies 280

Rectal bleeding 280

Red eyes 281

Refractive error 281

Renal colic 282

Renal dialysis 282

Renal failure, chronic 283

Renal stones 284

Renal vascular disorders 284

Respiratory system diseases 285

Respiratory system cancer (nasopharynx,
    larynx, tonsil and tongue) 285

Retention of urine, acute 286

Retracted nipples 287

Rheumatic fever 287

Rheumatoid arthritis 287

Ross River virus 288

Rubella 288

S

Salivary gland, stone 290

Scabies 290

Scarlet fever 291

Schizophrenia 291

Scrotal mass 292

Scrotal pain 293

Seborrhoeic keratoses 293

Septic arthritis 294

Septic shock 294

Sexually transmitted diseases 295

Shingles (herpes zoster) 296

Sinusitis 296

Skin problems 297

Slipped femoral epiphysis 298

Smoking 298

Snoring and sleep apnoea 299

Solar keratoses 300

Spleen disorders 301

Sprains 301

Staphylococcus aureus302

Stomach 302

Stomach cancer 302

Stroke 303

Sty 304

Sudden infant death syndrome 304

Sunburn 305

Sweating 305

Syphilis 306

Systemic lupus erythematosus 307

T

Tantrums 308

Tarsal tunnel syndrome 308

Tearduct blockage 308

Teething 309

Temporal arteritis 309

Temporomandibular joint 310

Tension headache 311

Testicular and epididymis infections 312

Testicular cancer and tumours 313

Testis, torsion 313

Testosterone, low (hypogonadism) 314

Tetanus 315

Thalassaemia 315

Thoracic outlet syndrome 316

Thrombophlebitis 316

Thrush 317

Thyroid cancer 317

Thyroid problems 318

Thyrotoxicosis 318

Tinea 318

Tiredness 319

Tonsillitis 319

Toxic diffuse goitre 320

Toxic nodular goitre 320

Toxic shock 320

Transient ischaemic attack (TIA) 320

Transplantation 321

Travel illness 322

Travel medicine 322

Travel sickness 323

Tremor 323

Tropical diseases 324

Tropical ear 325

Tuberculosis 325

Typhoid 326

U

Undescended testes 327

Urinary incontinence 328

Urinary tract infections 329

Uterus cancer 330

V

Vaginal bleeding 331

Vaginal discharge 332

Vaginitis, atrophic 334

Valvular disorders of the heart 335

Viral infections 336

Vision, sudden loss of 337

Visual acuity, problems 337

Vomiting blood (haematemesis) 338

W

Warts or human papilloma virus (HPV) 339

Weight management problems 339

Whooping cough 341

X

X-linked conditions 342

X-rays 342

Xanthelasma 342

Y

Yellow fever 344

ACKNOWLEDGEMENTS

This book would not have been possible without the help and support that I received during its conception and development.

I would first and foremost like to acknowledge the part which my family has played in those years leading up to the production of this book, including my husband, Colonel Keith Ford, for his constant love, support and encouragement; my sister, Dr Anne O'Malley, for her constructive and critical appraisal; and my mother, Mrs Isabel O'Malley, for the role she has played in the development, not only of my writing and medical career, but also in my formative years.

During the writing of this book I have enjoyed the advice, company and feedback of my good and dear friends Mrs Dianne Hermans and Mrs Julie Healy, who are themselves accomplished professionals in the fields of physiotherapy and nursing respectively. I also wish to thank Mrs Hermans for introducing me to Mrs Patsy Rowe, my friend and mentor at New Holland Publishers who has believed in my ability as an unknown author. My thanks also go to Martin Ford and Fiona Schultz at New Holland.

I would also like to thank the following for their technical support and services during this time: Ms Katherine O'Malley, Mr Killian O'Malley, Mr Simon Guthrie and Mrs Kay Ganley who have constantly been on hand to lend their assistance.

To my colleague and lifelong friend Professor Major General John Pearn, my thanks for writing the foreword for this book.

Last, but not least, thanks go to my faithful companions Grace and Bella for their presence and unconditional devotion at my feet.